PERCEPTUAL ORGANIZATION IN VISION
BEHAVIORAL AND NEURAL PERSPECTIVES

CARNEGIE MELLON SYMPOSIA ON COGNITION

David Klahr
Series Editor

Anderson
Cognitive Skills and Their Acquisition

Carroll and Payne
Cognition and Social Behavior

Carver and Klahr
Cognition and Instruction: Twenty-Five Years of Progress

Clark and Fiske
Affect and Cognition

Cohen and Schooler
Scientific Approaches to Consciousness

Cole
Perception and Production of Fluent Speech

Farah and Ratcliff
The Neuropsychology of High-Level Vision: Collected Tutorial Essays

Granrud
Visual Perception and Cognition in Infancy

Gregg
Knowledge and Cognition

Just and Carpenter
Cognitive Processes in Comprehension

Kimchi, Behrmann, and Olson
Perceptual Organization in Vision: Behavioral and Neural Perspectives

Klahr
Cognition and Instruction

Klahr and Kotovsky
Complex Information Processing: The Impact of Herbert A. Simon

Lau and Sears
Political Cognition

MacWhinney
The Emergence of Language

MacWhinney
Mechanisms of Language Acquisition

McClelland and Siegler
Mechanisms of Cognitive Development: Behavioral and Neural Perspectives

Reder
Implicit Memory and Metacognition

Siegler
Children's Thinking: What Develops?

Sophian
Origins of Cognitive Skills

Steier and Mitchell
Mind Matters: A Tribute to Allen Newell

VanLehn
Architectures for Intelligence

PERCEPTUAL ORGANIZATION IN VISION
BEHAVIORAL AND NEURAL PERSPECTIVES

Edited by

Ruth Kimchi
University of Haifa, Israel

Marlene Behrmann
Carnegie Mellon University

Carl R. Olson
Carnegie Mellon University
University of Pittsburgh

LAWRENCE ERLBAUM ASSOCIATES, PUBLISHERS
2003   Mahwah, New Jersey   London

Lawrence Erlbaum Associates, Inc., Publishers
10 Industrial Avenue
Mahwah, New Jersey 07430

Cover design by Kathryn Houghtaling Lacey

Library of Congress Cataloging-in-Publication Data

Perceptual organization in vision : behavioral and neural perspectives / edited by Ruth Kimchi,
   Marlene Behrmann, Carl R. Olson.
      p.   cm.
   Includes bibliographical references and index.
   ISBN 0-8058-3872-4 (c. : alk. paper)—ISBN 0-8058-3873-2 (pbk. alk. paper)
   1. Visual perception—Congresses.   2. Behavioral optometry—Congresses.
   3. Cognition—Congresses.   I. Kimchi, Ruth.   II. Behrmann, Marlene.   III. Olson, Carl R.
RE960 .P474   2003
152.14—dc21   2002033868

Books published by Lawrence Erlbaum Associates are printed
on acid-free paper, and their bindings are chosen for strength
and durability.

Printed in the United States of America
10   9   8   7   6   5   4   3   2   1

Contents

Preface   **vii**

I. COGNITIVE APPROACHES TO PERCEPTUAL ORGANIZATION

1 Perceptual Organization and Grouping   **3**
       Stephen E. Palmer

2 Perceptual Grouping in Space and in Space-Time:
       An Exercise in Phenomenological Psychophysics   **45**
       Michael Kubovy and Sergei Gepshtein

3 On Figures, Grounds, and Varieties of Surface Completion   **87**
       Mary A. Peterson

4 Visual Perceptual Organization: A Microgenetic Analysis   **117**
       Ruth Kimchi

5 Visual Perception of Objects and Boundaries:
       A Four-Dimensional Approach   **155**
       Philip J. Kellman

II. DEVELOPMENT AND LEARNING IN PERCEPTUAL ORGANIZATION

6 The Development of Object Segregation
       During the First Year of Life   **205**
       Amy Needham and Susan M. Ormsbee

7 Learning to Perceive While Perceiving to Learn   **233**
       Robert L. Goldstone

III. NEURAL APPROACHES TO PERCEPTUAL ORGANIZATION

8 Neural Coding of Border Ownership: Implications for the Theory
       of Figure-Ground Perception   **281**
       Rüdiger von der Heydt, Hong Zhou and Howard S. Friedman

v

9   Neuronal Correlates of Perceptual Organization in the Primate
        Visual System   **305**
        Thomas D. Albright, Lisa J. Croner, Robert O. Duncan,
        and Gene R. Stoner

10 Visual Perceptual Organization: Lessons From Lesions   **337**
        Marlene Behrmann and Ruth Kimchi

11 Binding in Vision as a Multistage Process   **377**
        Glyn W. Humphreys

IV.   COMPUTATIONAL APPROACHES TO PERCEPTUAL
ORGANIZATION

12 Perceptual Completion and Memory   **403**
        David W. Jacobs

13 Neural Basis of Attentive Perceptual Organization   **431**
        Tai Sing Lee

Author Index   **459**

Subject Index   **471**

Preface

This volume is based on papers presented in June 2000 at the 31st Carnegie Symposium on Cognition. As is the case at all the Carnegie symposia, this meeting brought together a small group of leading scientists to explore an issue at the forefront of the study of cognition. The subject of this symposium was perceptual organization in vision.

The problem of perceptual organization is central to understanding visual perception. The visual world consciously perceived is very different from the retinal mosaic of intensities and colors that arises from external objects. We perceive an organized visual world consisting of discrete objects that are coherently arranged in space. Some internal processes of organization must be responsible for structuring the bits and pieces of visual information into the larger units of perceived objects and their relations to each other.

The Gestalt school of psychology was the first to raise the problem of perceptual organization during the first half of the 20th century, suggesting that organization is composed of grouping and segregation processes. Although the Gestaltists' work on perceptual organization has been widely credited with identifying crucial phenomena of perception, and their demonstrations of grouping appear in almost every textbook about perception, there has been relatively little theoretical and empirical emphasis on perceptual organization during the latter half of the 1900s. This may be, in part, because the study of visual perception has been dominated for several decades by the "early feature-analysis" view, according to which early perceptual processes analyze simple features and elements (e.g., oriented line segments) that are integrated later, somewhat mysteriously, into coherent objects. A major contributor to the popularity of this view has been earlier work on physiology of vision—most notably the work of Hubel and Wiesel—in the 1950s and 1960s, that has fostered the idea of a hierarchical system that proceeds from extracting simple properties to extracting more complex stimulus configurations in a strictly feedforward way. Despite all the valuable knowledge that has been gained by investigations within this framework, it is now becoming evident that organizational issues cannot be ignored and that solving the problem of perceptual organization is crucial for understanding vision. This change in attitude has been inspired in part by psychological and neurophysiological findings and in part by theoretical considerations.

This first Carnegie symposium of the 21st century celebrates the awakening of new interest in perceptual organization. In the last decade or so, there has been a growing body of research on perceptual organization, some of which defied several aspects of the traditional view of visual perception. Clear progress has been made, but many open questions and controversial issues that pose a vast array of challenges for vision science still remain. We requested that contributors to the symposium highlight new research, discuss difficulties in the interpretation of findings and gaps in existing theories, and explore new directions. In preparing for the symposium, all contributors were asked to address the following questions:

1. What are the processes involved in perceptual organization?
2. Where in the sequence of visual processing does organization occur? Is organization an early or late process?
3. What are the stimulus factors that engage the processes of organization?
4. How does perceptual organization develop? What is the role of learning and experience in perceptual organization?
5. What is the relation between perceptual organization and other cognitive processes, in particular, visual attention and object recognition?
6. What are the neural mechanisms underlying perceptual organization?

The issues raised by these questions provide recurrent themes in the chapters in this volume.

As indicated by the title of this volume, this symposium also celebrates perceptual organization becoming the subject of interdisciplinary research. Indeed, the central aim of the symposium was to exchange ideas emanating from behavioral, developmental, neurophysiological, neuropsychological, and computational approaches to the problem of visual perceptual organization. The symposium was intended to facilitate the dialogue between researchers from different disciplines to foster cross-fertilization and the use of converging operations to tackle research questions. We believe that this goal was met in the context of this symposium and that the speakers broke new common ground among these different approaches and perspectives. We hope that this volume will serve to further this goal. In it, we attempt not only to detail the current state of the art in the field but also to initiate an interdisciplinary approach to perceptual organization that will enhance our understanding of this important function of the visual system.

The symposium was divided into four main sessions corresponding to the different perspectives on the topic, and this volume follows that thematic organization. It is important to note, however, that several authors incorporate more than one perspective in their chapters, providing examples of an interdisciplinary approach to perceptual organization.

PART I: COGNITIVE APPROACHES TO PERCEPTUAL ORGANIZATION

This first part presents an overview by a number of renowned psychologists who laid out the problem of perceptual organization, different frameworks for understanding perceptual organization, and a state-of-the-art summary of the domain. Stephen Palmer has written a comprehensive and broad introductory chapter, which includes an historical perspective, a review of theoretical approaches to understanding perceptual organization (ecological, structural, computational, and neural), and a discussion of different methodological approaches (phenomenological demonstrations, quantified behavioral reports, and objective behavioral tasks) to studying grouping. Palmer then provides evidence for new principles of grouping and describes attempts to locate the level of visual processing at which grouping takes place, concluding that grouping operates both early and late in the course of visual processing, possibly at every level in which coherent representation is formed. Michael Kubovy and Sergei Gepshtein first present their elegant empirical and theoretical work on grouping by spatial proximity and grouping by spatiotemporal proximity, proposing that these two processes are inextricably entangled. They then provide a meta-methodological discussion concerning phenomenological and objective methods, arguing forcefully that experimental phenomenology has much power and yields valuable information. Mary Peterson discusses her recent work on figure-ground organization. She presents data suggesting that—contrary to traditional assumptions—input from object memories is among the configural cues that determine figural status. According to her parallel interactive model of configural analyses (PIMOCA), cooperation between configural cues on the same side of a border and competition between configural cues on opposite sides of a border produce the perception of definite shape on one side and shapelessness on the other side. Peterson then reports findings concerning three-dimensional displays, suggesting that figure-ground segregation is not a stage of processing but rather one possible outcome of the interactions among cues to shape and depth. Ruth Kimchi describes her recent work using mainly a microgenetic approach. She presents data establishing the time course of perceptual grouping, evaluating the power of different grouping factors, demonstrating the role of past experience in grouping, and examining the role of attention in organization. In discussing the implications of her findings, Kimchi suggests that early perceptual processing involves organizational processes providing more complex structures than has been assumed by traditional views of perception, and that these organizational processes rely on lower level and higher level cues and vary in their time course and attentional demands. The final chapter in Part I is by Phillip Kellman. Kellman suggests an overall framework for thinking about object perception, indicating the particular tasks that need to be accomplished. Within this framework he focuses on contour and surface interpolation and the formal notion of contour relatability. He then describes research showing that accounts of grouping and segmentation will need to incorporate all three spatial dimensions as well as time and that, with simple extensions, the geometry of contour relatability may account for contour interpolation not only in static, two-dimensional displays but also in three-dimensional and spatiotemporal (motion-based) object perception. Kellman concludes his chapter with a discussion of the unsettled issue concerning the role of local verses global factors in object perception.

PART II: DEVELOPMENT AND LEARNING IN PERCEPTUAL ORGANIZATION

One particularly provocative issue concerns the development and learning associated with perceptual organization. Questions concerning which organizational processes are hardwired in the perceptual system and which are acquired through experience, and how object perception relates to other aspects of cognition, are not only important in their own right but also shed light on our understanding of the processes involved in perceptual organization. Amy Needham and Susan M. Ormsbee describe a series of studies that investigate infants' early object segregation abilities, using a familiarization-type paradigm and manipulating the complexity of the displays. The information that infants extract from the visual display is inferred from the infants' reactions (as reflected by the length of their looking) to what they perceive to be novel. In interpreting these finding, Needham and Ormsbee suggest that infants use both featural and physical information to segregate objects, relying more on physical information when both types are available, and that the use of object features to define object boundaries develops in the 1st year of life as infants learn more about the relations between object features and object boundaries. In an attempt to understand perceptual learning and its bottom-up and top-down contributions, Robert Goldstone describes both empirical work and data from a computational model. His experiments exploit novel displays on which subjects make categorization judgments. Depending on the nature of the task assigned to the subjects and the set of stimuli, subjects come up with different interpretations and rules for their category assignment. The powerful influence of top-down effects on the segregation of the input at an early level is interesting and not well demonstrated to date. Consistent with this, the model demonstrates that there is not only a top-down contribution during perceptual organization but also that its very contribution alters the nature of the bottom-up processing.

PART III: NEURAL APPROACHES TO PERCEPTUAL ORGANIZATION

The chapters in this part describe attempts to understand the neural mechanisms underlying perceptual organization, using two different approaches: neurophysiological studies of single-cell recordings in awake, behaving monkeys and neuropsychological studies of brain-damaged human patients. Rudiger von der Heydt, Hong Zhou, and Howard Friedman review their recent neurophysiological work on the neural representation of border ownership. They describe recordings from the monkey cortical areas V1, V2, and V4 that show cells that not only code location and orientation of contours but also are influenced by information outside the classic receptive field—coding how these contours belong to adjacent regions. von der Heydt and his colleagues then offer a classic hierarchical model, proposing that figure-ground organization is accomplished in a feedforward fashion: Possible figure-ground solutions are computed in early visual areas on the basis of lower level cues and fed forward to higher levels, where a final solution is achieved by attentional processes. Thomas Albright and his colleagues examine the way in which motion is perceived and demonstrate this with elegant studies in monkey cortical area MT. In particular, they show that the responses of some MT neurons are influenced by the spatial context in which moving stimuli appear, implying that visual neurons have ready access to specific contextual information.

The next two chapters describe data from human adults who have sustained a lesion to the cortical system in adulthood and who, subsequently, are impaired in perceptual organization processing. Marlene Behrmann and Ruth Kimchi describe their recent work with two visual agnosic patients, examining the patients' perceptual organization and object recognition abilities. Based on their findings, they argue that perceptual organization is not a unitary phenomenon but rather involves a multiplicity of processes, some of which are simpler, operate earlier, and are instantiated in lower level areas of the visual cortex (e.g., grouping by collinearity). Other processes are more complex, operate later, and rely on higher order visual areas (e.g., configuring into a shape). The failure to exploit these latter configural processes adversely affects object recognition. Glyn Humphreys discusses the issue of binding—the process of integrating image features both between and within visual dimensions. He reports data from patients with selective brain lesions, suggesting that several forms of binding can operate in vision: binding of elements into a contour, binding contours into a shape, and binding shape to surface detail. Humphreys then proposes a multistage account of binding that distinguishes between the processes involved in binding shape information, presumably operating within the ventral system, and the processes involved in binding shape and surface detail that seem to depend on interactions between the dorsal and the ventral systems.

PART IV: COMPUTATIONAL APPROACHES TO PERCEPTUAL ORGANIZATION

A computational approach to the problem of perceptual organization in vision is adopted by two computational vision scientists in the last two chapters. David Jacobs proposes that perceptual organization is part of the processes of visual memory, which is, in turn, the process of bringing prior knowledge of the world into alignment with a current image of it. Perceptual organization, in this view, is the first step in this process. Jacobs then describes a concrete example of how a generic model, in the form of a Markov model, can be used for perceptual completion of illusory contours and for word completion. The chapter by Tai Sing Lee provides an example of an interdisciplinary approach to perceptual organization, addressing a wide range of organizational issues at both the computational and physiological levels. Lee describes findings from visual search, illusory contours, and object recognition using electrophysiological measures and describes their computational counterpart. He strongly emphasizes the interactivity in the visual system, instantiated via lateral connections in the cortex and via feedforward and feedback connections between more anterior and posterior regions.

ACKNOWLEDGMENTS

Generous funding for this symposium was contributed by the National Science Foundation and the National Institutes of Mental Health. The Department of Psychology at Carnegie Mellon University under the leadership of Dr. Roberta Klatzky also supported the conference in diverse ways as did the Center for Neural Basis of Cognition, a joint research institute of Carnegie Mellon University and the University of Pittsburgh, under the leadership of Dr. James McClelland. We benefited greatly from the advice and wisdom of Dr. Sharon Carver and Dr. David Klahr, both of whom have experience in organizing the Carnegie symposia. Numerous other individuals also contributed their time and effort enthusiastically, and we are grateful to them: Rochelle Sherman, Queenie Kravitz, Thomas McKeeff, and Bridget Boring.

We extend our deep appreciation to each of the symposium participants. All of them contributed a chapter to this volume as well as their time and effort in reviewing chapters of other contributors. The symposium benefited from the presence of 16 junior scientists—graduate students, postdoctoral students, and assistant professors—who were supported by funding from the National Science Foundation. These individuals contributed actively to the intellectual discourse during the symposium, and we are grateful to them for their keen interest.

Ruth Kimchi
Marlene Behrmann
Carl R. Olson

I

Cognitive Approaches
to Perceptual Organization

1   Perceptual Organization and Grouping

Stephen E. Palmer
University of California at Berkeley

The problem of perceptual organization is central to understanding vision. Its importance—and its difficulty—can perhaps be most easily appreciated by considering the output of the retinal mosaic at any moment in time as a numerical array in which each number represents the neural response of a single receptor. The main organizational problem faced by the visual nervous system is to determine the structure of the retinal image: What parts of this numerical array go together in the sense of corresponding to the same parts, objects, or groups of objects in the environment? These are such crucial issues in visual processing that it is hard to imagine how vision would be possible without organization.

Nevertheless, the topic of perceptual organization has had a rather uneven history. It was nearly unrecognized in the early days of perceptual inquiry. Gestalt psychologists first raised the organizational problem in its modern form during the first half of the 20th century. After the influence of Gestalt psychology diminished, however, organization in vision has received less attention than it deserves. This decline was precipitated in part by revolutionary developments in other areas of vision science, particularly single-cell recording techniques in primary visual cortex (e.g., Hubel & Wiesel, 1959) and the linear systems approach in visual psychophysics (e.g., Campbell & Robson, 1968). Vision scientists engaged in these programs of research largely ignored organizational issues until quite recently, apparently confident that organizational effects either did not matter or could be easily explained within the framework of their own theories.

Despite the abundance of knowledge uncovered by these research programs, it is now becoming evident that the theoretical constructs required to understand visual perception go beyond the limited vocabularies of linear systems and single-cell responses in area V1. Indeed, the next frontier of vision science will probably be to solve the problem of perceptual organization and to analyze its influences on other visual processes. Recent psychophysical work on organizational effects in basic visual processing has awakened new interest in a field that is now sometimes called mid-level vision (e.g., Adelson, 1993; Anderson, 1997; Gilchrist, Kossyfidis, Bonato, & Agostini, 1999; Nakayama & Shimojo, 1992). Organization is the key problem in mid-level vision, and it will not reveal its secrets unless we stop ignoring it in the vain hope that it will simply go away.

We should be clear, however, that solving the problem of perceptual organization will not be an easy task. If it were, we would surely have made more progress on it in the past 80 years than we have. Not only do we not have the answers yet, but it is not entirely clear what the proper questions are. I recently defined perceptual organization as "the processes by which the bits and pieces of visual information that are available in the retinal image are structured into the larger units of perceived objects and their interrelations" (Palmer, 1999, p. 255). This covers an enormous range of topics that can easily be construed to include almost all of vision. I will not attempt to address this entire domain but will focus instead on the more specific problem of visual grouping: determining what goes with what in the retinal image.

I begin with some general remarks about different kinds of theoretical approaches that one can take in understanding perceptual organization, with particular emphasis on grouping. These comments provide an historical backdrop not only for my own chapter but also for the contents of this entire volume. I then discuss different methodological approaches to studying grouping, with emphasis on a new paradigm that my colleagues and I recently developed. Next, I describe the evidence for some new principles of grouping that my colleagues and I identified using a variety of different methods. Then, I describe a series of experiments that we performed to discover the level of visual processing at which grouping is completed. I close by briefly considering the implications of these findings for my own theoretical views about the processes that underlie grouping and their relation to other processes of perceptual organization.

THEORETICAL APPROACHES

The theoretical issue I consider is how we are to understand organizational phenomena such as grouping. I briefly outline the four approaches that I find most important: structural, ecological, computational, and neural approaches. The first two concern the informational rationale for perceptual organization. The last two concern the metatheoretical level at which we seek explanations. I do not claim that these four approaches are mutually exclusive in any sense. Indeed, I will argue that they are largely compatible and complementary. Only by pursuing all four, as well as the relations among them, are we likely to reach a full and satisfying understanding of how visual perception is organized.

Structural Simplicity Approaches

Perhaps the most obvious theoretical approach to the problem of perceptual organization is the Gestalt approach, which is based on the notion of structural simplicity. Gestaltists believed that the key to understanding perceptual organization was to identify the kinds of structure in the retinal image to which the visual system was sensitive. Wertheimer's (1923/1950) well-known laws of grouping, for example, are most easily understood in terms of the visual system being tuned to detect the sameness (or similarity) of perceptual elements in terms of certain salient properties, such as their location, color, size, orientation, motion, continuity, and so forth. Later theorists, such as Garner (1974), Leeuwenberg (1971), and Palmer (1983, 1991), have followed Gestaltists by analyzing the kinds of structural regularities to which the visual system is sensitive.

Why should structure be so important? The Gestalt answer was that structural simplicity was the driving force behind all of perception. They expressed this view in their famous principle of Prägnanz: Perception will be as "good" as the prevailing conditions allow. The prevailing conditions refer to stimulus constraints on the perceptual interpretation. In the case of vision, these constraints are provided by the structure of the retinal image. But because retinal constraints are not generally sufficient to uniquely solve the problem of perceiving the environment, Gestaltists proposed that additional constraints could be understood as arising from the maximization of "goodness" or structural simplicity—or, alternatively, the minimization of complexity. Wertheimer's (1923/1950) original principles of grouping were very much along these lines, although he did not formulate them directly in terms of Prägnanz. The basic idea is that visual elements that are the same in color, motion, size, and so forth, are seen as grouped together because this organized perception is simpler than the alternative of seeing them as unorganized, independent elements. No further justification is required: These regularities simply are the particular kinds of stimulus structure to which the visual system is sensitive as a result of its underlying physiological mechanisms, whatever those might be.

Gestaltists never actually produced a well-defined theory of Prägnanz, however. A satisfying version of it was proposed several decades later by Dutch psychologist Emanuel Leeuwenberg in his coding theory of perception (Leeuwenberg, 1971), later renamed structural information theory (Buffart & Leeuwenberg, 1983; Van der Helm & Leeuwenberg, 1991). Leeuwenberg's theory provided (a) a language for describing patterns, (b) a set of rules for simplifying these pattern descriptions by eliminating structural regularities, and (c) a metric for measuring the complexity of pattern descriptions based on the number of free parameters they contained. Together, these principles are able to predict, with reasonable success, the probabilities that people will see different interpretations of the image over a range of different tasks and conditions.

There are other computational theories that fit within the mold of structural simplicity. Many are couched in the language of minimization solutions, such as minimizing energy or minimizing the length of a symbolic description. The chapter by Lee in this volume discusses some of these approaches. Minimization is a general approach that can be used to solve underconstrained problems in the visual domain, such as completion of partly occluded surfaces and depth from texture. The basic idea is that when many different codings or interpretations are possible for the same sensory data, the visual system will pick the one that minimizes some relevant cost or energy function. Kellman and Shipley (1991), for example, claimed that amodally completed contours are constructed by finding the completion that will connect the visible edges of the partly occluded surface with the minimum curvature. In a very different application, Horn (1975) proposed a computational solution to the problem of depth from shading that involved finding the surface of minimum energy that would satisfy the shading constraints in the image. These approaches are related to Gestalt notions of structural simplicity but not as directly as Leeuwenberg's coding theory.

Another modern computational approach that falls within the family of structural simplicity theories is minimal description length (MDL) coding (e.g., Rissanen, 1978). The underlying idea of the MDL approach to visual structure comes from two main sources. One is the conjecture, often attributed to Barlow (1961), Attneave (1954), or both, that the visual system recodes visual information optimally by eliminating redundancy in the structure of visual input. The other source of MDL theories is the mathematical theory of complexity, pioneered by Kolmogorov and Chaitin. Within this framework, the complexity of a given object or event can be measured by the length of the program required to generate it. Although this idea was initially applied to symbol strings (such as the 1s and 0s of numbers expressed in binary notation), it can be formulated to apply to two-dimensional image structures as well. The hypothesis is that the visual system recodes image information into the shortest possible description.

Ecological Approaches

Structural simplicity theories of perceptual organization provide explanations of at least some kinds of perceptual organization. But they leave unanswered the important question of why the visual system is sensitive to those particular kinds of structure. In some sense, the most obvious answer is an ecological one: This sensitivity is helpful to the organism in discovering the structure of the external world. Perhaps the most important task of perceptual grouping is to find out which parts of the projected image belong to the same environmental objects. It seems that there are objectively correct answers to this formulation of the problem of grouping, and, if there are correct answers, then the most straightforward approach to finding them is to do whatever will maximize the probability of this outcome. This makes sense from an evolutionary standpoint because the organism that can accurately determine which parts of an image correspond to the same environmental objects will have important advantages over an organism that cannot. This is the general rationale for an ecological approach to perceptual organization: Determine which parts of an image go together in whatever way is most likely to conform to the actual state of affairs in the external world.

Notice that by this statement of the problem, Gibson (1979) does not stand alone as an ecological theorist but stands alongside none other than his archenemy, Hermann von Helmholtz (1867/1925), whose likelihood principle is unabashedly ecological: The retinal image is interpreted as the most probable environment that could have projected that optical structure into the eye of the observer. This surprising juxtaposition of theorists arises because neither the statement of the organizational problem nor the nature of the ecological solution constrains how that solution is to be reached. Rather, they concern only the informational basis of the solution. What makes both Gibson and Helmholtz ecological theorists is that, faced with explaining an organizational phenomenon such as grouping, both would appeal to the utility of certain visual features because of the optically projected structure of the actual environment. Color similarity, for example, is a good cue to grouping because objects, their significant parts, or both, tend to be reasonably homogeneous in surface reflectance and therefore reasonably similar in the color of their projected images.

Two Philosophical Issues

The ecological rationale for perceptual organization is powerful and persuasive, but it suffers from at least two potential difficulties of a philosophical nature. First, there is an epistemological problem: How does the organism manage to get information about the actual state of the external world? This is a problem because if organizational process are optimized to conform with the state of the world, then implicitly or explicitly, the visual system must have knowledge about the actual state of the world. It is unclear how this occurs, however, because there is no unimpeachable sensory or perceptual access to the nature of the environment. An organism only has access to internal evidence available through its imperfect sensory systems, and it is unclear how this can legitimately be taken as accurately reflecting the state of the world.

The most promising answer to this objection is that environmental information is ultimately grounded in evolution via natural selection. The scenario is presumably that individuals who have some accurate, innate knowledge of the environment—or at least biases toward such knowledge—should have better chances of survival and reproduction than individuals who have none or who have inaccurate knowledge. Some particularly salient and powerful information about the external world would thus be inborn and could begin a bootstrapping process, as Spelke (1990) has argued for common fate in the development of object completion processes. Even so, it seems that most of the specific knowledge people have is learned during their lifetimes. How much is actually innate and how much is learned through interaction with the world is surely one of the most important developmental issues of visual perception. Needham's chapter in this volume presents some new and intriguing pieces of this complex puzzle.

The second problem for ecological theories of perceptual grouping is ontological and, in many ways, deeper than the epistemological problem: Is there really an objectively true organizational state of affairs in the environment to which an ecological account can appeal? In a purely physical sense, the universe is just a distribution of probability density clouds of elementary quantum particles over space-time. Where are the objects here? Are not they actually the result of our perceptions rather than their cause? Objects reside, it seems, not so much in the physical world as in an organism's ecological niche. I take a niche to be a functional projection by the organism onto the external world that results from its history of interaction with that world. In this view, objects are more accurately understood as constructions of the organism than as objective entities in the physical environment.

I hasten to add that I am not advocating radical skepticism about organization. The world does have structure, as Simon (1969) and Garner (1974) both have pointed out in their own unique ways. What I am questioning is the widely held belief that there is some single, real structure in the world that is revealed by our perceptions. Rather, there are presumably many possible organizations of the world, a few of which have much higher evolutionary utility for a particular organism than the rest, and these are the organizations that we actually perceive.

There is indeed structure in the world to support our perception of the objects and parts that we see. The probability density distribution of quantum particles over space-time does not behave randomly but with regularities that can be stated at macro as well as micro levels of physical description. And, just as surely, there are evolutionary benefits in our seeing the particular structure we do see as opposed to other possible structures. What we perceive as objects are subsets of the environment that typically move together when we push them, for example, or that move on their own relative to their surroundings. It makes great evolutionary sense for us to reflect such regularities in our perceptions, and this is presumably why common fate is such a salient factor in grouping. But the additional step of supposing that the perceptual organization that we see is really out there in the physical world may not be justified—except by reference to the operation of the visual system and the evolutionary benefit of this organization to an organism's fitness within its ecological niche.

From this perspective, objects and organization are properly considered ecological constructs rather than purely physical ones. That is, they reside in the interaction between organism and environment rather than simply in the environment per se. In this respect, Gibson is on firmer footing than Helmholtz, because Gibson's theoretical analysis appeals to the mutual effects of organism and environment on each other rather than on the organism simply inferring the true nature of the environment from optical information, as did Helmholtz (and later Marr, 1982).

It is worth noting that the structural-simplicity approach of Gestalt theory does not run into either of these philosophical problems. Because structural simplicity can be computed over internal representations without access to any external realities, it sidesteps the epistemological problem entirely. And because it does not presume there to be any true or objective organization in the external world, it does not run into the ontological problem either.

Relating Structural-Simplicity and Ecological Approaches

The question to which I now turn is how the structural-simplicity approach and the ecological approach might be related. Are they fundamentally incompatible, or might they both be part of some single, larger story?

It seems to me that they are actually complementary in a particularly interesting way. Ecological arguments are useful for understanding the evolutionary utility of perceptual organization, but they have trouble explaining how the requisite knowledge gets into the system to be used in the actual mechanisms. Structural-simplicity arguments are useful for understanding how the visual system can select among alternative interpretations based on internally available criteria, but it is unclear why these criteria are useful. The connection between them is this: The interpretation that is evolutionarily most useful in an ecological sense is usually the simplest in some structural sense. If there is a strong correlation between what is structurally simple and what is evolutionarily useful, simplicity can be used as a surrogate for reality. The hypothesis I am suggesting is that evolution may have built simplicity mechanisms into the visual system as a heuristic for likelihood.

This possibility is perhaps most compellingly understood through an analogy to eating behavior.[1] Evolutionarily speaking, it is advantageous for an organism to eat things that are nourishing and to avoid eating things that are poisonous. But we do not have veridical nourishment detectors or poison detectors in any sensory modality to trust in deciding what to eat and what not to eat. In other words, we don't have sensory access to the objective conditions that will help us versus

---

[1]I first heard this analogy from Michael Leyton.

harm us. Rather, the actual mechanism of selective consumption—the internal criterion of eating behavior, if you will—is that we eat things that taste good and avoid eating things that taste bad. This works because there is a high correlation between what tastes good and what is nourishing and between what tastes bad and what is nonnourishing or even poisonous. The correlation is not perfect, of course, because some nonnourishing things taste good (e.g., saccharine), and some nourishing things taste bad (e.g., liver, for some).

An intriguing possibility is that something similar may be going on in perceptual organization. Perhaps evolution built a simplicity heuristic into the visual system that correlates well enough with the relevant ecological realities of the physical world that it regularly provides us with useful information about the environment. It is at least food for thought, so to speak.

A different, but nevertheless important, relation between the ecological and structural aspects of perception concerns their interaction in determining the kind of organization to which we are actually sensitive. The key insight is that we perceive only the structure in the world that is evolutionarily important for us. The physiological structure of our perceptual systems predisposes us toward perceiving certain kinds of structure, only a subset of which is ecologically relevant. We are quite sensitive to bilateral symmetry in the visual domain, for example, because symmetry is a salient property of many visible objects in our environment, and it can therefore be used in organizational processes, such as grouping and figure-ground determination. Indeed, we are more sensitive to vertical symmetries of reflection than to those about other axes (e.g., Palmer & Hemenway, 1978), probably because there are more objects with vertical symmetry than other symmetries. In contrast, we appear to be quite insensitive to auditory symmetries (Dowling, 1972; Weber, 1993), probably because this is not a frequent property of acoustic events with respect to either reflections in frequency or in space-time. If they were ecologically frequent and relevant, we would probably be sensitive to them.

Computational Approaches

The computational approach to perceptual organization is orthogonal to the two just mentioned. It concerns the language in which theories of perceptual organization are stated, namely, computation. As we have already indicated, one can create computational theories of structural simplicity (e.g., Buffart & Leeuwenberg, 1981; Leeuwenberg, 1971), computational theories of ecological constraints (e.g., Kellman & Shipley, 1991; Waltz, 1975), or both. There are at least two different levels at which computational theories are relevant: the macro level of overall architecture and the micro level of particular mechanisms.

At the macro level, the goal of computational theories is to try to analyze perceptual organization in terms of the kinds of architectures suitable for computing the structure we see. The usual procedure is to analyze perceptual organization into a flowchart of simpler component processes, consistent with the assumptions of functional description and recursive decomposition (Palmer & Kimchi, 1986) for nearly decomposable systems (Simon, 1969). Although this general theoretical orientation has been around for more than 30 years, few systematic attempts have been made within the domain of perceptual organization.

Irvin Rock and I made one of the more direct and ambitious attempts in our 1994 article entitled "Rethinking Perceptual Organization" (Palmer & Rock, 1994a, 1994b). An important part of our motivation was to bring perceptual organization into a modern theoretical framework. It was a topic that had been largely ignored in modern vision science, and we thought it should be treated as the result of an information processing system. For primarily logical rather than empirical reasons, we argued for the structure depicted in Fig. 1.1. The three most important proposals that it embodies are the following:

1. There is an initial process that partitions an image into a set of connected regions of relatively uniform perceptual properties, such as color, texture, motion, and depth. We called the organizational principle underlying this process uniform connectedness (UC) and argued that it must logically precede all other organizational processes because it is the one that first articulates the image into discrete regions.

2. Next come those processes that specify figure-ground organization: the assignment of edges to the region on one side rather than the other. When figure-ground organization is viewed in this way, it is tantamount to perceiving the relative depth of surfaces, and it is not clear whether the classical figural factors, such as

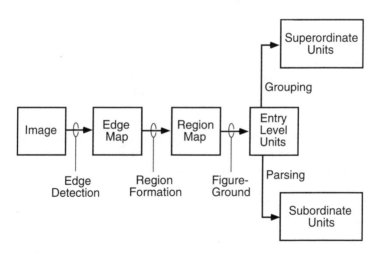

FIG. 1.1. Palmer and Rock's (1994a) process theory of perceptual organization. (See text for details.) From "Rethinking Perceptual Organization: The Role of Uniform Connectedness," by S. E. Palmer and I. Rock, 1994, *Psychonomic Bulletin and Review, 1*(1), p. 42, with permission from Psychonomic Society, Inc.

surroundedness, relative size, convexity, and symmetry, are really anything more than a set of pictorial cues to ordinal depth. The regions given figural status then become what we called entry level units, meaning that they are the first units to make contact with the part–whole hierarchy of perceptual organization.

3. Entry level units are then further organized by grouping and parsing operations into higher order superordinate perceptual units or lower level subordinate units, respectively. There is no logical priority for one versus the other process, so we supposed that they could proceed in parallel. In natural settings, grouping processes are probably more important for two reasons. First, few real-world objects constitute a single, uniform connected region in the optical image, so multiple regions must usually be grouped together to recover the organization of complex objects. Second, because two different objects seldom project to a single homogeneous region in an image, uniform connected regions seldom need to be split. Only in the latter situation is parsing of entry level units required, although this does occur under conditions of camouflage and when illusory contours are perceived.

Rock and I proposed this ordering of organizational processes not as a strict stage model, in which all processing at one level must be completed before that at the next level begins, but as an architectural structuring that is suggested by logical constraints of the task. The image must be partitioned into two-dimensional regions before the relative depth of those regions can be computed; relative depth must be determined before one can decide which regions are object candidates to be grouped into a single object or split into two or more objects. We actually conceived of the computational activity within this architecture as a cascade of processing (cf. McClelland, 1979), in which each level begins as soon as it receives any output from its input processes and as compatible with feedback connections going from higher level to lower level processes (Palmer & Rock, 1994b).

At a more molecular level of computational theorizing, the focus is on the particular computational elements and their interactions. One such computational approach that is particularly relevant for perceptual organization comes from recurrent connectionist networks: configurations of neuronlike elements that have feedback connections. They are of special interest because of their relation to the ideas of Gestalt theorists about physical Gestalts, as discussed by Köhler (1920/1950). Physical Gestalts are holistic physical systems that converge toward an equilibrium state of minimum energy. They are sometimes called soap bubble systems (e.g., Attneave, 1982) because of the analogy favored by Gestaltists to illustrate the concept. Free-floating soap bubbles have the intriguing property that, no matter what their initial shape, they evolve over time into a perfect sphere because that is a state of global stability in which the forces on the bubble's surface reach minimum physical energy. There are many other physical Gestalt systems defined by this property, and the Gestaltists hypothesized that the brain was among them.

Köhler (1920/1950) made the further conjecture that the brain's physical Gestalt was based on dynamic electromagnetic fields distributed throughout the cortex. He appears to have been wrong in his bold assertion—and this was surely one of the reasons why Gestalt theory fell out of favor—but it is now clear that re-current networks of neuronlike elements are a much more plausible implementation of the physical Gestalt hypothesis. Physicist John Hopfield (1982) clarified this possibility when he proved that symmetric recurrent networks (i.e., networks with equal weightings in both directions between any pair of units) will always converge to an equilibrium state that satisfies an informational constraint that is isomorphic to minimum energy in physics. This means that although the Gestaltists may have been wrong in detail about the brain being an electromagnetic Gestalt system, they may still have been correct at a more abstract level. Important models of organizational phenomena within recurrent networks have been proposed by Grossberg and others (e.g., Grossberg & Mingolla, 1985; Kienker, Sejnowski, Hinton, & Schumacher, 1986) and have many intriguing features.

Neural Approaches

Another approach to understanding perceptual organization theoretically is to analyze its underlying physiological mechanisms. The goal is to describe the nature of the actual neural events that cause organizational phenomena such as grouping to occur. Nobody has seriously challenged the value or validity of this kind of theorizing—except perhaps Gibson (1979), who often minimized its importance relative to ecological analysis—and some believe it to be the only valid approach. Even so, it is important to realize that, in reality, neural approaches rely heavily on computational approaches. No physiological theory is complete or compelling unless it specifies the function of the neural mechanisms it postulates, and these functions are usually described within a computational framework.

There is perhaps no better example of the interdependence of function and physiology than the debate that has evolved over the nature of simple cells in area V1 of visual cortex. Hubel and Wiesel (1959) described the receptive field structure of these cells nearly half a century ago, and although there have been some factual revisions in the intervening years (cf. De Valois & De Valois, 1988), their basic empirical work has withstood the test of time admirably. Even so, the functional interpretation of these cells is still unclear. Some claim that they are detectors of ecological features of natural images, particularly of lines and edges at different retinal orientations (e.g., Hubel & Wiesel, 1968; Marr, 1982) or perhaps of shading patterns on curved surfaces (Lehky & Sejnowski, 1988). Others claim that they are general filters for local spatial information at different orientations and spatial frequencies (e.g., Daugman, 1980; De Valois & De Valois, 1988). Still others claim that their function is to eliminate redundancies inherent in the statistical structure of natural images (e.g., Olshausen & Field, 1996). The important point for the present discussion is that this is an argument about what these cells are computing rather than about their basic physiology.

There are several different ways of attacking physiological problems methodologically, including single-cell physiology, functional brain imaging, and neuropsychological studies of brain-damaged patients. I will not say much about these approaches in this chapter simply because I do not do that sort of work myself, not because I am opposed to it. Surely it needs to be done, and it needs to be integrated with work at the more abstract computational level to understand the functional role of the physiological processes. The chapters in this volume by von der Heydt, Zhou, and Friedman, by Lee, and by Albright, Croner, Duncan and Stoner provide state-of-the-art presentations of single-cell recording research, and those by Behrman and Kimchi, and by Humphreys describe pioneering work in neuropsychology. All of them add significant further constraints to the organizational problem we are trying to solve.

METHODOLOGICAL APPROACHES

At this point I want to shift gears by considering the kinds of methods that can be used to study perceptual organization. I will concentrate on perceptual grouping because that is currently the main focus of my own research, but what I say is generally true for other organizational phenomena, such as figure-ground, illusory figures, and amodal completion. The three general methods I will discuss are phenomenological demonstrations, quantified behavioral reports of phenomenology, and performance on objective behavioral tasks. Each of these can be used alone, as in classical perceptual psychology, or they can be used together with different physiological measures of brain activity.

Phenomenological Demonstrations

Historically, principles of grouping have initially been established by phenomenological demonstrations that appeal directly to an observer's introspective experiences on viewing appropriately constructed visual displays. Wertheimer began this tradition in his seminal 1923 article on grouping, and it has been used to good effect by many other Gestaltists (e.g., Kanizsa, 1979; Metzger, 1953), including myself (Palmer, 1992; Palmer & Rock, 1994a). To illustrate the method, consider the drawings shown in Fig. 1.2, which are similar to Wertheimer's original demonstrations. The top row of figures (part A) shows equally spaced circles, which produce no differential grouping. Part B shows that elements that are spaced more closely group together more strongly, supporting the principle of proximity: All else being equal, closer elements are grouped together. Part C shows a similar demonstration of the principle of color similarity, part D shows a demonstration of size similarity, and so forth. To the extent that viewers of such displays agree with the phenomenological descriptions provided by the writer, viewers show the effect, thereby establishing the relevance of the factor that has been manipulated in the demonstration.

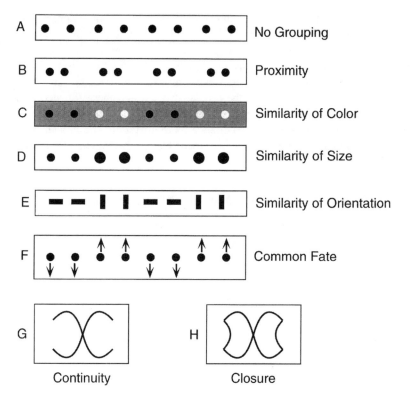

FIG. 1.2. Demonstrations of several of Wertheimer's (1923/1950) classical principles of grouping. From *Vision Science: Photons to Phenomenology*, by S. E. Palmer, 1999, p. 258, Cambridge, MA: MIT Press. Copyright 1999 by MIT Press. Reprinted with permission.

Such demonstrations are virtually indispensable because they give the reader the experiential feel of the phenomenon in a way that no report of experimental results can ever do. This is of paramount importance because it defines the phenomenon itself, the very thing we are trying to explain. Nevertheless, such demonstrations have several serious drawbacks from a scientific viewpoint that limit their usefulness. One is that they are purely qualitative: They generate no numerical data. Some viewers actually may not show the effect, but because they are not counted, nobody knows how widespread this outcome might be. For the same reason, the size of various different organizational effects cannot easily be compared in such demonstrations, and they therefore cannot be used to test quantitative theories of perceptual organization. A related problem is that only robust organizational effects can be effectively established in this way. If there is any serious ambiguity, something more than a demonstration is required.

A different problem is that phenomenological demonstrations of organizational outcomes rest on subjective rather than objective foundations. The experimenter cannot say whether one or another grouping is right or wrong, except by fiat. Phenomenological demonstrations are also notoriously sensitive to uncontrolled bias and strategic effects. Observers usually read or hear what they are supposed to see before they even look at the critical display, and these instructions may have large, systematic effects on what observers actually experience. As a result of these considerations, phenomenological demonstrations are crucial methods for establishing basic organization phenomena but relatively blunt instruments for further analysis.

Quantified Behavioral Reports of Phenomenology

Some of the problems of phenomenological demonstrations can be overcome simply by asking observers to provide overt behavioral reports of some aspect of their phenomenology, which can then be quantified. In the central column grouping task that I developed several years ago (Rock, Nijhawan, Palmer, & Tudor, 1992), observers see a square or rectangular array of discrete elements and are asked to say whether the central column groups to the left or to the right by pressing the corresponding button on a response box. The proportion of observers who report grouping to one side or the other can then be used as a quantitative measure of the strength of the grouping due to the factors that are manipulated in the displays. Observers can also be instructed to make subjective ratings of the strength of the grouping they experience to provide a finer grained measure.

I will have a lot more to say about results using this kind of method later in this chapter. For now, I only want to make clear which problems of phenomenological demonstrations such methods solve and which they do not. Obviously, it solves the quantification problem. This means that effect sizes of different factors or combinations of factors can be compared and that quantitative models can be tested against its results. Among the most elegant examples of this methodological approach are the experiments by Michael Kubovy and his collaborators of grouping in dot lattice displays, some of which are described in Kubovy and Gepshtein's chapter of this volume.

Quantification does not solve the other major problem of phenomenological demonstrations, however, which is its subjective basis. The reason is that it is still based on introspective reports about a phenomenon that has no objectively correct answer. This difficulty is related to the ontological problem of perceptual organization that I mentioned earlier: The organization of the environment into objects, parts, and other groupings of visual experience is difficult to define objectively in terms of the external world. True performance-based measures of subjective grouping are therefore not possible because there is no objective standard in the stimulus that can be used as a yardstick. For this reason, measuring perceived grouping appears to be fundamentally different from measuring perceived size or perceived distance, which have well-defined objective measures against which people's behavioral reports can be compared for accuracy. This problem can be overcome but only by changing what is actually being studied from subjective grouping to something else.

Performance on Objective Behavioral Tasks

To remedy the subjectivity of phenomenological reports, one can ask observers to report on some other aspect of perception that is objective, yet sensitive enough to subjective grouping effects that it provides an indirect measure of them. There are many ways to do this. Perhaps the most direct approach is to define a particular organization as correct by fiat in different instructional conditions. As I will report later when I describe the experiments by Palmer and Nelson (2000), we used central column grouping displays that involved illusory figures, but we told our subjects on some trials to respond according to grouping by the illusory figures themselves and on other trials to respond according to grouping by the inducing elements. Here the objective task is at least about grouping. However, it is not about spontaneously achieved grouping and therefore does not measure exactly the same thing as quantified reports of subjective grouping.

It is also possible to study a very different behavioral task that is sensitive to grouping effects. One example of such an objective, but indirect, method is the Repetition Discrimination Task (or RDT) that Diane Beck and I have developed (Beck & Palmer, 2002; Palmer & Beck in preparation). In our studies using the RDT, we show subjects simple linear arrays of elements like the ones shown in Fig. 1.3. Each display consists of a row of squares and circles that alternate, except for a single adjacent pair in which the same shape is repeated. The subject's task on each trial is to determine whether the adjacent repeated pair is composed of squares or circles. They indicate the answer by pressing one button for squares or another for circles as quickly as they can.

Response times are measured in three different conditions. In the within-group trials, a grouping factor (proximity in part A) biases the target pair to be organized as parts of the same group. In the between-group trials (part B), the same factor biases the target pair to be organized as part of two different groups. In the neutral trials (part C), the factor does not bias the pair one way or the other. The expectation is that the target pair will be detected more quickly when it is part of the same group than when it is part of different groups. The difference in these two reaction times can then be used as a measure of the strength of the grouping effect. Similar stimuli can be constructed for other grouping factors, such as color similarity, as shown in parts D, E, and F.

The results of one such experiment are shown in Fig. 1.3 in parentheses on the right side. They reveal large differences in reaction times due to grouping by the classical principles of proximity and color similarity. The proximity stimuli, for example, produced responses that were about 400 ms slower on the between-group

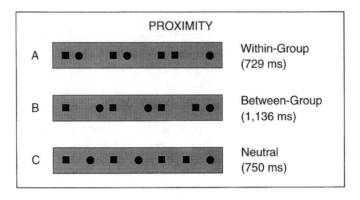

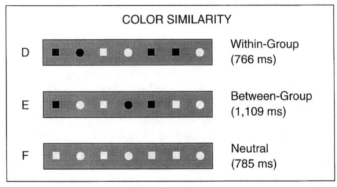

FIG. 1.3. Stimuli and results for an experiment using the RDT to study grouping effects. (See text for details.)

trials than on the within-group trials, which were about the same speed as on the neutral trials. At first, it seemed somewhat surprising that the within-group trials were not reliably faster than the neutral trials. On further reflection, however, it makes sense because the target pair in the neutral condition tends to be grouped together by shape similarity, even in the absence of other grouping factors.

The same pattern of results was obtained for discriminating target pairs when they were grouped by color similarity. The latter case shows that the reaction time difference between grouping conditions in the proximity stimuli is not simply an effect of relative distance because there are no differences in distance for the color stimuli (see Fig. 1.3, parts D and E). That we found such differences in the RDT for the same factors that determine grouping thus supports the hypothesis that grouping is being measured, albeit indirectly, in this task.

Performance in objective behavioral tasks has certain advantages over phenomenological measures, but it also has certain drawbacks. The main advantage is that it allows precise measurements through objective performance. The dependent measure does not have to be processing speed; it could just as well be accuracy. The displays in Fig. 1.3, for instance, could be presented briefly and then masked so that performance on the discrimination task was about 75% correct in the neutral condition. With the same stimulus parameters, performance on the between-group trials should then be measurably less accurate than on the within-group trials.

The main drawback of objective tasks is that they can only measure subjective organizational effects indirectly. Participants in the RDT, for example, do not make any overt response to the grouping they might perceive in the display; they respond only to the shape discrimination task. This leaves the results open to the objection that they are not actually measuring grouping at all. Perhaps proximity and color similarity merely have their own independent effects on this particular task, quite apart from their effects on grouping.

The remedy to this objection is to use indirect, objective measures as part of a set of converging operations to study organizational effects. If the same factors that affect phenomenological demonstrations, behavioral reports of phenomenology, or both, also affect an indirect, objective task, then the most plausible interpretation of the indirect results is that they are also caused by organizational effects. The RDT, for example, is influenced by all the grouping factors we have tried, and it is affected in corresponding ways by differences in the parameters of such grouping factors, such as different degrees of proximity (Palmer & Beck, in preparation). We therefore argue that it is actually measuring grouping, albeit indirectly.

In the remainder of this chapter, I describe some empirical contributions that have been made in my own laboratory toward understanding the specific organizational phenomena of grouping using a mixture of all three of the methods that I just described. I organize this research under two broad headings: extensions of the classical principles of grouping and attempts to locate grouping within an information-processing framework.

EXTENSIONS OF GROUPING PRINCIPLES

Max Wertheimer formulated the problem of perceptual grouping in his famous 1923 paper. At the same time he took the first step toward answering it by means of phenomenological demonstrations like the ones shown in Fig. 1.2. The results of his investigations are the famous Gestalt laws (perhaps better termed principles or factors) of grouping, such as proximity, similarity, and common fate. They are among the best known, yet least understood, phenomena of visual perception. Recent findings from my own laboratory have added three new principles of grouping, which we have called common region (Palmer, 1992), element connectedness (Palmer & Rock, 1994a), and synchrony (Palmer & Levitin, in preparation).

Common Region

Common region is the tendency for elements that lie within the same bounded area to be grouped together. It is evident phenomenologically in viewing Fig. 1.4, part A, when one then sees the black circles as grouped into pairs that lie within the

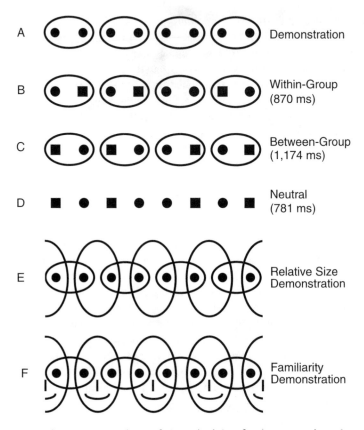

FIG. 1.4. Demonstrations of the principle of common region plus stimuli and results for an RDT experiment on common region.

same ovals, as most observers spontaneously do. Theoretically, the structural basis for common region appears to come from the fact that all the elements within a given region share the topological property of being inside of or contained by some larger surrounding contour. In this respect it is similar to several other grouping principles based on similarity, such as similarity of color, orientation, and size. In this case it is similarity of containment, if you will. Common region also appears to have an ecological rationale arising from textures. When a bounded region encloses a number of image elements, they are likely to be texture elements on the surface of a single object, such as a leopard's spots, rather than independent objects that just happen accidentally to lie within the bounding contour.

Objective evidence for the existence of common region as a grouping factor comes from studies using the RDT method (Palmer & Beck, in preparation). Within-group, between-group, and neutral displays for this factor are shown in parentheses in Fig. 1.4, parts B, C, and D, respectively. They produced the mean response times shown on the right side of Fig. 1.4, demonstrating that within-group response times are much shorter than between-group response times. Interestingly, response times in the neutral trials are even faster than those in the within-group trials. This probably reflects, at least in part, a complexity effect that arises because the neutral trials contain no ovals at all and therefore can be processed more quickly.

An important advantage of quantitative methods such as the RDT is that they allow precise measurement of grouping effects, even when phenomenology is unclear. Beck and I used it, for example, to determine whether small or large ovals produce stronger grouping by common region when they conflict within the same display. In the common region paper, I suggested that smaller regions dominate grouping using demonstration displays like the one shown in Fig. 1.4, part E, but admitted that this claim was phenomenologically equivocal (Palmer, 1992). Using the RDT, Beck and I showed that small ovals do indeed have a much stronger effect than large ovals, at least when they conflict in the same display, as in Fig. 1.4, part E. We further showed that this difference is due to an interaction between the size of the ovals and their orientation. The stimuli were constructed so that size and orientedness were varied orthogonally to form the 2 × 2 design shown in Fig. 1.5. Below each type of display are the mean response times for performing the RDT when the pair of adjacent shapes were within versus between the smaller ovals, horizontal ovals, or both. As the reader can see, there are small effects of both size and orientation alone, but the combination of smaller ovals and horizontal

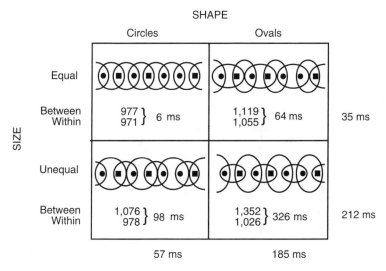

FIG. 1.5. Stimuli and results for an RDT experiment on the effects of relative size and orientation of enclosing regions on grouping by common region.

orientation produces a much bigger effect, more than twice as large as the sum of the two simple effects alone. This kind of precision is impossible to achieve with phenomenological demonstrations.

Element Connectedness

Element connectedness is the tendency for elements that are connected to be grouped together, as illustrated in Fig. 1.6, part A, using a Wertheimer-type display. The important structural basis for this form of grouping is the topological property of connectedness. Connectedness can be considered the limiting case of the classical factor of proximity, but Rock and I argued that framing it this way puts the cart before the horse (Palmer & Rock, 1994a). The compelling rationale is ecological: Pieces of matter that are actually connected to each other in three-dimensional space are the primary candidates for being parts of the same object, presumably because they tend to behave as a single unit. The eraser, metal band, wooden shaft, and lead point of a pencil, for example, constitute a single object in large part because of their connectedness, as demonstrated when you push one part, which makes the other parts move with it in rigid motion.

Again, Beck and I used the RDT to establish the effectiveness of element connectedness in an objective behavioral task. The within-group, between-group, and neutral displays are illustrated in Fig. 1.6, parts B, C, and D, respectively. The results of an RDT experiment using these figures as stimuli are shown in parentheses on the right side of the same figure. As was the case for all other grouping factors we have studied, within-group displays produced reliably faster responses than between-group displays. And, like common region, we found that response times to the neutral displays were even faster than to the within-group displays. This effect can be explained in the same way as for the common region results: The neutral displays may be processed faster just because they are simpler, lacking the additional connecting elements that the element connected conditions contain.

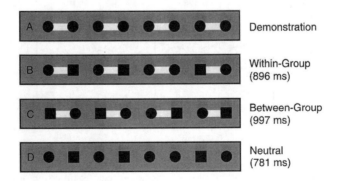

FIG. 1.6. A demonstration of the principle of element connectedness plus stimuli and results for an RDT experiment on this principle.

Another behavioral result that strikingly supports the importance of element connectedness in perceptual grouping comes from a neuropsychological study by Humphreys and Riddoch (1992). Their patient was afflicted with Balint's syndrome, a condition resulting from bilateral damage to parietal cortex. These lesions result in a serious perceptual deficit in which the patient remains fixated on a single object. The inability to shift attention from one object to another is so severe that Balint's patients are unable to discriminate between arrays containing many circles of just one color (either all red or all green) and arrays in which half of the circles are red and the other half green. This result suggests that such patients are only able to perceive one object (a single circle) in the visual field. However, if pairs consisting of one red circle and one green circle are connected by lines, the same patient is able to make the discrimination between one-color and two-color arrays. Unifying a pair of circles through element connectedness thus appears to enable these patients to perceive them as a single perceptual object so that they could see two circles at once. This feat was impossible for them in the absence of the connecting line.

Synchrony

Synchrony is the tendency for elements that change at the same time to be grouped together. It is related to common fate, but the simultaneous changes do not have to involve motion as in classical examples of common fate. Indeed, the changes do not have to be common in any sense because they occur for synchronous changes even in different perceptual dimensions. Grouping by synchrony can occur, for example, when some elements change color and others change shape or size, as long as the changes are simultaneous. Unfortunately, I cannot provide demonstrations in this chapter.

Daniel Levitin and I have been studying grouping by synchrony experimentally using reports of phenomenal grouping in the central column task I described briefly previously in this chapter. In the initial experiment, subjects see a square 7 × 7 array of randomly dark and light elements that change their lightness levels discretely over time as shown in Fig. 1.7. The task is to say whether the central column appears to group with the columns to the left, the columns to the right, or neither. Subjects then rate the strength of the grouping they perceive on a 3-point scale. All of the elements in the three left columns change their state at the same time, including both light-to-dark and dark-to-light transitions. All the elements in the three right columns likewise change their state at the same time but in counterphase with the ones in the left three columns. The elements in the central column change synchronously with those either on the left side or (as in Fig. 1.7) on the right side. The principle of synchrony predicts that observers will see them group with the synchronous side.

The results are shown as the curve labeled "Brightness (ISI = 0)" in Fig. 1.8. This graph plots the average rating of grouping strength as a function of stimulus onset asynchrony (SOA), where positive ratings indicate that the central column

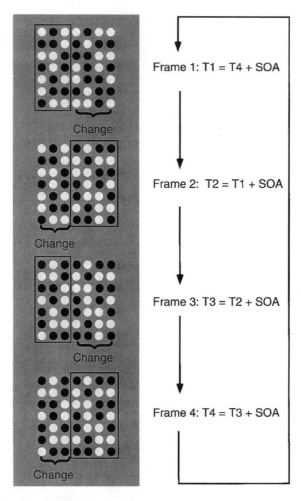

FIG. 1.7. Stimulus sequences for studying grouping by synchrony. (See text for details.)

was grouped with the synchronous side and negative ratings indicate grouping with the asynchronous side. Clearly, there is strong evidence for grouping by synchrony for SOAs of about 30 ms or more, as indicated by the highly positive ratings.

We also investigated whether the synchronous changes need to be along the same dimension or not. In the two other conditions I will describe here, the central column of circles always changed in brightness. On some trials the flanking elements on both sides were squares that changed in size, and on other trials they were triangles that changed in orientation from upward to downward. Both of these cross-dimensional cases produced grouping by synchrony that was just as strong as the within-dimensional case, as shown in Fig. 1.8.

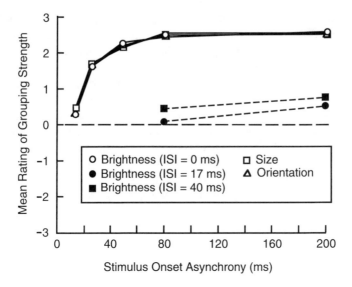

FIG. 1.8. Results of two experiments on grouping by synchrony. (See text for details.)

We discovered one manipulation that virtually obliterates grouping by synchrony, however. When we presented a brief blank interval between the successive arrays—an interstimulus interval (ISI) of 13 or 40 ms—spontaneous grouping by synchrony disappeared almost completely, as indicated by the two dashed lines connecting solid symbols near the zero-line in Fig. 1.8. We actually expected this result, based on the recent findings of change blindness (e.g., Rensink, O'Regan, & Clark, 1997). If the visual system cannot register changes in an object over a blank interval unless it is focally attended, then it follows that the visual system should not be able to group objects based on such changes. This is precisely what we found.

Returning to the theoretical framework with which I began, the structural basis for grouping by synchrony is clear enough: the sameness in time of changes in visible properties. Such grouping makes perfect sense from a purely structural point of view because it reflects a very strong temporal regularity in the stimulus events. It is far less clear what the ecological rationale for this form of grouping might be, however. Objects in the natural environment seldom change their properties in different directions or along different dimensions in temporal synchrony. Indeed, I am hard-pressed to come up with any plausible examples of the ecological utility of this principle of grouping, except for special cases such as common motion or the simultaneous brightening or darkening that occurs when shadows disappear or appear in a scene. The most general case, however, is ecologically unlikely.

Several alternative rationales are possible. One is that temporal synchrony of changes drives grouping because synchrony is the mechanism by which the brain codes grouping (e.g., Blake & Yang, 1997; Gray & Singer, 1989; Milner, 1974; von der Malsburg, 1987). Note that this is essentially a computational or physiological explanation rather than a structural or ecological one. One ecological possibility is that there is some general nonaccidentalness detection mechanism in the visual system, possibly connected to the perception of causality, as discussed by Michotte (1946/1963). The idea is that the temporal coincidence of several such changes is too unlikely to be due to chance alone, so it must have some common underlying cause. A third possibility is that it is a by-product of the operation of some other perceptual mechanism, such as the third-order motion perception system (e.g., Lu & Sperling, 1996). The idea here is that there are good ecological reasons for the visual system to be able to perceive the other property (e.g., motion based on attentional tracking of object features), and this system is engaged by the stimuli we have used even though they are not ecologically typical.

Uniform Connectedness

The final new principle I want to mention is more controversial and represents a more radical change in Gestalt ideas about perceptual organization. Irvin Rock and I proposed that there may be an earlier organizational process that operates before any of the classical grouping processes (Palmer & Rock, 1994a). We suggested this in large part because Wertheimer (1923/1950) never actually said where the elements themselves came from. Presumably he believed that they were somehow derived from the grouping principles he articulated, but we argued that they arise from a different kind of organizational principle that we call uniform connectedness (UC).

Uniform connectedness is the principle by which the visual system partitions an image into connected regions having uniform (or smoothly changing) properties, such as luminance, color, texture, motion, and depth. Fig. 1.9 shows an example of a

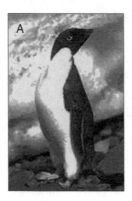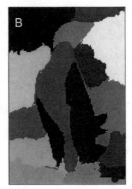

FIG. 1.9. A demonstration of Shi and Malik's (1997) algorithm for global partitioning of an image (A) into a set of mutually exclusive connected regions (B).

scene containing a penguin that has been segregated into a reasonably small number of UC regions. We did not specify the mechanism through which such a partitioning might be accomplished. It could be local edge detection (e.g., Marr & Hildreth, 1980), some more global process of image segmentation (e.g., Shi & Malik, 1997), or some other as-yet-undiscovered algorithm. But, however it happens, its effect is to partition the image into a set of nonoverlapping regions, like a stained-glass window, each of which has uniform or slowly changing visual properties. The empirical status of this proposal is weak (see Kimchi's chapter in this volume), but the logic of there being some process to divide images into regions seems almost unavoidable.

IS GROUPING AN EARLY OR LATE PROCESS?

In the final section of this chapter, I want to ask where grouping might occur in the stream of visual information processing. I should be clear at the outset that I am not asking a physiological question but a computational one. I want to know where grouping occurs relative to other perceptual processes (e.g., before vs. after stereoscopic depth perception or lightness constancy or illusory contour formation), not where it occurs in the visual nervous system (e.g., in V1, V2, or V4). My impression is that grouping has generally been presumed to be a relatively primitive, low-level operation that works on some early, two-dimensional representation and creates an initial set of discrete elements on which subsequent perceptual and attentional operations can be performed (e.g., Marr, 1982; Neisser, 1967; Treisman, 1988). This is ultimately an empirical issue, however, that can only be settled by doing the relevant experiments.

Stereoscopic Depth

An early study was performed by Rock and Brosgole (1964), who asked whether proximity grouping operated at the level of two-dimensional retinal distance or perceived three-dimensional distance. They presented a two-dimensional array of luminous beads in a dark room (see Fig. 1.10, part A), either in the frontal plane (Fig. 1.10, part B) or slanted in depth (Fig. 1.10, part C) so that the horizontal dimension was foreshortened. The beads were actually closer together vertically than horizontally so that when they were viewed in the frontal plane, observers always reported seeing them organized in columns rather than rows. The crucial question was how the beads would be grouped when the same lattice was slanted in depth so that the beads were now retinally closer together in the horizontal direction but perceptually closer together in the vertical direction.

Observers still reported seeing them grouped into vertical columns. These results and those of a variety of clever control conditions showed compellingly that grouping is based on the phenomenally perceived distance between the beads rather than on their retinal distance. It therefore supports the conclusion that final

GROUPING AND STEREOSCOPIC DEPTH

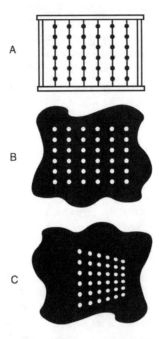

FIG. 1.10. Stimuli used by Rock and Brosgole (1964) to study the effects of stereoscopic depth perception on grouping by proximity. (See text for details.) From *Vision Science: Photons to Phenomenology*, by S. E. Palmer, 1999, p. 258, Cambridge, MA: MIT Press. Copyright 1999 by MIT Press. Reprinted with permission.

grouping occurs after what Rock and I called a postconstancy representation that includes information from stereoscopic depth perception.

Lightness Constancy

Rock and I wanted to determine the generality of this conclusion in other domains, and we decided to look next at lightness constancy. Using cast shadows and translucent overlays to decouple pre- and postconstancy aspects of lightness perception, Rock, Nijhawan, Palmer and Tudor (1992) investigated whether the important factor in grouping by lightness similarity is preconstancy retinal luminance or postconstancy perceived lightness.

Observers were shown displays containing five columns of squares (as in Fig. 1.11, part A) and were asked to report whether the central column grouped with those to the left or right. This display was carefully constructed so that

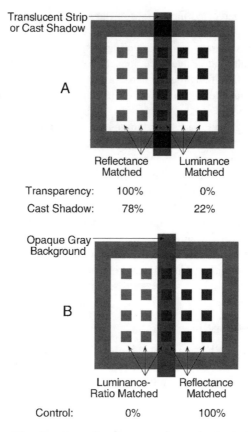

FIG. 1.11. Stimuli and results of an experiment by Rock, Nijhawan, Palmer, and Tudor (1992) to study the effects of lightness constancy on grouping. Data below figures are the percentages of trials on which subjects reported that the central column of squares grouped with the ones on the side indicated. (See text for details.)

the central squares were identical in reflectance to those on the left because they were made of the same shade of gray paper. They were seen behind a strip of translucent plastic, however, such that their retinal luminance was identical to the squares on the right. Thus, if grouping were based on retinal luminance, the central squares should be grouped with the luminance-matched ones on the right. If it were based on processing after transparency perception had been achieved, they would group with the reflectance-matched ones on the left. In another condition, the same luminances were achieved by casting a shadow over the central column of squares. The results for both the transparency and shadow conditions supported the postconstancy hypothesis: Grouping was based on the perceived lightnesses of the squares rather than on their retinal luminances.[2]

We also studied perception of a similar display (see Fig. 1.11, part B) that eliminated some alternative interpretations. One possible explanation of the results described previously is that observers grouped the elements based on the luminance of the squares relative to their immediate surrounds (i.e., based on local luminance ratios). If this were the case, observers' responses to Fig. 1.11, part B would be the same as for Fig. 1.11, part A. But there is an important difference in Fig. 1.11, part B that blocks the shadow/transparency interpretation: The vertical rectangle around the central squares completely occludes the border behind it rather than merely attenuating the light coming from it. This difference causes observers to perceive this rectangle as an opaque strip behind the central squares, which are then seen as having the same reflectance as the squares on the right rather than the ones on the left. Thus, the postconstancy hypothesis predicts that the perceived grouping of the central column in Fig. 1.11, part B, will be the reverse of that for Fig. 1.11, part A. This is precisely what we found, demonstrating that local luminance ratios cannot account for the results. The postconstancy hypothesis is therefore supported.

Amodal Completion

In another experiment, Palmer, Neff, and Beck (1996) examined whether grouping is influenced by amodal completion of partly occluded objects. When a simple object is partly occluded by another, its shape is often completed perceptually behind the occluding object. We asked whether grouping by shape similarity would be determined by the retinal shape of uncompleted elements, as predicted by the early view, or by the perceived shape of completed elements, as predicted by the late view.

Again using the central column grouping task, we examined grouping when a central column of half circles could be perceived as whole circles completed behind an occluding strip, as shown in the upper left quadrant of Fig. 1.12. An early view of grouping predicts that the central elements will group with the half circles on the right; a late view predicts that they will group with the full circles on the left. The situation is complicated by the presence of common region due to the occluding rectangle that breaks the display into two different regions such that the central elements would be expected to group with the ones in the same region (i.e., also to the left in the upper left display). We were able to disentangle the effects of amodal completion and common region by using a stimulus design that orthogonally combined these two grouping factors (see Fig. 1.12). We found

---

[2]The reader is warned that they may not experience the same outcome from the two-dimensional display shown in Fig. 1.11, part A. The lack of real shadows or transparency substantially diminishes the tendency to group according to the postconstancy predictions.

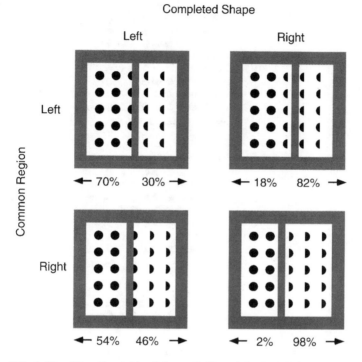

FIG. 1.12. Stimuli used by Palmer, Neff, and Beck (1996) to study the effects of shape completion on grouping by shape similarity. Data under the figures are the percentages of trials on which subjects reported that the central column of figures grouped with ones on the side indicated. (See text for details.)

that both factors had significant effects and that they were approximately additive. Grouping by shape similarity therefore also appears to be strongly influenced by the perceived shape of partly occluded objects in the three-dimensional environment, again supporting the postconstancy hypothesis.

Illusory Figures

Illusory figures are perceived where inducing elements, such as the notched ovals in Fig. 1.13, part B, are positioned so that their contours align to form the edges of a closed figure. Under the right circumstances, observers then perceive an opaque figure with about the same reflectance as the background surface in front of and partly occluding the black elements, which are then amodally completed behind the illusory figure. The question at hand is whether final grouping occurs before the perception of such illusory figures, as would be predicted by the early, preconstancy view, or whether it occurs afterwards, as expected from a late, postconstancy view.

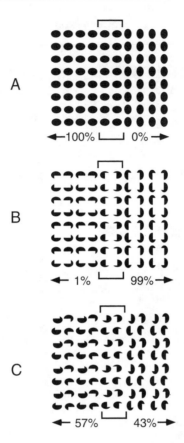

FIG. 1.13. Stimuli and results of an experiment by Palmer and Nelson (2000) on the effects of illusory figures on grouping. Data show the percentage of subjects who reported perceiving the central region to group with the left or right sides.

Rolf Nelson and I studied this question using the central column method (Palmer & Nelson, 2000). The inducing elements were horizontal ovals in the left six columns and vertical ovals in the right four columns, as shown in Fig. 1.13, part A. Here, the central two columns of ovals unequivocally group to the left. Fig. 1.13, part B, shows that when these same inducing elements are notched so that illusory rectangles are perceived, the central column of vertical illusory rectangles groups strongly to the right with the other vertical illusory rectangles and opposite to the grouping of the inducing elements themselves. To be sure that this is not due simply to the nature of the notched elements themselves, Fig. 1.13, part C, shows a control condition containing the same elements as in Fig. 1.13, part B, but slightly rearranged to disrupt the formation of illusory contours and figures. Here the grouping is very weak, with about equal numbers of observers seeing the central columns group to the left and to the right. The striking difference between the grouping evident in Fig. 1.13, parts B and C, can therefore be attributed to the strong effect of illusory figures on grouping.

To show that this particular display is not unique, we also studied three other displays: two line-induced illusory figures and one edge-induced illusory figure, like Fig. 1.13, part B. All three other examples supported the same conclusion. We also noted that the same effects are not found for all stimulus displays of these general types because it depends on the right balance of parameters. Nevertheless, we argued that the existence of any examples is sufficient to rule out the hypothesis that grouping occurs exclusively before the perception of illusory contours.

To be sure that the effects we found were due to obligatory perceptual processing rather than some optional bias or cognitive judgment, Palmer and Nelson (2000) also studied speeded performance in an objectively defined grouping task using the same kinds of stimuli. In some blocks of trials subjects had to determine with which side the central columns grouped according to characteristics of the illusory figures; in other blocks they had to determine the grouping based on characteristics of the inducing elements. We found that subjects' grouping responses were faster and more accurate when they performed the grouping task based on illusory figures rather than based on inducing elements (i.e., the lower two vs. the upper two curves in Fig. 1.14).[3] We also found that responses were generally faster when the groupings by illusory figures and the inducing elements were consistent with each other (conditions not shown in the displays in Fig. 1.13) than when they conflicted (as in Fig. 1.13, part B). Moreover, this difference was much larger for the element-directed trials than for the figure-directed trials. This pattern of results implies that grouping by illusory contours is faster and more automatic than grouping by the inducing elements, at least for the stimuli we studied.

Attention

Another issue for which we have attempted to address the question of the temporal priority of grouping effects is attention. Beck and Palmer (2002), used the RDT to determine whether grouping is subject to strategic attentional effects. The view that grouping is relatively early and automatic suggests that it should be impervious to attentional strategies. Against this hypothesis is the (possibly erroneous) intuition that many people have of being able to exert some degree of voluntary control over grouping of ambiguous stimuli: Simply attending selectively to a certain subset of elements seems to increase the probability that it will be perceived as a group.

We investigated these and related issues by measuring probability effects in the RDT. The rationale is that if subjects can intentionally ignore and attend to

---

[3]The data in Fig. 1.14 include all four illusory figure conditions, not just the single type shown in Fig. 1.13

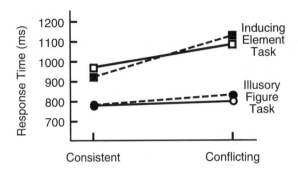

FIG. 1.14. Response time results for a grouping task in which subjects were forced to group the central region of displays like the one
in Fig. 1.13, part B, according to the illusory figures or inducing elements under conditions in which these two factors were either consistent (not shown in Fig. 1.13) or conflicting (as shown in Fig. 1.13,
part B).

grouping factors, then their performance in the RDT should change systematically
as a function of the percentage of within-group trials. More specifically, when
they are told that a given block of trials contains 75% between-group displays and
only 25% within-group trials, they should ignore the grouping factor, if they can.
When they are told that a given block contains 75% within-group trials and only
25% between-group trials, however, they should selectively attend to the grouping
factor, if they can.

Fig. 1.15 shows some characteristic results from these studies. For the
proximity-based conditions, there is the expected main effect of within- versus
between-group trials (i.e., the basic RDT grouping effect) and only a minor pertur-
bation due to probability. For common region, however, there is a strong interaction
between the grouping factor and probability. Subjects are apparently able to at least
partly ignore or attend to common region information when it is advantageous to
do so.

At first we thought that this difference was due to the nature of these particular grouping factors—specifically, that proximity is an intrinsic grouping factor,
whereas common region is an extrinsic one (see Palmer, 1992)—but later experiments led us conclude that the critical factor is probably the overall difference
in processing time. The proximity displays are processed more quickly than the
common region displays, and the extra time required for the latter conditions apparently gives the system enough additional time for strategic processing to have
an effect. This, in turn, suggests that there may be an initial bottom-up, feedforward
phase of grouping that is not affected by strategy, followed by a later, top-down
feedback phase that is. If performing the required task takes long enough for the
top-down attentional effects to manifest themselves, they influence performance
in the task by enhancing or reducing the magnitude of the grouping effect.

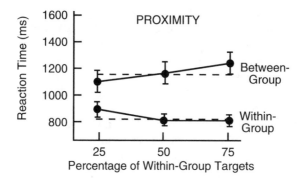

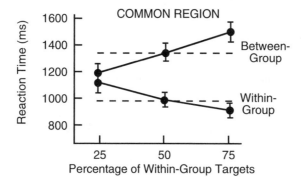

FIG. 1.15. Results of an RDT experiment on strategic effects in grouping in which the percentage of the target pair being within (vs. between) a single group was varied. (See text for details.) From "Top-Down Influences on Perceptual Grouping," by D. M. Beck and S. E. Palmer, 2002, *Journal of Experimental Psychology: Human Perception and Performance, 28*(5), pp. 1071–1084. Copyright 2002 by APA. Reprinted with permission.

Theoretical Implications

All of the effects I have just described point to the same conclusion: Phenomenally perceived grouping is ultimately governed by the structure of relatively late, postconstancy and postattentional perceptions. This fact categorically rules out the possibility of an early-only view, in which grouping occurs just at a two-dimensional, preconstancy level. Three alternatives remain. First, grouping may happen only after constancy has been achieved. I do not believe this to be a viable hypothesis for reasons I will explain shortly. Second, grouping may occur in two (or more) phases, both before and after the perception of depth and the achievement of constancy. Third, grouping might begin prior to constancy operations but receive postconstancy feedback that alters the initial grouping. In both of the latter cases, early grouping at the image-processing level would provide a preliminary organization that could be used to bootstrap the higher level processes involved in constancy. The results of these constancy computations would then be used to modify the provisional two-dimensional organization that resulted from image-based grouping processes so that the final organization conformed to the perceived, postconstancy properties.

Further groupings and organization might well be determined even later, when the objects in the display are recognized as members of meaningful categories. Fig. 1.4, part F, illustrates this possibility in that the circles tend to be grouped within the large ovals when observers recognize the schematic faces. Beck and I have actually looked for such effects using the RDT but have not yet managed to find them with this indirect perceptual measure.

Grouping and Figure-Ground Organization

If grouping has some early effects as well as later ones, grouping should influence depth perception, various constancy operations, or both, and should also be affected by them. Recently, Joseph Brooks and I examined the effect of grouping factors on figure-ground organization and relative depth, which Palmer and Rock (1994a) argued occur before grouping operations (see Fig. 1.1). Palmer and Rock thus predict that grouping should not affect either figure-ground organization or relative depth.

The most fundamental aspect of figure-ground organization is that the contour belongs to or is assigned to the figural region, thus giving it shape. The ground region extends shapelessly behind the figural region. Figure-ground perception is also closely allied with pictorial depth perception because of its implication that the figural region is closer than the ground region. It occurred to me that this idea of a contour belonging to the figural region was actually very close to a statement that the contour is grouped with the figural region. That, in turn, suggested that grouping factors might influence figure-ground organization. Although not all of the grouping principles are relevant to this situation, some of them are. Brooks and I therefore investigated its effect in a recent experiment (Palmer & Brooks, in preparation).

We constructed ambiguous figure-ground stimuli with vertical contours between a black region and a white region, as shown in Fig. 1.16, part A. The texture elements could move back and forth in common fate with each other, with the edge between the regions, or both. We showed subjects such displays and asked them to indicate which region they saw as the figure (left or right) and to rate the strength of that perception on a scale from 1 (*weakly figural*) to 3 (*strongly figural*). The hypothesis that grouping influences figure-ground perception predicts that when the texture on one side moves with the contour, that region should be perceived as figural. And so it is, as indicated by the nearly perfect ratings for that condition in Fig. 1.16, part B. To be sure that this is not just due to the motion of the texture elements making that region look figural, we also studied the condition in which

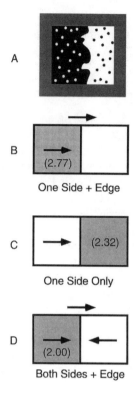

FIG. 1.16. Stimuli and results for an experiment showing the effect of common fate on figure-ground organization. Displays like the one in part A were moved as shown schematically in parts B, C, and D, where texture motion is represented by the arrows within the boxes and edge motion by the arrows above the edges. In each case, the side predicted by the grouping hypothesis (shaded) was perceived as figure and rated as strongly figural.

only the texture on one side moved so that the edge and the texture on the other side were both stationary (Fig. 1.16, part C). By our grouping hypothesis, the moving side should now be seen as ground because the edge would be grouped with the stationary side by static common fate. And so it is, as indicated by the high ratings for the unmoving side in Fig. 1.16, part B. We also included a condition in which both sides moved in opposite directions, with the contour moving in common fate with just one of them (Fig. 1.16, part D). Again, the side whose texture elements were moving in common fate with the edge between them was seen as figural, although the magnitude of this effect was not quite as great as for the other two cases (Fig. 1.16, parts B and C).

We have also begun to look for effects on figure-ground organization of other kinds of grouping factors, such as proximity, color similarity, and synchrony.

Preliminary results suggest that they, like common fate, affect figure-ground organization, as predicted by the grouping hypothesis, although their effects are not as strong.

Palmer and Rock's Theory Revisited

That grouping influences figure-ground organization constitutes evidence against Palmer and Rock's 1994 theory (see Fig. 1.1). How might this theory be revised in light of such results? Perhaps the most promising alternative is to view grouping operations not as a unitary phenomenon that operates at a single level in the process of visual perception (as depicted in Fig. 1.1) but as an interactive influence that occurs at every level throughout the system. The basic idea is that visual representations are subject to grouping at every point along the cascade of visual processing. If so, every coherent representation that gets constructed would be subject to the influence of grouping operations based on the properties that are available in that representation. Fig. 1.17 illustrates how such a structure might be realized.

In this view, two-dimensional grouping would occur at an image-based, pre-constancy representation, such as the region maps shown in Fig. 1.17. Here, early grouping would be governed by factors such as two-dimensional proximity, image luminance, projected shape, retinal motion, and so forth. In most cases this would yield valuable structure that would be used by later depth and constancy processes. This provisional structure would be subject to revision at later stages that depend on the results of depth and constancy processes, however, producing

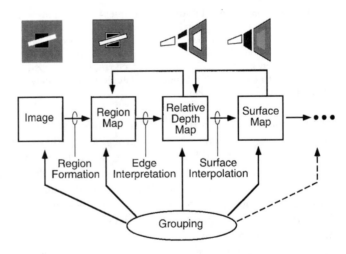

FIG. 1.17. A revised theory of perceptual organization. Rather than operating at one specific point, as in Fig. 1.1, grouping processes are hypothesized to operate on every representation that is constructed as new information becomes available.

amended organizations in the relative depth map and surface map representations indicated in Fig. 1.17.

As another example, consider the possible role of common fate in lightness constancy (Palmer, 2002). Grouping by common fate could be used to help discriminate illumination edges from reflectance edges because they behave differently when an object is moved. If luminance edges within a locally smooth surface move in common fate with the occluding depth edges that bound the surface, they are likely to be caused by changes in surface reflectance, as when the internal edges of a checkerboard move rigidly with its outer edges as the whole board is moved. If luminance edges within a locally smooth surface move in a different way than its depth edges, however, they are likely to be due to a cast shadow or translucent overlay, as when an object of uniform reflectance moves relative to another object that casts a shadow over it.

These early effects of grouping on depth and constancy processing may not operate as a unitary set of principles but as domain-specific factors that apply selectively to particular constancy problems (cf. Rensink & Enns, 1995). If so, the fact that common fate strongly influences lightness constancy would not necessarily mean that proximity, similarity, and every other grouping factor will also influence it in the same way—although they might. Such effects are likely to be governed by the ecological relevance of the factors in question to the constancy problem.

For present purposes, the key proposal is that once processing has constructed a new representation of later, three-dimensional surfaces or objects, grouping can occur again using these later, more sophisticated results. Moreover, there is no reason why grouping should stop at the object-based level because the categorization of objects as instances of familiar types may—indeed should—induce further reorganization based on stored knowledge about the structure of object categories.

CONCLUSION

I hope to have convinced you that organizational phenomena, including the grouping effects on which I have concentrated, are central to visual perception and that there are many complementary ways of understanding them, both theoretically and methodologically. I also hope to have demonstrated that the factors that govern these phenomena are not restricted to the particular closed set that Gestalt psychologists described many years ago but are an open set in which new and important variables have yet to be discovered. I hope to have convinced you further that such grouping effects are ubiquitous in visual processing. They are clearly influenced by high-level perceptual processes, such as stereoscopic depth perception, shadow and transparency perception in lightness constancy, illusory figures, and amodal completion, but they also appear to influence these same processes. The most likely conclusion is that some form of grouping occurs at many different levels of visual processing, perhaps at every level in which a coherent representation is constructed.

How are we to understand the mechanisms underlying these grouping effects? Can they be explained by low-level, linear responses of individual cells in area V1? It seems unlikely to me, unless there is extensive nonlinear feedback from higher level cortical systems as Lee suggests in his chapter of this volume. We must look toward finding these more complex mechanisms whose function is to detect and encode structural invariances of surface-based and object-based representations in addition to the structure of image-based representations on which so much energy has been concentrated to date. How much of this organizational story can be understood in purely computational terms and how much will require knowledge of the actual neural mechanisms is not yet clear, but I am willing to bet that we will find out more quickly by pursuing both directions at once, as I believe the interdisciplinary nature of this symposium demonstrates.

ACKNOWLEDGMENT

The research described in this chapter and this chapter's preparation were supported in part by Grant 1-R01-MH46141 from the National Institutes of Mental Health to the author.

REFERENCES

Adelson, E. H. (1993). Perceptual organization and the judgment of brightness. *Science, 262,* 2042–2044.

Anderson, B. L. (1997). A theory of illusory lightness and transparency in monocular and binocular images: The role of contour junctions. *Perception, 26*(4), 419–453.

Attneave, F. (1954). Some informational aspects of visual perception. *Psychological Review, 61,* 183–193.

Attneave, F. (1982). Prägnanz and soap bubble systems: A theoretical exploration. In J. Beck (Ed.), *Representation and organization in perception* (pp. 11–29). Hillsdale, NJ: Lawrence Erlbaum Associates.

Barlow, H. B. (1961). The coding of sensory messages. In W. H. Thorpe & O. L. Zangwill (Eds.), *Current problems in animal behavior.* Cambridge, UK: Cambridge University Press.

Beck, D., & Palmer, S. E. (2002). Top-down effects on perceptual grouping. *Journal of Experimental Psychology: Human Perception & Performance.*

Blake, R., & Yang, Y. (1997). Spatial and temporal coherence in perceptual binding. *Proceedings of the National Academy of Sciences, 94,* 7115–7119.

Buffart, H. F. J. M., & Leeuwenberg, E. L. J. (1983). Structural information theory. In H. G. Geissler, H. F. J. M. Buffart, E. L. J. Leeuwenberg, & V. Sarris (Eds.), *Modern issues in perception* (pp. 48–71). Berlin, Germany: VEB Deutscher Verlag der Wissenschaften.

Campbell, F. W., & Robson, J. G. (1968). Application of Fourier analysis to the visibility of gratings. *Journal of Physiology, 197,* 551–566.

Daugman, J. G. (1980). Two-dimensional spectral analysis of cortical receptive field profiles. *Vision Research, 20*(10), 847–856.

De Valois, R. L., & De Valois, K. K. (1988). *Spatial vision.* New York: Oxford University Press.

Dowling, W. J. (1972). Recognition of melodic transformations: Inversion, retrograde, and retrograde-inversion. *Perception & Psychophysics, 12,* 417–421.

Garner, W. R. (1974). *The processing of information and structure.* Hillsdale, NJ: Lawrence Erlbaum Associates.

Gibson, J. J. (1979). An ecological approach to visual perception. Boston: Houghton Mifflin.

Gilchrist, A., Kossyfidis, C., Bonato, F., & Agostini, T. (1999). An anchoring theory of lightness perception. *Psychological Review, 106,* 795–834.

Gray, C. M., & Singer, W. (1989). Stimulus-specific neuronal oscillations in orientation columns of cat visual cortex. *Proceedings of the National Academy of Sciences, USA, 86,* 1698–1702.

Grossberg, S., & Mingolla, E. (1985). Neural dynamics of form perception: Boundary completion, illusory figures, and neon color spreading. *Psychological Review, 92*(2), 173–211.

Helmholtz, H. von (1867/1925). Treatise on physiological optics. (3rd ed., vol. III). New York: Dover Publications.

Hopfield, J. J. (1982). Neural networks and physical systems with emergent collective computational abilities. *Proceedings of the National Academy of Sciences, USA, 79*(8), 2554–2558.

Horn, B. K. P. (1975). Obtaining shape from shading information. In P. H. Winston (Ed.), *The psychology of computer vision* (pp. 115–156). New York: McGraw-Hill.

Hubel, D. H., & Wiesel, T. N. (1959). Receptive fields of single neurons in the cat's striate cortex. *Journal of Physiology, 148,* 574–591.

Hubel, D. H., & Wiesel, T. N. (1968). Receptive fields and functional architecture of monkey striate cortex. *Journal of Physiology, 195,* 215–143.

Humphreys, G. W., & Riddoch, J. (1992). Interactions between object and space systems revealed through neuropsychology. In D. E. Meyer & S. Kornblum (Eds.), *Attention and performance* (pp. 143–162). Cambridge, MA: MIT Press.

Kanizsa, G. (1979). *Organization in vision: Essays on Gestalt perception.* New York: Praeger.

Kellman, P. J., & Shipley, T. F. (1991). A theory of visual interpolation in object perception. *Cognitive Psychology, 23*(2), 141–221.

Kienker, P. K., Sejnowski, T. J., Hinton, G. E., & Schumacher, L. E. (1986). Separating figure from ground with a parallel network. *Perception, 15*(2), 197–216.

Köhler, W. (1950). Physical Gestalten. In W. D. Ellis (Ed.), *A sourcebook of Gestalt psychology* (pp. 17–54). New York: The Humanities Press. (Original work published 1920)

Leeuwenberg, E. L. (1971). A perceptual coding language for visual and auditory patterns. *American Journal of Psychology, 84*(3), 307–349.

Lehky, S. R., & Sejnowski, T. J. (1988). Network model of shape-from-shading: Neural function arises from both receptive and projective fields. *Nature, 333*(6172), 452–454.

Lu, Z.-L., & Sperling, G. (1996). Three systems for visual motion perception. *Current Directions in Psychological Science, 5*(2), 44–53.

Marr, D. (1982). *Vision: A computational investigation into the human representation and processing of visual information.* San Francisco: W.H. Freeman.

Marr, D., & Hildreth, E. C. (1980). Theory of edge detection. *Proceedings of the Royal Society of London: Series B, 207,* 187–217.

McClelland, J. L. (1979). On the time relations of mental processes: An examination of systems of processes in cascade. *Psychological Review, 86*(4), 287–330.

Metzger, F. (1953). *Gesetze des Sehens.* Frankfurt-am-Main, Germany: Waldemar Kramer.

Michotte, A. (1946/1963). The perception of causality (T. R. Miles & E. Miles, Trans.). London: Methuen.

Milner, P. M. (1974). A model for visual shape recognition. *Psychological Review, 81,* 521–535.

Nakayama, K., & Shimojo, S. (1992). Experiencing and perceiving visual surfaces. *Science, 257*(5075), 1357–1363.

Neisser, U. (1967). *Cognitive psychology.* Englewood Cliffs, NJ: Prentice Hall.

Olshausen, B. A., & Field, D. J. (1996). Emergence of simple-cell receptive field properties by learning a sparse code for natural images. *Nature, 381,* 607–609.

Palmer, S. E. (1983). The psychology of perceptual organization: A transformational approach. In J. Beck, B. Hope, & A. Baddeley (Eds.), *Human and machine vision* (pp. 269–339). New York: Academic Press.

Palmer, S. E. (1991). Goodness, Gestalt, groups, and Garner: Local symmetry subgroups as a theory of figural goodness. In G. R. Lockhead & J. R. Pomerantz (Eds.), *The perception of structure: Essays in honor of Wendell R. Garner* (pp. 23–39). Washington, DC: American Psychological Association.

Palmer, S. E. (1992). Common region: A new principle of perceptual grouping. *Cognitive Psychology, 24*(3), 436–447.

Palmer, S. E. (1999). *Vision science: Photons to phenomenology.* Cambridge, MA: Bradford Books/MIT Press.

Palmer, S. E. (2002). Perceptual grouping: It's later than you think. *Current Directions in Psychological Science. 11*(3), 101–106.

Palmer, S. E., & Beck, D. (in preparation). The repetition discrimination task: A quantitative method for studying grouping.

Palmer, S. E., & Brooks, J. L. (in preparation). Effects of grouping factors on figure-ground organization.

Palmer, S. E., & Hemenway, K. (1978). Orientation and symmetry: Effects of multiple, rotational, and near symmetries. *Journal of Experimental Psychology: Human Perception & Performance, 4*(4), 691–702.

Palmer, S. E., & Kimchi, R. (1986). The information processing approach to cognition. In T. J. Knapp & L. C., Robertson (Eds.), *Approaches to cognition: Contrasts and controversies.* Hillsdale, NJ: Lawrence Erlbaum Associates.

Palmer, S. E., & Levitin, D. (2002). *Synchrony: A new principle of perceptual organization.* Manuscript submitted for publication.

Palmer, S. E., Neff, J., & Beck, D. (1996). Late influences on perceptual grouping: Amodal completion. *Psychonomic Bulletin & Review, 3*(1), 75–80.

Palmer, S. E., & Nelson, R. (2000). Late influences on perceptual grouping: Illusory contours. *Perception & Psychophysics, 62,* 1321–1331.

Palmer, S. E., & Rock, I. (1994a). On the nature and order of organizational processing: A reply to Peterson. *Psychonomic Bulletin & Review, 1,* 515–519.

Palmer, S. E., & Rock, I. (1994b). Rethinking perceptual organization: The role of uniform connectedness. *Psychonomic Bulletin & Review, 1*(1), 29–55.

Rensink, R. A., O'Regan, J. K., & Clark, J. J. (1997). To see or not to see: The need for attention to perceive changes in scenes. *Psychological Science, 8,* 368–373.

Rensink, R. A., & Enns, J. T. (1995). Preemption effects in visual search: Evidence for low-level grouping. *Psychological Review, 102,* 101–130.

Rissanen, J. J. (1978). Modeling by shortest data description. *Automatica, 14,* 465–471.

Rock, I., & Brosgole, L. (1964). Grouping based on phenomenal proximity. *Journal of Experimental Psychology, 67,* 531–538.

Rock, I., Nijhawan, R., Palmer, S., & Tudor, L. (1992). Grouping based on phenomenal similarity of achromatic color. *Perception, 21*(6), 779–789.

Shi, J., & Malik, J. (1997). *Normalized cuts and image segmentation.* Paper presented at the Proceedings of the IEEE Conference on Computation: Vision and Pattern Recognition, San Juan, Puerto Rico.

Simon, H. A. (1969). *The sciences of the artificial.* Cambridge, MA: MIT Press.

Spelke, E. S. (1990). Principles of object perception. *Cognitive Science, 14*(1), 29–56.

Treisman, A. (1988). Features and objects: The Fourteenth Bartlett Memorial Lecture. *Quarterly Journal of Experimental Psychology: Human Experimental Psychology, 40*(2), 201–237.

Van der Helm, P. A., & Leeuwenberg, E. L. (1991). Accessibility: A criterion for regularity and hierarchy in visual pattern codes. *Journal of Mathematical Psychology, 35*(2), 151–213.

von der Malsburg, C. (1987). Synaptic plasticity as a basis of brain organization. In J. P. Chaneaux & M. Konishi (Eds.), *The neural and molecular bases of learning* (pp. 411–432). New York: Wiley.

Waltz, D. (1975). Understanding line drawings of scenes with shadows. In P. H. Winston (Ed.), *The psychology of computer vision* (pp. 19–92). New York: McGraw-Hill.

Weber, J. (1993). *The detection of temporal regularity in hearing and vision.* Unpublished PhD dissertation, Psychology Department, University of California, Berkeley.

Wertheimer, M. (1950). Untersuchungen zur Lehre von der Gestalt. *Psychology Forschung, 4,* 301–350. (Original work published 1923)

2 Perceptual Grouping in Space and in Space-Time: An Exercise in Phenomenological Psychophysics

Michael Kubovy and Sergei Gepshtein
University of Virginia

Perceptual organization lies on the border between our experience of the world and unconscious perceptual processing. It is difficult to study because it involves both bottom-up and top-down processes and because it is—like respiration—a semivoluntary process. For example, when we first glance at a Necker cube, we usually see a cube below eye level. Over this response we have no control; it is spontaneous and automatic. But as soon as we have seen the cube reverse, we seem to have some control over our interpretation of the drawing.

In this chapter we summarize our work on grouping in static and dynamic stimuli. In this work we have developed new methodologies that have allowed us to explore perceptual organization more rigorously than had hitherto been possible. These methodologies rely on the spontaneity and the multistability of grouping, while taking care to minimize the effects of whatever voluntary control observers might have over what they see.

The first two sections of this chapter deal with empirical and theoretical studies of grouping. The third is metamethodological. This third section is needed because our methods are phenomenological: They rely on the reports of observers about their phenomenal experiences. They also are psychophysical: They involve systematic exploration of stimulus spaces and quantitative representation of perceptual responses to variations in stimulus parameters. In short, we do phenomenological psychophysics. Because the observers' responses are based on phenomenal experiences, which are still in bad repute among psychologists, we fear that some may doubt the rigor of the research and seek other methods to supplant ours. So we conclude the chapter with an explication of the roots of such skeptical views and show that they have limited validity.

A CLARIFICATION OF TERMS

Grouping by spatial proximity is the process by which temporally concurrent regions of a scene become perceptually linked across space. Small-scale regions are customarily called elements. Fig. 2.1, part A, shows two such elements—❶ and ❷—being connected into a larger-scale entity. The two elements in Fig. 2.1, part A, could persist at their locations; in that case, they would be depicted as horizontally elongated ovals in the space-time diagram.

If ❶ and ❷ are not concurrent (❶ appears at Time 1, and ❷ appears at Time 2), to perceive ❶ and ❷ as a single element in motion (Fig. 2.1, part B), vision must link them across space and across time, a process we call grouping by spatiotemporal proximity (Gepshtein & Kubovy, 2001).

Now consider a more complicated display: two elements at Time 1 (❶ and ❷) and two elements at Time 2 (❸ and ❹). When motion is seen, one of two things happens: (1) ❶ may be linked with ❹, and ❷ is likely to be linked with ❸ so that the elements are matched independently (Fig. 2.1, part C[i]), or (2) the elements may form a grouping and be seen as a single moving entity (❶❷——→❸❹, Fig. 2.1, part C[ii]). In the latter case, the motion of the elements is the same as the motion of the group (Fig. 2.1, part C[iii]). In this process the visual system establishes a correspondence between elements visible at successive instants; the successive visual entities that undergo grouping by spatiotemporal proximity are called correspondence tokens (Ullman, 1979). Grouping by spatiotemporal proximity is also known as matching; the entities are then called matching units.

The representation of entities by dots in Fig. 2.1 should not be taken too literally. Research on perceptual grouping is not only about the perception of displays that consist of elements that are discrete in time and space. In the next section we discuss several examples of grouping between regions that at every instant appear

———→

FIG. 2.1.   A. Grouping by spatial proximity, B. grouping by spatiotemporal proximity, and C. their interactions. The configurations in C(i) and (ii) were introduced by Ternus (1936) who described two kinds of percepts: (i) element-motion, ❶——→❹ and ❷——→❸, and (ii) group-motion: ❶❷——→❸❹. (iii) Ullman (1979) argued that what looks like group-motion (iii) may actually be element-motion ❶——→❸ and ❷——→❹ (see also Fig. 2.16).

A. Grouping by Spatial Proximity

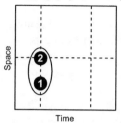

B. Grouping by Spatiotemporal Proximity

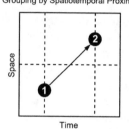

C. Interactions

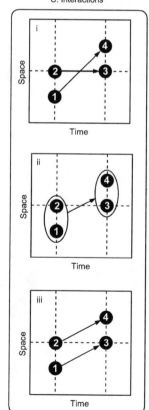

connected but that behave as separate matching units in grouping by spatiotemporal proximity. In general, we prefer to think of grouping as a process that causes us to see certain regions of the scene as being connected (whether they are physically connected or not) rather than a process that causes us to see the connections among discrete entities.

GROUPING BY SPATIAL PROXIMITY

The Gestalt psychologists' accounts of grouping were vague and qualitative. This need not be the case. When one pays attention to demonstrations of grouping, one becomes aware of the differential strength of certain effects. For example, in Fig. 2.2, part A, one spontaneously sees horizontal grouping. Even in Fig. 2.2, part B, one can see horizontal grouping, but with some difficulty. The tendency to see horizontal grouping is weaker in part B of Fig. 2.2 than in part A. Such observations are the seed of a quantitative theory.

More than 30 years elapsed between Wertheimer's formulation of the grouping principles and the emergence of the idea that the strength of grouping might

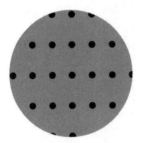

(A) Horizontal grouping by proximity.

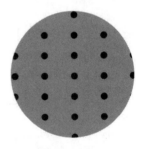

(B) Vertical grouping by proximity.

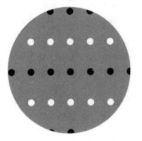

(C) Proximity and similarity in concert.

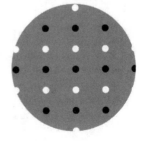

(D) Proximity and similarity in opposition.

FIG. 2.2. Examples of grouping by proximity and of the interaction of grouping by proximity and similarity.

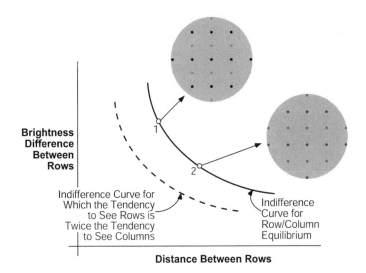

FIG. 2.3. Two grouping indifference curves. Only the solid curve is achievable by methods such as Hochberg's (illustrated here for the trade-off between grouping by proximity and grouping by similarity) and Burt and Sperling (1981; for the trade-off between grouping by spatial proximity and grouping by temporal proximity). Our method allows us to plot a family of indifference curves.

be measurable. Hochberg and his associates thought that the way to measure the strength of grouping by proximity was to pit it against the strength of grouping based on another principle, such as similarity. They used 6 × 6 rectangular lattices of squares (Hochberg & Silverstein, 1956) or 4 × 4 rectangular lattices of dots (Hochberg & Hardy, 1960). They determined which values of proximity and luminance were in equilibrium with respect to their grouping strength. For instance, while the spacing between columns remained constant, observers were asked to adjust the spacing between the rows of different luminance (Fig. 2.2, part D) until they found the spacing for which their tendency to see rows and columns was in equilibrium. Using this method, Hochberg and Hardy (1960) plotted what microeconomists call an indifference curve (Krantz, Luce, Suppes, & Tversky, 1971).[1] When Hochberg reduced the luminance difference between the rows, the distance between rows for which observers reported an equilibrium between rows and columns increased (Fig. 2.3). We call this a grouping indifference curve because the observer is indifferent among the ⟨luminance-difference, row-distance⟩ pairs that lie on it: They are all in equilibrium.

---

[1] Imagine a consumer who would be equally satisfied with a market basket consisting of 1 lb of meat and 4 lb of potatoes and another consisting of 2 lb of meat and 1 lb of potatoes. In such a case, the ⟨meat, potato⟩ pairs ⟨1, 4⟩ and ⟨2, 1⟩ are said to lie on an indifference curve.

Unfortunately, this method can give us only one indifference curve: the equilibrium indifference curve. We cannot tell where to place a grouping indifference curve for which all ⟨luminance difference, row distance⟩ pairs are such that the tendency to see rows is twice as strong as the tendency to see columns (dashed curve in Fig. 2.3). Can we measure the strength of grouping by proximity without reference to another principle of grouping? We have found that if we use a suitable class of stimuli, we can.

Generalizing the Gestalt Lattice

The suitable class of stimuli is dot lattices (Fig. 2.2 parts A and B) These are arrays of dots similar to those used by the Gestalt psychologists in their classic demonstrations. In most previous demonstrations and experiments, such arrays have been rectangular, with one direction vertical. Our dot lattices differ in two ways: The two principal directions of grouping are not always perpendicular, and neither principal orientation of the lattice need be vertical or horizontal.

A dot lattice is an infinite collection of dots in the plane. It is characterized by two (nonparallel) translations, represented by vectors **a** and **b** (Fig. 2.4). The idea of the two translations can be understood as follows. Suppose you copied the lattice onto a transparent sheet, which was overlaid on top of the original lattice so that the dots of the overlay were in register with the dots of the original lattice. You could pick up the overlay and shift it in either the direction **a** by any multiple of the length of **a**, |**a**|, and the dots of the overlay would once again be in register with the dots of the original lattice. The same is true of **b**. In other words, translating the lattice by **a** or **b** leaves it unchanged, invariant. Operations that leave a figure unchanged are called symmetries of the figure. Therefore, these two translations are symmetries of the lattice.

The two translation vectors **a** and **b** are not the only ones that leave the lattice invariant. In addition, the vector difference of **a** and **b**, **a** − **b** (which we denote **c**, Fig. 2.4), and the vector sum of **a** and **b**, **a** + **b** (which we denote **d**), are also symmetries of the lattice.[2] Any dot in the lattice has eight neighbors. Its distance from a neighbor is either **a**, **b**, **c**, or **d**. Another way to think about a dot lattice is to consider its building block: the basic parallelogram, $ABCD$ in Fig. 2.5. Its sides are **a** and **b**; its diagonals are **c** and **d**.

Any lattice can be defined by specifying three parameters: the lengths of the two sides of the basic parallelogram, |**a**| and |**b**|, and the angle between them, γ. If we do not care about the scale of a lattice, and are concerned only with its shape, only two parameters are needed: $|\mathbf{b}|/|\mathbf{a}|$ and γ.[3] Furthermore, these parameters are somewhat constrained. The distances between dots are constrained by the inequalities |**a**| ≤ |**b**| ≤ |**c**| ≤ |**d**|, and the angle γ is bounded, such that $60° \leq \gamma \leq 90°$ (Kubovy, 1994).

---

[2]There is an infinity of others, but they need not concern us here.

[3]Let |**a**| = 1.0. Then $|\mathbf{c}| = \sqrt{1 + |\mathbf{b}|^2 - 2|\mathbf{b}|\cos\gamma}$ and $|\mathbf{d}| = \sqrt{1 + |\mathbf{b}|^2 + 2|\mathbf{b}|\cos\gamma}$.

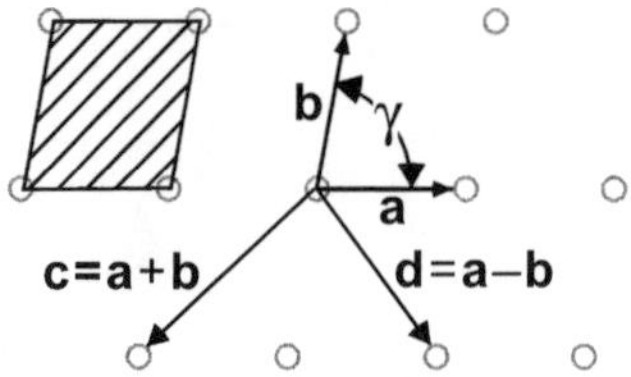

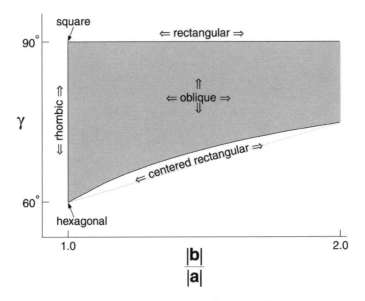

FIG. 2.4.   The features of a dot lattice (see text).

FIG. 2.5.   The space of dot lattices (see Fig. 2.6).

The two-parameter space of lattices is depicted in Fig. 2.5. This space can be partitioned into six classes, whose names appear in Fig. 2.5. The differences among these classes are portrayed in Fig. 2.6, where each class occupies a column.[4] In the top row of each column is the name of the lattice class. In the second row we show a sample lattice. In third row we show the basic parallelogram of the lattice. In the fourth row we compare the lengths of the four vectors. A dashed line connecting two bars means that they are of the same length. In the fifth row we depict the important properties of the lattice, which determine its symmetries. We spell out these properties symbolically at the bottom of each column. Two of these classes consist of just one lattice: the hexagonal lattice and the square lattice.

---

[4]Bravais (1866/1949), the father of mathematical crystallography, found five classes: According to his scheme, centered rectangular and rhombic lattices belong to the same class. The taxonomy proposed by Kubovy (1994) has six classes because he did not only consider the symmetries of dot lattices (as did Bravais) but also their metric properties.

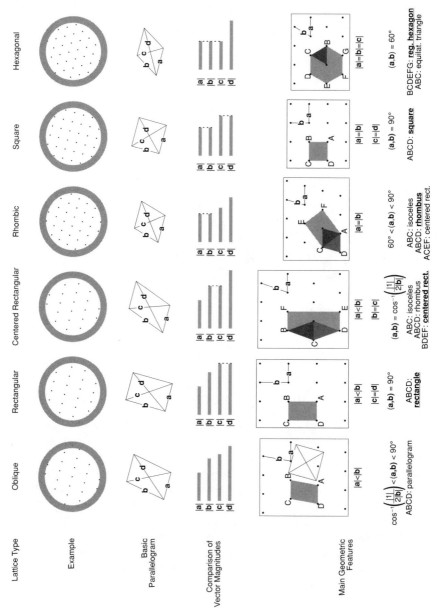

FIG. 2.6. The six classes of dot lattice according to Kubovy (1994).

The left to right order of the lattice classes in Fig. 2.6 is determined by their expected degree of ambiguity:[5]

- **Oblique:** No two vectors are of equal length. Therefore, these lattices have only two symmetries (disregarding the identity): the two translations.
- **Rectangular:** Because $|\mathbf{c}| = |\mathbf{d}|$, lattices in this class have three more symmetries than oblique lattices: two mirrors (one that bisects **a** and one that bisects **b**) and a rotation of 180° (also known as twofold rotational symmetry, or a half turn).
- **Centered rectangular:** Because $|\mathbf{b}| = |\mathbf{c}|$, you can always draw a rectangle that skips a row and a column (such as $BDEF$). This means that lattices in this class have two additional symmetries, called glide reflections. Imagine a horizontal axis between two adjacent rows of the lattice. Now reflect the entire lattice around this axis, while translating it over a distance $|\mathbf{a}|/2$. This transformation is similar to the relation between the right and left footprints made by a person walking on wet sand. There is also a vertical glide reflection in these lattices.
- **Rhombic:** The symmetries of this class of lattices are the same as those of centered rectangular lattices. Nevertheless these symmetries are more salient because $|\mathbf{a}| = |\mathbf{b}|$.
- **Square:** Here we have two equalities: $|\mathbf{a}| = |\mathbf{b}|$ and $|\mathbf{c}| = |\mathbf{d}|$. These add two mirrors along the diagonals of the basic parallelogram and fourfold rotational symmetry instead of the twofold rotational symmetry that the preceding classes inherited from the rectangular lattice.
- **Hexagonal:** Here we have a triple equality: $|\mathbf{a}| = |\mathbf{b}| = |\mathbf{c}|$. This means that this lattice has six mirrors and sixfold rotational symmetry.

The phenomenology of each lattice is determined by the symmetries we have just described. We might expect that the more symmetries a lattice has, the more unstable it is. We discuss this idea in the next section.

The Instability of Lattices

Kubovy and Wagemans (1995) conducted an experiment to measure the instability of grouping in dot lattices, which amounts to measuring their ambiguity. On each trial they presented 1 of 16 dot lattices (Fig. 2.7), sampled systematically (Fig. 2.8) from the space shown in Fig. 2.5 The screen was divided into two regions, the aperture and the black mask around it (Fig. 2.9A). The lattices, which consisted of a large number of yellow dots, were visible in the blue region of the screen only. Observers saw each lattice in a random orientation, for 300 ms. They were told that each lattice could be perceived as a collection of

---

[5]The reader who wishes to know more about the mathematics of patterns would do well to consult Martin (1982) and Grünbaum and Shepard (1987).

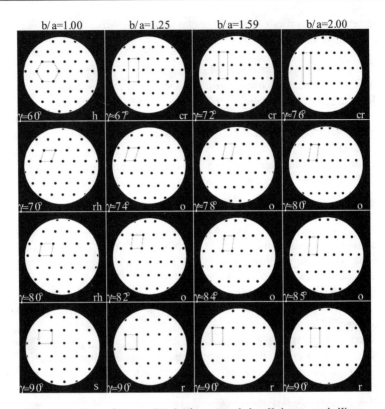

FIG. 2.7. The sixteen dot lattices used by Kubovy and Wagemans (1995): h—hexagonal; cr—centered rectangular; s—square; r—
rectangular; o—oblique. At the top of the figure, the |**b**|/|**a**| ratio. In
the lower lefthand corner of each panel, the value of γ.

parallel strips of dots and that the same lattice could have alternative organizations. They used a computer mouse to indicate the perceived organization of the
lattice (i.e., the direction of the strips) by selecting one of four icons on the response screen (Fig. 2.9B). Each icon consisted of a circle and one of its diameters.
The orientation of the diameter corresponded to the orientation of one of the four
vectors of the lattice just presented. Because the task involved a four-alternative
forced choice (4AFC) but no incorrect response, it is an example of phenomenological psychophysics (see discussion of phenomenological psychophysics in
the section "Subjectivity and Objectivity in Perceptual Research," later in this
chapter).

Some Theory.   Kubovy and Wagemans (1995) wanted to better understand the nature of Gestalts. They chose to formulate the least Gestaltlike model
they could and see where the data deviated from their predictions. We develop these

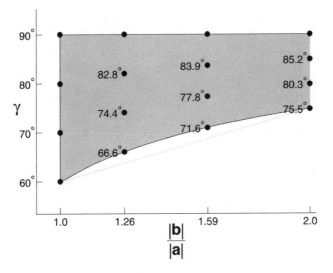

FIG. 2.8. How the sixteen stimuli were sampled from the space of dot lattices (see Fig. 2.5).

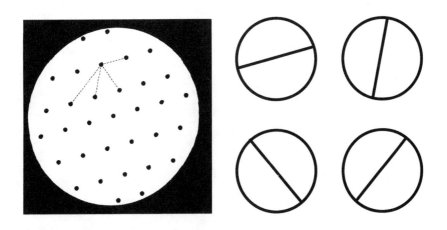

(A) A stimulus with four vectors.

(B) The four response alternatives.

Clockwise, from upper left: *a, b, d, c.*

FIG. 2.9. The Kubovy and Wagemans (1995) experiment.

ideas in a way that differs somewhat from the presentation in Kubovy and Wagemans.

Suppose that grouping is the product of interpolation mechanisms, and suppose that the visual system provides a number of independent orientation-tuned interpolation devices (OTID). Let us suppose that the **a**, **b**, **c**, and **d** vectors in the lattice excite four of these devices—α, β, γ, and δ—and that the others remain quiescent. The activated OTIDs will produce outputs that depend on the distance between dots in the four directions. We call these outputs grouping strengths, and we label them $\phi(\alpha)$, $\phi(\beta)$, $\phi(\gamma)$, $\phi(\delta)$. To make this function independent of scale, we use relative rather than absolute interdot distances (e.g., $^{|\mathbf{b}|}/_{|\mathbf{a}|}$, where $|\mathbf{a}|$ is the shortest distance between dots), rather than $|\mathbf{b}|$:

Grouping strength   If **v** is a general element of the set of lattice vectors, $\{\mathbf{a}, \mathbf{b}, \mathbf{c}, \mathbf{d}\}$, and υ is a general element of the set of OTIDs, $\{\alpha, \beta, \gamma, \delta\}$, then

$$\phi(\upsilon) = e^{-s\left(\frac{|\mathbf{v}|}{|\mathbf{a}|} - 1\right)}. \tag{1}$$

This means that grouping strength is a decaying exponential function of the distance between dots in the direction parallel to **v**, $|\mathbf{v}|$, relative to the shortest distance between dots, $|\mathbf{a}|$. The computation of $\phi(\upsilon)$ is illustrated in Fig. 2.10.

Choice probability   The four OTIDs are active concurrently, but the observer sees only one organization because the lattice is multistable. So we must distinguish overt responses from internal states; we do so by using italic characters to refer to responses (i.e., v represents the observers' indication that the lattice appears organized into strips parallel to **v**). Following Luce (1959) we assume that grouping strength is a ratio scale that determines the probability of choosing v, $p(v)$, in a simple way:

$$p(v) = \frac{\phi(\upsilon)}{\phi(\alpha) + \phi(\beta) + \phi(\gamma) + \phi(\delta)}. \tag{2}$$

The computation of $p(v)$ is illustrated in Fig. 2.11.

Entropy.   Having proposed their model of grouping, Kubovy and Wagemans (1995) were in a position to predict the instability of the organization of any dot lattice. To test this prediction they used the model to calculate the expected entropy (also known as the average uncertainty) of the responses to each lattice (Garner, 1962). The reader will recall that the entropy of a discrete random variable **x**, with sample space $X = \{x_1, \ldots, x_N\}$ and probability measure $P(x_n) = p_n$, is

$$H(\mathbf{x}) = -\sum_{n=1}^{N} p_n \log(p_n). \tag{3}$$

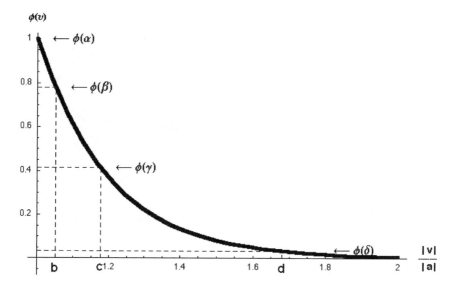

FIG. 2.10. Grouping strength in the theory proposed by Kubovy and Wagemans (1995). Here we have set the slope of the grouping strength function to $s = 5$. We also illustrate how one calculates the four grouping strengths for an oblique lattice in which $^{|b|}/_{|a|} = 1.05$ and $\gamma = 70°$. To indicate the inter-dot distances in this lattice we have placed the letters b, c, and d at $^{|b|}/_{|a|} = 1.05$, $^{|c|}/_{|a|} \approx 1.18$ and $^{|c|}/_{|a|} \approx 1.68$. The corresponding values of ϕ are $\phi(\beta) \approx 0.78$, $\phi(\gamma) \approx 0.41$, and $\phi(\delta) \approx 0.034$ ($\phi(\alpha)$ is always 1.0).

If the base of the logarithm is 2, the entropy is measured in bits (binary digits). Turning now to the predicted entropy of dot lattices, we have the following:

$$H = -\sum_{w \in W} p(w) \log_2 p(w), \qquad (4)$$

where $W = \{a, b, c, d\}$. These predictions are shown in Fig. 2.12.

The results, were encouraging (Fig. 2.13) but not entirely satisfactory. The model underestimated the amount of entropy in the responses to the most unstable lattices (i.e., those with the highest predicted entropy). That is one reason why Kubovy, Holcombe, and Wagemans (1998) revisited these data.

The Pure Distance Law

Kubovy et al. (1998) did not reanalyze the Kubovy and Wagemans (1995) data merely to improve the model but to address a fundamental question. Did the data deviate from the model because the anti-Gestalt assumptions of

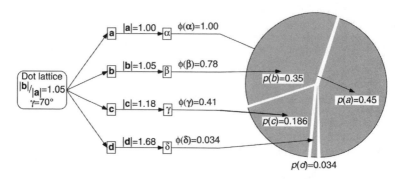

FIG. 2.11. How $p(v)$ is computed, according to the model of Kubovy and Wagemans (1995). The parameters are the same as those in Fig. 2.10.

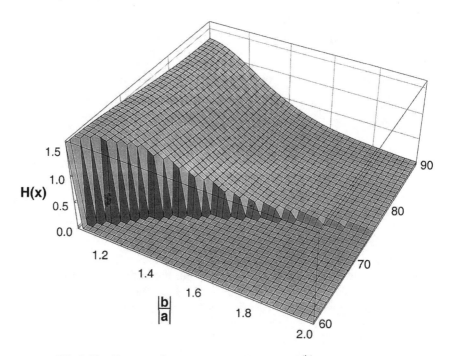

FIG. 2.12. Entropy of responses as a function of $^{|b|}/_{|a|}$ and γ, as predicted by Kubovy and Wagemans (1995). The x and y axes are the same as in Fig. 2.5. Note that where entropy is not defined (outside the curved boundary of the space of dot lattices) we let $H(x) = 0$. The value of s ($= 5$) is the same as in Fig. 2.10.

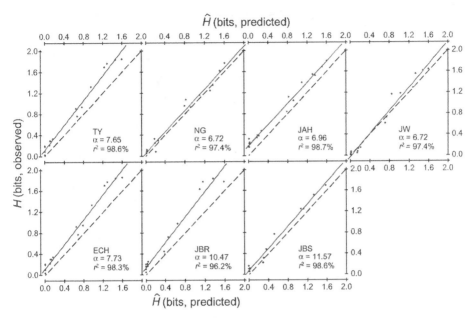

FIG. 2.13. Observed entropy of responses as a function of entropy predicted by Kubovy and Wagemans's model (1995) for seven observers. (Figure after Kubovy & Wagemans, 1995, Fig. 11.)

the model were false? Did they contain a clue to an interesting Gestaltish interaction?

The data collected by Kubovy and Wagemans (1995) were ideally suited to answering these questions. The stimuli had been sampled (Fig. 2.8) so that each type of lattice was represented multiple times (except for the hexagonal and the square, of course, which are points in the space of lattices, Fig. 2.5). As the reader will recall (see Fig. 2.6), the different classes of lattices have different symmetries and therefore have the potential to be organized differently. Kubovy et al. (1998) reasoned that if they could show that the probability of choosing a vector v depended on γ, or on the identity of the vector ($\mathbf{a}$, $\mathbf{b}$, $\mathbf{c}$, or $\mathbf{d}$), perhaps these dependencies would lead to a formulation of the Gestalt component of grouping in lattices.

They first noted that the data use four probabilities—$p(a)$, $p(b)$, $p(c)$, and $p(d)$. Because there are only three degrees of freedom in these data, they reduced them to three dependent variables: $p(b)/p(a)$, $p(c)/p(a)$, and $p(d)/p(a)$ (or $p(v)/p(a)$ for short). In addition, because in the data the range of these probability ratios was large, they used $\log[p(v)/p(a)]$ as their dependent variable(s).

The intricacies of the analyses conducted by Kubovy et al. (1998) are beyond the scope of this article. To make a long story short, they faced two problems, both of which were most severe when $|\mathbf{b}|$ was large: low probabilities for responses c and d and larger probabilities for response d than for response c. There was little they

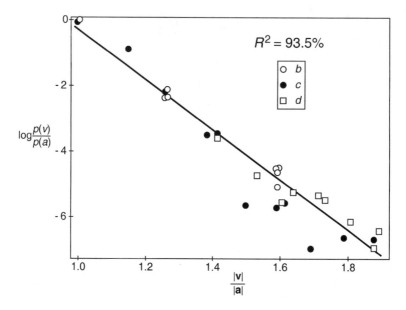

FIG. 2.14. The pure distance law for dot lattices. Average data for the seven observers.

could do about the first problem.[6] They were able to remedy the second problem, however, which was an unforeseen consequence of the geometry of lattices. If one holds $|\mathbf{a}|$ and γ constant and one increases the length of $\mathbf{b}$, the angle between $\mathbf{b}$ and $\mathbf{d}$ decreases. Thus the likelihood that an observer will respond d when he or she intended to choose b increases with $|\mathbf{b}|$. (Of course the observer will also respond b when he or she intended to choose d, but these are rare cases.) By carrying out an auxiliary experiment they were able to estimate the probability of this confusion and to develop a multinomial model that corrected for these errors.

Fig. 2.14 shows the results. This linear function, which we call the attraction function, whose slope is $s = 7.63$, accounts for 93.5% of the variance. Notice the three different data symbols: They represent the data for the log odds of choosing, b, c, or d relative to a. The fact that all these observation fall on the same linear function supports our theory and shows that the probability of choosing a vector v does not depend on γ or on the identity of the vector ($\mathbf{a}$, $\mathbf{b}$, $\mathbf{c}$, or $\mathbf{d}$). In other words, we have a pure distance law. This is a quantitative law of grouping by proximity, which states that grouping follows a decaying exponential function of relative interdot distances. We refer to this empirical relationship as a law because our evidence implies that it holds for all vectors in all possible dot lattices.

---

[6]We have since settled on a rule of thumb: not to use dot lattices in which $p^{(b)}/p(a) \geq 1.5$.

Where's the Gestalt?   The Gestalt psychologists were interested in emergent properties, in phenomena where the whole is different from the sum of the parts. Grouping by proximity is indeed an emergent property: It is not a property that holds for sets of dots smaller than say a 4 × 4 lattice. Nevertheless, the pure distance law is as simple a law as we can imagine. We can model the law by assuming that the lattice activates four independent units whose outputs jointly determine the probability of a winner-take-all percept (we see only one organization at a time). This independence is not in the spirit of the complex interactive processes we have come to associate with Gestalt-like theorizing.

GROUPING BY PROXIMITY IN SPACE-TIME

In the preceding section we saw that grouping by spatial proximity is decomposable into separable mechanisms and does not require the kind of holistic system the Gestalt psychologists proposed. Now we turn to the study of apparent motion (AM), a prototypical Gestalt concern (Wertheimer, 1912). Is AM decomposable into separable mechanisms: grouping by spatial proximity and grouping by spatiotemporal proximity?[7] The answer is no.

Sequential and Interactive Models

What is the relation between grouping by spatial proximity and grouping by spatiotemporal proximity? In this section of our chapter we consider two mutually exclusive classes of models:

Sequential models (SMs)   Grouping by spatial proximity and grouping by spatiotemporal proximity are separable and serial so that matching units are determined by their spatial proximity, independently of their spatiotemporal proximity. As we will see, this model can account for many phenomena of AM and is often tacitly taken as the default model.

Interactive models (IMs)   Grouping by spatial proximity and grouping by spatiotemporal proximity are inseparable: The latter can override former; matching units are sometimes derived by the combined operation of both processes.

Although many phenomena of AM are consistent with SMs, we will review evidence (including an experiment of our own) that shows that AM is better described by IMs than by SMs.

We assume (following McClelland, 1979) that in processing a scene the visual system constructs a cascade (a hierarchical set) of spatial representations. In such

---

[7]We defined these terms and others that we will need in the section "A Clarification of Terms" (p. 46).

a cascade more complex representations may contain entities from less complex ones, and each representation may interact both with more and less complex representations. Alternative representations emerge concurrently and can be accessed in parallel, as soon as they become available.

In SMs, mechanisms of temporal grouping can access alternative spatial representations in parallel so that the most salient spatial organization becomes a matching unit. Matching units can be thought of as sliders along the cascade of spatial perceptual organization because spatial entities of arbitrary complexity can serve as matching units (Fig. 2.15, part A). The most salient spatial organization determines what is seen to move.

The IM implies that both spatial and temporal grouping determine the level of spatial organization at which matching units arise. Competition occurs between the outputs of parallel motion matching operations applied to different

A. Sequential Model

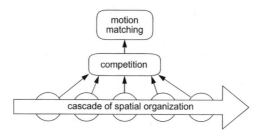

B. Interactive Model

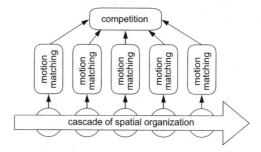

FIG. 2.15.   A. In the SM, alternative spatial representations compete so that the most salient one undergoes temporal grouping. Spatial grouping alone determines what is moving. B. In IMs, outputs of motion matching operations compete so that both spatial and temporal grouping determine the spatial complexity of matching units. (The horizontal arrows in A and B correspond to the direction of increasing complexity of spatial organization in the cascade.)

levels in the cascade of spatial organization (Fig. 2.15, part B). Thus, the salience of both spatial and temporal grouping contributes to the formation of matching units.

It is obvious that IMs preclude giving primacy to grouping by spatial proximity or grouping by spatiotemporal proximity. It may not be as obvious that SMs do not require giving priority to grouping by spatial proximity. For example, according to Neisser's (1967) early account of AM, motion perception integrates successive snapshots of the scene: Grouping by spatial proximity has priority— it alone determines which visual elements undergo motion matching. But this cannot be the whole story: Motion matching may precede grouping by spatial proximity. This is the case in random-dot cinematograms (RDCs), where each frame contains a different random texture. If we introduce a correlation between successive frames, so that a compact region of elements, f, moves from one frame to the next while retaining its texture (and the remaining dots are uncorrelated between frames), we see f segregated from the rest of the display, even though none of the individual frames is distinguishable from random texture. This is possible only if motion matching can occur before grouping by spatial proximity. The Gestalt psychologists referred to such phenomena as grouping by common fate (Wertheimer, 1923, who did not, however, have such unambiguous examples as RDCs).

Evidence That Seems to Favor Interactive Models, but Doesn't

As the exploration of AM progressed, increasingly complex motion displays were studied. We now review some of these and show that the complexity of an AM display does not count as evidence against SMs.

SMs and Ullman's Theory of Matching Units.
Our first illustration is Ullman's (1979) broken wagon wheel demonstration (Fig. 2.16). Every other spoke is interrupted in the middle. The angle between the neighboring spokes is α (Fig. 2.16, left). If between frames we rotate the spokes counterclockwise by an angle $\beta > \frac{\alpha}{2}$, one sees three rotating objects. The outer segments of the spokes are seen moving clockwise. The same is true of the inner segments of the spokes. In addition one sees a counterclockwise motion of the gaps. This result could be taken as evidence against SMs because entities that are not present in the static image are created in the AM display. However, we should not commit the isomorphism error, the error of thinking that what we experience is necessarily isomorphic with the underlying process. If we follow Ullman (1979) and assume that the visual system considers the line to be a collection of short line segments or dots, which it uses as matching units, and that the visual system chooses the shortest path between successive matching units to solve the correspondence problem, we can explain

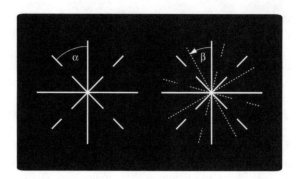

FIG. 2.16. The broken wagon wheel demonstration of Ullman (1979).

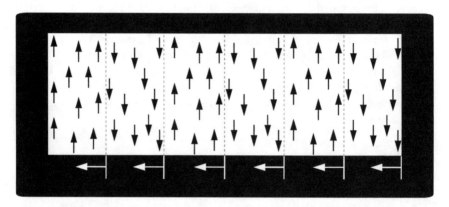

FIG. 2.17. Second-order motion as an example of recursive grouping (Cavanagh & Mather, 1990).

this effect in the spirit of SMs. (As we will see, Ullman's model is probably too restrictive because complex organizations can serve as matching units.)

The second illustration is the aperture problem (Hildreth, 1983; Wallach, 1935; Wallach & O'Connell, 1953). Whenever a line moves behind an aperture that occludes its endpoints, we see motion orthogonal to the line (illustrated on the left side of Fig. 2.18). This observation raises two problems:

1. Any segment on the line at time t_i may match any segment on the line at time t_{i+1}. This is the correspondence problem.
2. The size of these segments is unknown. This is the matching unit problem.

Ullman's (1979) model, which is a SM, can predict the visual system's solution to the aperture problem (e.g., Fig. 2.16).

A similar analysis applies to other displays. For example, Wallach, Weisz, and Adams (1956) observed that if one rotates an ellipse about its center, under some circumstances it is seen as a rigid rotating object and under others it is seen as an object undergoing elastic (nonrigid) transformation. The closer the ellipse aspect ratio is to 1 (i.e., the more closely it approximates a circle), the more likely we are to see an elastic transformation. In keeping with Ullman's view, Hildreth (1983) assumed that the matching units are fragments of the contour of the ellipse. She then showed that the effect of aspect ratio is predicted by a system that finds the smoothest velocity field that maps successive contour fragments onto each other.

According to Ullman (1979) and Hildreth (1983) the first stage of the matching process locates spatial primitives, which then become matching units: This is a SM; temporal grouping can have no influence on this process. Although the Ullman-Hildreth approach is parsimonious, the data for which it accounts are not inconsistent with IMs.

Recursive Grouping.   Matching units can be derived by the grouping by spatial proximity of entities that in turn are derived by grouping by spatiotemporal proximity. Such matching units are part of a hierarchical perceptual organization in which elements move within moving objects. Such cases are easily described by SMs.

One such example is grouping by common fate (Wertheimer, 1923): Elements extracted by grouping by spatiotemporal proximity are segregated from the background and form a moving figure. It occurs for both translation (Wertheimer, 1923) and rotation (Julesz & Hesse, 1970). The resulting elements may be subject to further spatial organization, which might produce, for example, a three-dimensional object (shape-from-motion; Ullman, 1979). This phenomenon is consistent with SMs because the matching units are derived by grouping by spatial proximity alone (S_1), which is followed by grouping by spatiotemporal proximity (T_1). T_1 determines the directions and the velocities of the elements, which are used by a subsequent grouping by spatial proximity (S_2) to derive the object's shape. The recursive operation is $S_1 \longrightarrow T_1 \longrightarrow S_2$.

Cavanagh and Mather (1990) produced another instance of recursive grouping. They created a stimulus composed of a set of adjacent vertical bands, in each of which randomly positioned short-lived elements moved vertically. Adjacent bands contained elements moving in opposite directions (Fig. 2.17). The boundaries between these bands were easily visible. When they were made to drift to the left, observers readily saw the motion. A recursive SM would describe the phenomenon as follows:

S_1. The short-lived random elements are output by grouping by spatial proximity, which cannot do much grouping because the elements in each frame are random.

T_1. The elements in each frame are matched by grouping by spatiotemporal proximity and identified as dots moving up or down.

S_2. Dots moving in the same direction undergo grouping by spatial proximity (grouping by common fate) to generate the different moving strips, as a result of which we see boundaries between them. These boundaries, which from frame to frame are translated to the left, serve as input to T_2.

T_2. Compares successive boundaries and detects their leftward motion (called second-order motion by Cavanagh & Mather, 1990). The output of T_2 does not depend on the boundaries between the strips being derived by T_1, which is a grouping by spatiotemporal proximity. These boundaries could have been produced by grouping in space by luminance or color. The recursive SM is $S_1 \longrightarrow T_1 \longrightarrow S_2 \longrightarrow T_2$.

Matching of Groupings.   We have seen that matching units can be spatial primitives or spatial aggregates of similar moving spatial primitives. Can SMs account for cases when grouping by spatial proximity organizes visual primitives into groupings that become matching units?

Adelson and Movshon (1982) showed observers two superimposed moving gratings through a circular aperture (Fig. 2.18). When either moving grating is presented alone, it is seen moving at right angles to the orientation of its bars, which is the visual system's solution of the aperture problem. When the superimposed gratings are identical (as in Fig. 2.18, part A), the gratings are fused and seen as a single plaid moving in an orientation different from the motion of the individual gratings. However, when the superimposed gratings are sufficiently different (as in Fig. 2.18, part B), they are not fused; they are seen as two overlaid gratings, each moving at a right angle to the orientation of its bars. Thus, from the appearance of the static displays we can infer the output of the spatial grouping by similarity that derives the matching units—the gratings or the plaids—is independent of grouping by spatiotemporal proximity. This is consistent with a SM.

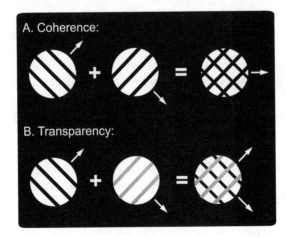

FIG. 2.18.   The Adelson and Movshon (1982) plaids.

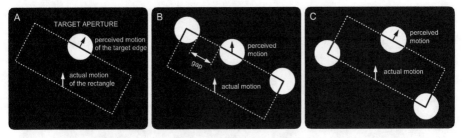

FIG. 2.19. An outline of a rectangle (the white dotted outline in the diagrams) moves vertically behind an opaque screen (Ben-Av & Shiffrar, 1995). Panel B: the only configuration that produces veridical motion perception.

SMs are applicable even when the components of a figure do not overlap but still group in space. Consider, for example, displays (Shiffrar & Pavel, 1991) in which a rectangle moves vertically behind an opaque screen, seen through circular apertures (Fig. 2.19; Ben-Av & Shiffrar, 1995). When only one edge of the rectangle is visible (the black solid line in Fig. 2.19, part A) through the circular aperture (labeled "target aperture"), its motion is orthogonal to its orientation, the default solution of the aperture problem. When a single corner is visible, it is seen to move vertically. Ben-Av and Shiffrar asked whether the motions of the corners can capture (or disambiguate) the motion of the edge when two corners and an edge are visible. They found that the motion of the corners did capture the motion of the edge (and produce veridical vertical motion) when the visible corners were collinear with the edge and when the distance between the corners and the edge (the "gap" in Fig. 2.19, part B) was short. When the corners were collinear but remote, or when they were not collinear, no matter how close (Fig. 2.19, part C), the motion of the edge was not affected by the motion of the corners; the edge appeared to move orthogonal to its orientation. The findings of Ben-Av and Shiffrar are consistent with SMs: Corners and edges group into matching units. When the visible components of the rectangle are collinear and close to each other, they group in space so that grouping by spatiotemporal proximity occurs between the composite matching units.

Matching of High-Level Units. Organizations more complex than aggregates of similar elements can become matching units. These phenomena too are consistent with SMs. For example, Shepard and Judd's (1976) rapid alternation of two images of a three-dimensional object (such as in Fig. 2.20) looks like the object is rotating in depth. To derive this motion, grouping by spatiotemporal proximity must match homologous parts of the object, rather than small spatial primitives (Rock, 1988, p. 33–57). According to SMs, it was the grouping by spatial features of the frames that derived the complex matching units in the displays of Shepard and Judd.

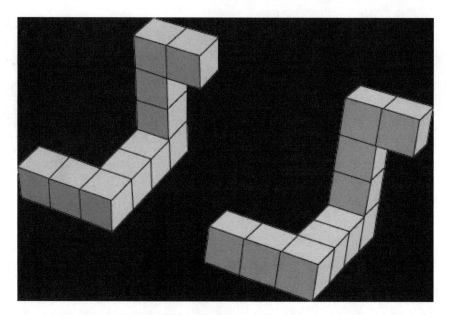

FIG. 2.20. When the two images are shown in rapid alternation, observers see a rotating three-dimensional object (Shepard & Judd, 1976).

The Shepard and Judd displays suggest that if grouping by spatiotemporal proximity had matched small-scale entities, the percept would have been different. Ramachandran, Armel, and Foster (1998) created a display that showed just that. They created pairs of fragmented patterns, called Mooney faces, that are sometimes seen as faces, and sometimes as a random patterns (Fig. 2.21). Observers who saw the pattern as a face, experienced motion in a different direction from the one specified by matching the individual fragments. As in Shepard and Judd's display (1976), the grouping by spatial features within the frames derives complex matching units, and hence this phenomenon is consistent with a SM. However, Ramachandran et al. go further: They show that the familiarity of the nascent object can facilitate the grouping by spatial features of elements into complex matching units and thus determine the level in the cascade of spatial organization, which is accessed by grouping by spatiotemporal proximity. (Others have shown interactions between object familiarity and grouping by spatiotemporal proximity, including McBeath, Morikawa, & Kaiser, 1992; Shiffrar & Freyd, 1990; Tse & Cavanagh, 2000.)

Form and AM. AM has been commonly studied using displays of spatial shapes, spatially well-segregated from the rest of the scene. In these displays the spatial distance between the successive shapes has usually been much greater

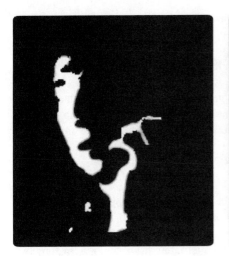 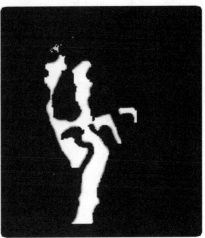

FIG. 2.21. The two images of Mooney faces are shown in rapid alternation. When observers see a face, they perceive it rotating in depth. When they do not, they perceive incoherent motion in the picture plane (Ramachandran et al., 1998).

than the distance between concurrent elements within the shapes. Under such conditions, the grouping by spatial proximity between the concurrent elements of a shape is much stronger than the grouping by spatiotemporal proximity between the elements of the shape in successive views. Hence, grouping by spatiotemporal proximity is given little chance to compete with the grouping by spatial proximity between the concurrent elements. Such displays always support SMs.

SMs have also been assumed in studies of the interaction of form and AM. In this literature, researchers assume that vision derives the form of an object before the grouping by spatiotemporal proximity between the objects takes place. Because of this bias in favor of SMs, the question of form-motion interaction has been generally posed in a way that excludes IMs: Do form properties of moving objects affect grouping by spatiotemporal proximity? An answer to this question has been sought in two directions: the similarity of an object's form across successive views of it (e.g., Burt & Sperling, 1981; Kolers, 1972; Orlansky, 1940; Oyama, Simizu, & Tozawa, 1999) and the transformational relations between successive forms (e.g., Eagle, Hogervorst, & Blake, 1999; Warren, 1977). In neither of these directions has a consensus been reached regarding the sensitivity of grouping by spatiotemporal proximity to form differences of the grouped entities.

The distinction between SMs and IMs has consequences for research on form and AM. If IMs are correct, the question of whether grouping by spatiotemporal proximity and object form affect each other should be explored under conditions where the strength of grouping by spatiotemporal proximity of objects is comparable with the strength of grouping by spatial proximity between the concurrent elements. Only then we find the conditions under which the form of nascent objects affects the interactions between concurrent and successive elements.

In a study we presently describe, Gepshtein and Kubovy (2000) show that spatial form affects motion matching when the spatial distances between concurrent elements are large enough to compete with the spatial distances between successive elements. One could also demonstrate the influence of spatial form on AM by reducing the spatial distances between successive elements, to the point that successive elements overlap. This approach has been adopted in the ingenious "transformational AM" displays by Tse and colleagues (Tse, Cavanagh, & Nakayama, 1998; Tse & Logothetis, 2002).

Seeming Evidence Against SMs. The Ternus display has been offered as evidence against the SM. In this section we show that it is not. In this display (Ternus, 1936) dots occupy three equally spaced collinear positions (Fig. 2.1C[i]–[iii]). These displays consist of two rapidly alternating frames, represented by two vertical dotted lines in Fig. 2.1. The dots in one frame are ❶ and ❷; the dots in the other frame are ❸ and ❹. This display can give rise to two percepts: (1) element motion (*e*-motion), which occurs when a single dot appears to move between the positions ❶ and ❹, and dot ❷ appears immobile when replaced by dot ❸ (Fig. 2.1C[i]), and (2) group motion (*g*-motion), which occurs when two dots appear to move back-and-forth as a group, from ❶❷ to ❸❹ (Fig. 2.1C[ii]).

The longer the interstimulus interval (ISI; interframe interval in this context), the higher the likelihood of *g*-motion (Kramer & Yantis, 1997; Pantle & Picciano, 1976). This phenomenon is called the ISI effect. According to Kramer and Yantis (1997) the ISI effect implies that grouping by spatiotemporal proximity between successive elements affects the grouping by spatial proximity between concurrent elements, thus supporting the IM. Kramer and Yantis assumed that the shorter the ISI, the stronger the grouping by spatiotemporal proximity. Thus, when ISI is short, grouping by spatiotemporal proximity overrides the grouping by spatial proximity of the concurrent dots, and *e*-motion is likely. As ISI grows, the strength of grouping by spatiotemporal proximity drops and allows concurrent dots to group within the frames, thus increasing the likelihood of *g*-motion.

We hold that the ISI effect is not inconsistent with SMs for two reasons:

1. Longer ISIs could have two effects: They could weaken grouping by spatiotemporal proximity, as Kramer and Yantis assumed, or they could allow more time for grouping by spatial proximity to consolidate the organization of concurrent dots. If the latter is true, we could attribute the ISI effect to grouping by spatial proximity, rather than to grouping by spatiotemporal proximity, and conclude that the ISI effect is consistent with SMs.
2. If an observer sees *g*-motion, one cannot tell whether the matching units were dots or dot groupings because in either case matching yields motion

in the same direction (Fig. 2.1C[iii]). Therefore, the group motion percept may actually be the result of matching of individual dots, just as in *e*-motion; different spatial distances would favor different kinds of *e*-motion (Braddick, 1974; Burt & Sperling, 1981; Korte, 1915). (Ullman, 1979, also explained the percept of *g*-motion in the Ternus display in terms of the grouping by spatiotemporal proximity of individual elements.)

Evidence for Interactive Models

The only types of motion perception in the current literature that truly undermine the generality of SMs involves overlapping objects and surfaces whose relation is changing dynamically, which we call dynamic superposition. The perception of dynamic superposition poses a challenge to SMs because grouping by spatial proximity alone cannot derive matching units when objects and surfaces are revealed gradually.

Take, for example, the perception of kinetic occlusion (Kaplan, 1969; Michotte, Thinès, & Grabbé, 1964), where a hitherto visible (or invisible) part of the scene is perceived to become occluded by (or revealed from behind) an opaque object or surface (Kellman & Cohen, 1984; Sigman & Rock, 1974; Tse et al., 1998). In such cases a simple correspondence between successive views is impossible because one frame has a different number of elements than the next frame or because the elements in successive frames are markedly different. Likewise, if the moving object or surface is transparent (Cicerone, Hoffman, Gowdy, & Kim, 1995; Shipley & Kellman, 1993), finding correspondence is hampered because the appearance of the covered region changes as it becomes covered.

Perhaps the most dramatic demonstration of perception under dynamic superposition is anorthoscopic form perception (Rock, 1981), where observers can perceive the form of an object revealed successively through a narrow slit in the occluder. The visual system must accumulate information over time to produce a percept that is the most likely cause of the observed optical transformations.

Although the evidence of perception under dynamic superposition undermines SMs, it is too specific to carry the burden of refuting SMs in favor of IMs. Displays of dynamic superposition contain characteristic clues, which may trigger specialized mechanisms. For example, two clues present in kinetic occlusion are the accretion of texture (as the textured object emerges from behind the occluder; Kaplan, 1969) and the presence of T-junctions between the contours of the occluder and of the occluded object. These cues may trigger a mechanism specialized in dealing with dynamic superposition or a high-level inferential mechanism designed to construct a plausible interpretation of the scene in a process of thoughtlike problem solving (von Helmholtz, 1962; Kanizsa, 1979; Rock, 1983).

To refute the class of SMs, we must demonstrate that grouping by spatial proximity and grouping by spatiotemporal proximity interact, even when a simple correspondence between the successive frames is possible and no specialized, or inferential, mechanism is required. Thus, we conducted a study (Gepshtein & Kubovy, 2000) in which we tested SMs using spatiotemporal dot lattices, called motion lattices.

Motion Lattices. Motion lattices allowed us to independently vary the strength of grouping by spatial proximity and grouping by spatiotemporal proximity by manipulating spatial proximity between concurrent and successive dots (Fig. 2.22).

As we observed earlier (with regard to Ternus displays), the duration of the ISI does not necessarily determine the strength of grouping by spatiotemporal proximity because grouping by spatial proximity may consolidate as the ISI grows and because longer ISIs may favor matching over a different spatial range. Therefore, in our motion lattices we held ISI constant and varied the strength of grouping by spatiotemporal proximity by manipulating the spatial proximity between successive dots.

Why not use other AM displays? First, consider Ternus displays, in which—as in motion lattices—either element motion (*e*-motion) or group motion (*g*-motion) can be seen. In Ternus displays, however, the directions of *e*-motion and *g*-motion do not differ. In motion lattices the direction of *e*-motion is determined by matching individual dots in successive frames of the display, whereas the direction of *g*-motion is determined by the matching of dot groupings (strips of dots, or virtual objects) in successive frames. In motion lattices the direction of *g*-motion is orthogonal to the orientation of the objects, which is different from the direction of *e*-motion.

Second, consider displays introduced by Burt and Sperling (1981), who presented observers with a succession of brief flashes of a horizontal row of dots. Between the flashes, they displaced the row both horizontally and downward so that under appropriate conditions observers saw it moving downward and to the right (or to the left). Burt and Sperling studied the trade-off between space and time in motion matching and the effect of element similarity on matching. But their stimulus did not allow them to explore the effect of relative proximity between

---

$\longrightarrow$

FIG. 2.22. The design of motion lattices. Two frames of a motion lattice are shown schematically in A and B; the frames are superimposed in C. Distances *b* and *s* correspond to the shortest inter-dot distances within the frames (shown in A and B). Vectors m_1 and m_2 (shown in C) are the most likely *e*-motions (i.e., motions derived by matching of individual elements). When vision derives motion by matching dot groupings (called virtual objects), rather than dots themselves, motion orthogonal to the virtual objects is seen (*g*-motion). In C, *g*-motion is horizontal (notated *orth*) because the virtual objects are vertical.

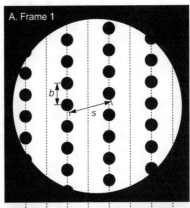

A. Frame 1

$$r_s = \frac{s}{b}$$

Static Ratio
controls spatial grouping within the frames

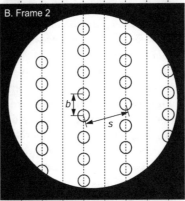

B. Frame 2

$$r_m = \frac{|m_2|}{|m_1|}$$

Motion Ratio
controls competition between e-motions m_1 and m_2

$$r_b = \frac{b}{|m_1|}$$

Baseline Ratio
controls competition between e-motion and g-motion

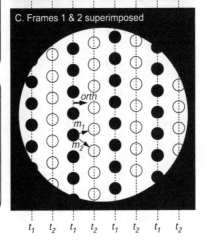

C. Frames 1 & 2 superimposed

t_1 t_2 t_1 t_2 t_1 t_2 t_1 t_2

concurrent and successive dots. Motion lattices allowed us to set up a competition between alternative spatial organizations within a frame because in these stimuli each frame contains a two-dimensional pattern of dots. We thus could ask whether grouping by spatiotemporal proximity affects grouping by spatial proximity.

A Critical Test of the SM.   According to the SM, the propensity of elements to form virtual objects within frames, and thus yield g-motion, is independent of the determinants of grouping by spatiotemporal proximity (i.e., grouping between successive dots). As Kubovy, Holcombe, and Wagemans (1998b) showed, grouping by spatial proximity within static dot lattices is only determined by relative proximity between the concurrent dots. That is, the angles between alternative organizations of the lattice and its symmetry properties do not affect its organization. Gepshtein and Kubovy (2000) used this property of static dot lattices to test the SM by asking whether the likelihood of g-motion is affected by variations in the proximity between successive dots when the proximity between concurrent dots is held constant.

Fig. 2.22 describes our motion lattices. We obtained them by splitting static lattices into two frames so that every frame contains every other column (or row) of the original lattice (we call them two-stroke motion lattices, $\mathcal{M}^2$). When the frames of a motion lattice are shown in rapid alternation with the appropriate spatial and temporal parameters, observers see a flow of AM. When they report dots flowing in a direction of matching between individual dots, we say that they are seeing e-motion. When they report dots flowing in a direction orthogonal to virtual objects formed within the frames, we say that they are seeing g-motion.

In Fig. 2.22, the dots are likely to group into vertical virtual objects within frames. If grouping by spatiotemporal proximity across frames occurs between virtual objects, rather than between dots, observers see motion orthogonal to the virtual objects (i.e., horizontal motion in Fig. 2.22). Fig. 2.23 (parts A–B) shows frames from $\mathcal{M}^2$ in which horizontal g-motion is likely. If we arrange dots within the frames so that virtual objects are less salient, g-motion is less likely. For example, the two frames shown in panels C–D of Fig. 2.23 belong to an $\mathcal{M}^2$, where g-motion is less likely than in the $\mathcal{M}^2$ whose frames are shown in panels A–B.

According to SMs, the likelihood of seeing g-motion rather than e-motion depends on the propensity of concurrent dots (within the frames) to form virtual objects and does not depend on grouping by spatiotemporal proximity. Because SMs hold that matching units are derived by grouping by spatial proximity alone, only spatial proximities between concurrent dots determine the likelihood of whether e-motion or g-motion is seen. In contrast, IMs hold that the grouping by spatial proximity of dots within frames is affected by grouping by spatiotemporal proximity between successive dots.

To pit the models against each other, we measured the relative frequency of reports of e-motion and g-motion under conditions of equivalent spatial grouping within frames (Fig. 2.24). Within frames, the salience of virtual objects cannot

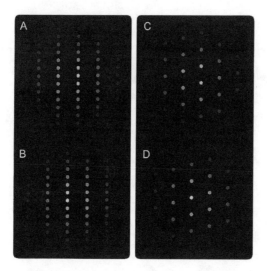

FIG. 2.23. Frames of motion lattices (not to scale). A–B. Two frames of a lattice in which *g*-motion is likely (high r_s and low r_b). C–D. Two frames of a lattice in which *e*-motion is likely (low r_s and high r_b).

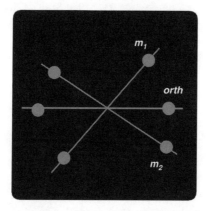

FIG. 2.24. A response screen corresponding to the lattice shown in Fig. 2.23 C–D (not to scale). Observers click on a circle attached to the radial line parallel to the perceived direction of motion. (Response labels m_1, m_2, and *orth* did not appear on the response screen.)

change as long as the ratio between relevant spatial distances is invariant. Thus, as long as $r_s = \frac{s}{b}$ (Fig. 2.22) does not change, the propensity of dots to form vertical virtual objects does not change. In our experiment we held r_s constant while varying the strength of grouping by spatiotemporal proximity. Under these conditions, according to SMs, the likelihood of seeing *g*-motion rather than *e*-motion should not change, but according to IMs the likelihood of *g*-motion should drop.

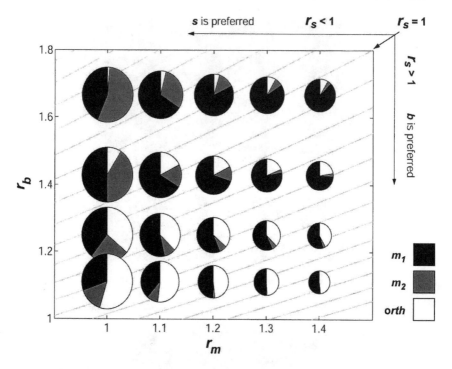

FIG. 2.25.   Results of our experiment. The pie charts show the distributions of three responses (m_1, m_2, and *orth*) for 20 configurations
of motion lattices. The gray lines in the background are iso-r_s lines;
within these lines the salience of spatial virtual objects is invariant
(see text). Gepshtein, S. & Kubovy, M. (2000). The emergence of visual objects in space-time. *Proceedings of the National Academy
of Sciences, 97,* 8186–8191. Copyright 2000 National Academy of
Sciences, U.S.A.

Our experiments supported IMs. The pie charts in Fig. 2.25 show the distributions of three responses—m_1, m_2, and *orth*—for different configurations of motion
lattices. Three trends in these data are noteworthy:

1. The frequency of m_1 motion grows as a function of r_m.
2. The frequency of *orth* motion drops as r_b grows.
3. The frequency of *orth* motion varies within the sets of iso-r_s conditions,
   marked with oblique gray lines.

We can explain the third observation in two steps:

1. We constructed a statistical model of the data shown in Fig. 2.25. (The model
   accounted for 98% of the variance in the data.)

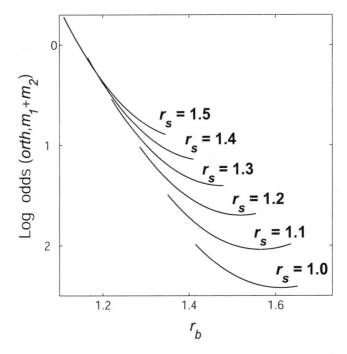

FIG. 2.26. Results of our experiment. The relative likelihood of *g*-motion (*orth* responses) and *e*-motion (*m$_i$* responses) changes within the iso-*r$_s$* sets of conditions, in contrast to the prediction of the sequential model (see text). Gepshtein, S. & Kubovy, M. (2000). The emergence of visual objects in space-time. *Proceedings of the National Academy of Sciences, 97,* 8186–8191. Copyright 2000 National Academy of Sciences, U.S.A.

2. We interpolated motion frequencies within the iso-*r$_s$* sets of parameters. A result of this computation is shown in Fig. 2.26, where each curve plots the relative frequency of *g*-motion and *e*-motion within a corresponding *r$_s$* set.

Fig. 2.26 shows that when *r$_s$* is big (i.e., when *s* ≫ *b*, as in the top iso-*r$_s$* curves), grouping by spatial proximity within the frames tends to derive vertical virtual objects (vertical in the coordinate system used in Fig. 2.22 and 2.23), and horizontal *g*-motion is likely. When *r$_s$* decreases (*s* approaches *b*, as in the bottom iso-*r$_s$* curves), the salience of vertical virtual objects drops, and the likelihood of *g*-motion decreases. Critically, the fact that the frequency of *g*-motion changes within the iso-*r$_s$* sets indicates that it is not only the spatial proximities within the frames that determine what is seen to move in motion lattices. This demonstrates the validity of IMs.

Where's the Gestalt?   AM is an emergent property, just as is grouping by proximity. We have found that it is impossible to decompose motion perception into two successive grouping operations: grouping by spatial proximity and grouping by spatiotemporal proximity. This complexity is more in the spirit of Gestalt theories than the Kubovy and Wagemans model presented in the first part of this chapter.

IN PRAISE OF PHENOMENOLOGICAL PSYCHOPHYSICS

Subjectivity and Objectivity in Perceptual Research

Palmer (this volume) opens his discussion of methodological approaches to the study of perceptual organization with Fig. 1.2, in which he shows several demonstrations of grouping. His discussion of such demonstrations concludes that the "phenomenological demonstration is a useful, but relatively blunt instrument for studying perceptual organization." We wholeheartedly concur. Two reasons Palmer gives for worrying about phenomenological demonstrations are they do not produce quantifiable results, and they have a subjective basis. Palmer believes that the quantification problem can be overcome by using what he calls quantified behavioral reports of phenomenology, an approach we prefer to call phenomenological psychophysics.[8] All the experiments we describe in this chapter belong to this category.

Although phenomenological psychophysics may solve the quantification problem, does it solve the problem of subjectivity? Twenty years ago, when Pomerantz and Kubovy (1981) wrote the overview chapter of *Perceptual Organization,* they did not think so:

> The pragmatic streak in American psychology drives us to ask what role... experiences, however compelling their demonstration, play in the causal chain that ends in action. Thus we ask whether such phenomenology might not be a mere epiphenomenon, unrelated to behavior. (p. 426)

Palmer's skepticism is very much in line with this position. His solution to the problem—to use objective behavioral tasks—is also in agreement with Pomerantz and Kubovy (1981):

> If we can set up situations in which we ask subjects questions about the stimulus that have a correct answer, and if organizational processes affect their judgments

---

[8]We prefer our term because we think that the data produced by such a method should be called quantified only if they have been described by a metric mathematical model. In phenomenological psychophysics, responses of different kinds can be counted, and therefore statistics may be applicable. They may or may not lend themselves to mathematical modeling.

(and so their answers), then the experimentalists' skepticism about the importance of organizational phenomena should be dispelled. This book presents a wealth of organizational phenomena that can be demonstrated by both the phenomenological method and by objective experimental techniques. (p. 426)

We have come to disagree with Pomerantz and Kubovy's views on this matter and therefore disagree with Palmer's. First, there is the matter of the contrast between phenomenological and objective. It is tendentious to use the terms subjective or objective in this context, for two reasons. First, because subjectivity is widely thought to be inconsistent with the scientific method, whereas objectivity is its hallmark. Second, because objectivity bespeaks unbiasedness; in current English it has an honorific connotation.

When we study perceptual organization we are studying perceptual experiences that are phenomenal but not idiosyncratic. The *Merriam-Webster Dictionary* gives several definitions for the adjective *subjective,* two of which are relevant here:

Subjective = phenomenal. "A characteristic of or belonging to reality as perceived rather than as independent of mind."
Subjective = idiosyncratic. "Peculiar to a particular individual... arising from conditions within the brain or sense organs and not directly caused by external stimuli."

One source of the concern with the subjectivity of the phenomena of perceptual organization is the conflation of these two senses. Judging that something is red is accompanied by a subjective experience that is phenomenal but is not idiosyncratic. One can easily find an object and viewing conditions under which an overwhelming majority of people would agree that the object is red. Judging that an object is beautiful is also accompanied by a subjective experience, but this experience is both phenomenal and idiosyncratic. It is not so easy find an object and viewing conditions under which an overwhelming majority of people would agree that the object is beautiful.

That is why, when we study perceptual experiences that are phenomenal but not idiosyncratic, we say that we are doing experimental phenomenology rather than studying subjective experience. We recommend that the discipline eschew the use of the terms objective and subjective to characterize perceptual research methods. They can only lead to confusion.

The Role of Traditional Psychophysical Tasks

What about the concern voiced then by Pomerantz and Kubovy (1981) and now by Palmer: Can one determine whether an experience is epiphenomenal (perhaps Palmer would call it purely subjective)? We take this concern seriously. After all, "measuring perceived grouping is fundamentally different from measuring perceived size or perceived distance, which have well-defined objective measures against which people's behavioral reports can be compared for accuracy"

(Palmer, this volume). Perceived size can be studied by the traditional methods of psychophysics. Can perceptual organization be studied by embedding it in an experimental task for which responses can be judged to be correct or incorrect (i.e., a traditional psychophysical task)? This involves, to quote Palmer, "changing what is actually being studied from subjective grouping to something else" (this volume).

We will now show just what this transformation of one task into another entails and what it achieves. Then, we will show what role phenomenological psychophysics can play in the study of perceptual organization.

As opposed to phenomenological psychophysics, traditional psychophysical tasks are indirect. This idea is illustrated in Fig. 2.27, parts A and B. In natural viewing conditions, as well as in the tasks used in phenomenological psychophysics, certain aspects of the visual scene ("stimulus" in the figure) lead to a corresponding percept by means of a private perceptual process. The latter is labeled "spontaneous perceptual process" in the figure to emphasize that the process occurs naturally, just as it does when the observer views the stimulus outside the laboratory. The hatched regions in Fig. 2.27 are private in the sense that only the observer enjoys immediate access to the outcomes of this process; this experience is made public (i.e., accessible to others) by means of a report. The experimental phenomenologist strives to devise experimental conditions such as to make the report as close as possible to how observers would describe their experiences outside of the laboratory but in a highly controlled environment. We will refer to such reports as phenomenological.[9]

In traditional psychophysics the natural perceptual experience is transformed. It is transformed by asking observers to judge certain aspects of the stimulus, which engages mechanisms normally not involved in the perception of natural scenes. Or the perception of the stimulus is hindered, either by adding external noise to the stimulus or by presenting the stimulus at the threshold of visibility. We question whether such transformations of perceptual experience are indispensable in the studies of perceptual organization.

As an illustration of traditional psychophysics applied to the research of perceptual organization, consider the experiments in which Palmer and Bucher (1981) studied the pointing of equilateral triangles (Fig. 2.27, part C). An equilateral triangle appears to point about equally often at 60°, 180°, or 300° (Fig. 2.27, part C, left). If you align three such equilateral triangles along a common axis of mirror symmetry tilted 60° (Fig. 2.27, part C, right), they appear to point most often at 60°. Palmer and Bucher used a two-alternative forced choice (2AFC) procedure; they asked observers to decide whether the triangle(s) could be seen pointing right or left (0° or 180°; Fig. 2.27, part C left). Obviously, these triangles cannot point to the right (0°). We have seen that the isolated triangle appears to point

---

[9]We recommend that the term for an indirect report be descriptive, such as correct/incorrect task, rather than evaluative, such as objective task.

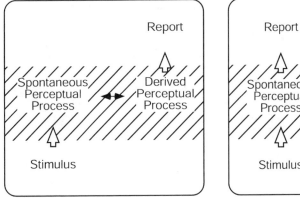

(A) Traditional psychophysical procedure.

(B) Phenomenological psychophysical procedure.

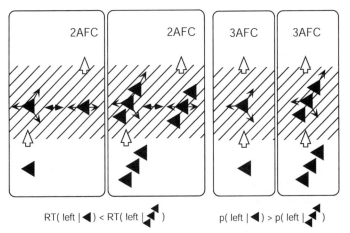

RT(left | ◀) < RT(left | ◀)

p(left | ◀) > p(left | ◀)

(C) The Palmer and Bucher (1981) experiment as a traditional psychophysical procedure (2 AFC). RT stands for reaction time.

(D) Hypothetical study of the pointing using phenomenological report (3AFC).

FIG. 2.27. Comparison of the processes that take place in an observer engaged in different types of experimental procedures. The hypothetical events that are not public are marked by hatched band. The procedures of traditional psychophysics force the observer to do perceptual work (horizontal double arrows; i.e., to transform their experience to meet the requirements of the procedure). Thus they engage additional perceptual processes compared to the procedures of phenomenological psychophysics. In that sense the latter are more direct than the former.

81

spontaneously in all directions equally, but when axis-aligned, it tends to point at 60°. As a consequence, in the configuration shown in Fig. 2.27, part C, right panel, observers were slower to decide whether the axis-aligned triangles pointed to the right or to the left than to decide whether the isolated triangle did. (RT in Fig. 2.27, part C, stands for reaction time.) We will say that the pointing induced by the common axis forced the observers in the experiments of Palmer and Bucher to do "perceptual work": The observers had to overcome the automatic effect of alignment on pointing to focus on the properties of each triangle and give a correct answer. Perceptual work is a transformation of spontaneous experience; it is represented in Fig. 2.27, part C, by double horizontal arrows. It is this perceptual work that persuades us that the effect of common axis is not epiphenomenal (or purely subjective).

After one has established that the effect of common axis on pointing is not epiphenomenal, one could explore the effect directly, without forcing observers to do perceptual work (Fig. 2.27, part D, right).[10] For example, one could use phenomenological psychophysics procedure with a three-alternative forced-choice (3AFC), in which the observer's task is to report (by pressing one of three keys) in which direction the middle (or single) triangle is pointing (in Fig. 2.27(d) "p(X)" stands for the probability of percept X). This is a phenomenological report because the three report categories offered to the observers agree with the three likely spontaneous organizations of the stimulus.

The inferences involved in the interpretation of psychophysical studies of perceptual organization would make no sense without assuming the existence of a covert spontaneous organization, which under the appropriate eliciting circumstances would have led to the phenomenological report. Psychophysical studies of perceptual organization are no more than an indirect assessment of the effects of grouping. Hence, when available, we prefer experimental phenomenology.

This is not to say that tasks that have correct and incorrect responses can only serve to examine the epiphenomenality of a Gestalt phenomenon. When an organizational phenomenon is subtle or complex, such tasks may give us valuable information about underlying processes. Yet we hope that we have persuaded the reader that indirect psychophysical methods do not have an intrinsic advantage over phenomenological methods. Indeed, one of our goals in this chapter was to demonstrate the power of experimental phenomenology.

ACKNOWLEDGMENTS

This chapter supported by NEI grant R01 EY 12926–06.

---

[10]Palmer (1980) used a similar procedure to the one we are recommending.

REFERENCES

Adelson, E. H., & Movshon, J. A. (1982). Phenomenal coherence of moving visual patterns. *Nature, 300,* 523–525.

Ben-Av, M. B., & Shiffrar, M. (1995). Disambiguating velocity estimates across image. *Vision Research, 35*(20), 2889–2895.

Braddick, O. (1974). A short-range process in apparent motion. *Vision Research, 14,* 519–1527.

Bravais, A. (1949). *On the systems formed by points regularly distributed on a plane or in space.* New York: Crystallographic Society of America. (Original work published 1866)

Burt, P., & Sperling, G. (1981). Time, distance, and feature tradeoffs in visual apparent motion. *Psychological Review, 88,* 171–195.

Cavanagh, P., & Mather, G. (1990). Motion: The long and short of it. *Spatial Vision, 4,* 103–129.

Cicerone, C. M., Hoffman, D. D., Gowdy, P. D., & Kim, J. S. (1995). The perception of color from motion. *Perception & Psychophysics, 57,* 761–777.

Eagle, R. A., Hogervorst, M. A., & Blake, A. (1999). Does the visual system exploit projective geometry to help solve the motion correspondence problem? *Vision Research, 39*(2), 373–385.

Garner, W. R. (1962). *Uncertainty and structure as psychological concepts.* New York: Wiley.

Gepshtein, S., & Kubovy, M. (2000). The emergence of visual objects in space-time. *Proceedings of the National Academy of Sciences, 97,* 8186–8191.

Gepshtein, S., & Kubovy, M. (2001). The weights of space and time in the perception of visual motion [abstract]. *Journal of Vision, 1,* 243a. Retrieved December 12, 2001 from http://journalofvision.org/ 1/3/243, DOI 10.1167/1.3.243

Grünbaum, B., & Shepard, G. C. (1987). *Tilings and patterns.* New York: W. H. Freeman.

Hildreth, E. C. (1983). *The measurement of visual motion.* Cambridge, MA: MIT Press.

Hochberg, J., & Hardy, D. (1960). Brightness and proximity factors in grouping. *Perceptual and Motor Skills, 10,* 22.

Hochberg, J., & Silverstein, A. (1956). A quantitative index of stimulus-similarity: Proximity versus differences in brightness. *American Journal of Psychology, 69,* 456–458.

Julesz, B., & Hesse, R. I. (1970). Inability to perceive the direction of rotation movement of line segments. *Nature, 225,* 243–244.

Kanizsa, G. (1979). *Organization in vision: Essays on gestalt perception.* New York: Praeger.

Kaplan, G. A. (1969). Kinetic disruption of optical texture: The perception of depth at an edge. *Perception & Psychophysics, 6,* 193–198.

Kellman, P. J., & Cohen, M. H. (1984). Kinetic subjective contours. *Perception & Psychophysics, 35,* 237–244.

Kolers, P. A. (1972). *Aspects of motion perception.* Oxford, UK: Pergamon.

Korte, A. (1915). Kinematoskopische untersuchungen [Kinematoscopic investigations]. *Zeitschrift für Psychologie, 72,* 194-296.

Kramer, P., & Yantis, S. (1997). Perceptual grouping in space and time: Evidence from the Ternus display. *Perception & Psychophysics, 59,* 87–99.

Krantz, D. H., Luce, R. D., Suppes, P., & Tversky, A. (1971). *Foundations of measurement Vol. I. Additive and polynomial representations.* New York: Academic Press.

Kubovy, M. (1994). The perceptual organization of dot lattices. *Psychonomic Bulletin & Review, 1*(2), 182–190.

Kubovy, M., Holcombe, A. O., & Wagemans, J. (1998). On the lawfulness of grouping by proximity. *Cognitive Psychology, 35*(1), 71–98.

Kubovy, M., & Wagemans, J. (1995). Grouping by proximity and multistability in dot lattices: A quantitative gestalt theory. *Psychological Science, 6*(4), 225–234.

Luce, R. D. (1959). *Individual choice behavior.* New York: Wiley.

Martin, G. E. (1982). *Transformation geometry: An introduction to symmetry.* New York: Springer-Verlag.

McBeath, M. K., Morikawa, K., & Kaiser, M. K. (1992). Perceptual bias for forward-facing motion. *Psychological Science, 3*(6), 362–367.

McClelland, J. L. (1979). On the time relations of mental processes: An examination of systems of processes in cascade. *Psychological Review, 86,* 287–330.

Michotte, A., Thinès, G., & Grabbé, G. (1964). Les compléments amodaux des structures perceptives. In *Studia psychologica.* Louvain, Belgium: Publications Universitaires de Louvain. [Translation into English in A Michotte's Experimental Phenomenology of Perception G, Thinees, A Costall, G, Butterworth (Eds.) (1991; Hillsdale, NJ: Lawerence Erlbaum Associates)]

Neisser, U. (1967). *Cognitive psychology.* New York: Appleton Century Crofts.

Orlansky, J. (1940). The effect of similarity and difference in form on apparent visual movement. *Archives of Psychology (Columbia University), 246,* 1–85.

Oyama, T., Simizu, M., & Tozawa, J. (1999). Effects of similarity on apparent motion and perceptual grouping. *Perception, 28*(6), 739–748.

Palmer, S. E. (1980). What makes triangles point: Local and Global effects in configurations of ambiguous triangles. *Cognitive Psychology, 12,* 285–305.

Palmer, S. E., & Bucher, N. M. (1981). Configural effects in perceived pointing of ambiguous triangles. *Journal of Experimental Psychology: Human Perception and Performance, 7,* 88–114.

Pantle, A. J., & Picciano, L. (1976). A multistable movement display: Evidence for two separate motion systems in human vision. *Science, 193,* 500–502.

Pomerantz, J. R., & Kubovy, M. (1981). Perceptual organization: An overview. In M. Kubovy & J. Pomerantz (Eds.), *Perceptual organization* (pp. 423–456). Hillsdale, NJ: Lawrence Erlbaum Associates.

Ramachandran, V. S., Armel, C., & Foster, C. (1998). Object recognition can drive motion perception. *Nature, 395,* 852–853.

Rock, I. (1981). Anorthoscopic perception. *Scientific American, 244,* 145–153.

Rock, I. (1983). *The logic of perception.* Cambridge, MA: MIT Press.

Rock, I. (1988). The description and analysis of object and event perception. In K. R. Boff, L. Kauffman, & J. P. Thomas (Eds.), *Handbook of perception and human performance* (Vol. 2, pp. 33-1–36-71). New York: Wiley.

Shepard, R. N., & Judd, S. A. (1976). Perceptual illusion of rotation of three-dimensional objects. *Science, 191,* 952–954.

Shiffrar, M., & Freyd, J. F. (1990). Apparent motion of the human body. *Psychological Science, 1*(4), 257–264.

Shiffrar, M., & Pavel, M. (1991). Percepts of rigid motion within and across apertures. *Journal of Experimental Psychology: Human Perception and Performance, 17*(3), 749–761.

Shipley, T. F., & Kellman, P. J. (1993). Optical tearing in spatiotemporal boundary formation: When do local element motions produce boundaries, form, and global motion? *Spatial Vision, 7,* 323–339.

Sigman, E., & Rock, I. (1974). Stroboscopic movement based on perceptual intelligence. *Perception, 3,* 9–28.

Ternus, J. (1936). The problem of phenomenal identity. In W. D. Ellis (Ed.), *A source book of Gestalt psychology* (pp. 149–160). London: Routledge & Kegan Paul. (Original work published 1926)

Tse, P., Cavanagh, P., & Nakayama, K. (1998). The role of parsing in high-level motion processing. In T. Watanabe (Ed.), *High-level motion processing* (pp. 249–266). Cambridge, MA: MIT Press.

Tse, P. U., & Cavanagh, P. (2000). Chinese and Americans see opposite apparent motions in a Chinese character. *Cognition, 74*(3), B27–B32.

Tse, P. U., & Logothetis, N. K. (2002). The duration of 3D form analysis in transformational apparent motion, *Perception & Psychophysics, 64*(2), 244–265.

Ullman, S. (1979). *The interpretation of visual motion.* Cambridge, MA: MIT Press.

von Helmholtz, H. (1962). *Treatise on physiological optics* (Vol. III). New York: Dover Publications. (Original work published 1867)

Wallach, H. (1935). Uber visuell wahrgenommene bewegungsrichtung [On the visually perceived direction of motion]. *Psychologische Forschung, 20,* 325–380.

Wallach, H., & O'Connell, D. N. (1953). The kinetic depth effect. *Journal of Experimental Psychology, 45,* 205–207.

Wallach, H., Weisz, A., & Adams, P. A. (1956). Circles and derived figures in rotation. *American Journal of Psychology, 69,* 48–59.

Warren, W. H. (1977). Visual information for object identity in apparent movement. *Perception & Psychophysics, 21*(3), 264–268.

Wertheimer, M. (1912). Experimentelle studien über das sehen von bewegung [Experimental studies on seeing motion]. *Zeitschrift für Psychologie, 61,* 161–265.

Wertheimer, M. (1923). Untersuchungen zur Lehre von der Gestalt, II [Investigations of the principles of Gestalt, II]. *Psychologische Forschung, 4,* 301–350.

3 On Figures, Grounds, and Varieties of Surface Completion

Mary A. Peterson
University of Arizona

FIGURE-GROUND SEGREGATION: UNANSWERED QUESTIONS

Two regions can be defined for each edge in the visual field, one lying on each side. Typically, the edge appears to shape only one of these two regions, and figure-ground segregation is said to occur. Figures are regions of the visual field that appear to have a definite shape, a shape bestowed in part by their bounding contour (i.e., their edge). If figures are familiar objects, they can be identified (barring brain damage or the imposition of external noise). The region adjacent to the figure is locally shapeless near the edge it shares with the figure; this shapeless region is called the ground (short for background) because it often appears to complete amodally behind the figure. Although figure-ground segregation is a venerable topic in visual perception (cf. Rubin, 1915/1958), a number of questions about figures and grounds remain unanswered.

One critical longstanding question is, Why can figures be identified if they are familiar, whereas grounds cannot? A traditional answer to this question is that the determination of figure versus ground precedes access to object memories and that figures, not grounds, are matched to object memories. On this view, grounds cannot be identified because they are not matched to object memories. The observation

87

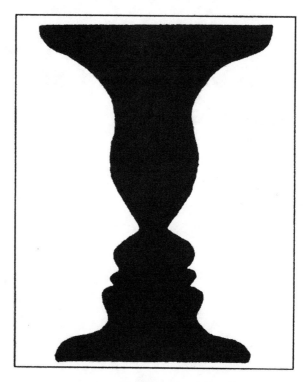

FIG. 3.1. The Rubin vase-faces display.

that identifiability is coupled to figural status has been taken as support for this figure-ground first assumption.

Consider Fig. 3.1. When the black region appears to be the figure, it can be identified as a vase; the white regions appear shapeless near the borders of the vase and seem to continue behind the vase. Alternatively, when the white regions appear to be the figures, they can be identified as face profiles, whereas the black region appears to be shapeless near the borders of the faces, apparently continuing behind them. The coupling between identifiability and figural status does not constitute support for the figure-ground first assumption, however, because couplings cannot support inferences of causality (Peterson, 1999a). Many theorists adopt the causal approach for functional reasons, arguing that it would be computationally inefficient to match against object memories those regions that will ultimately appear shapeless. However, when arguments regarding computational inefficiency are raised, it is worth pointing out that the design features of vision are not necessarily those that are deemed efficient a priori.

A second question concerning figure-ground segregation, related to the first question, is, Why is the region adjacent to the figure shapeless? Some have answered this question by claiming that one-sided contour assignment is obligatory

(Driver & Baylis, 1996) and that a region lacking a contour (as the ground does) is necessarily shapeless. But one-sided contour assignment is not obligatory. It has long been known that certain contours shape both adjacent regions and that others shape neither region (Kennedy, 1974, p. 96). Moreover, it is generally agreed that the two regions on either side of a contour (or edge) are assessed for the Gestalt configural cues of symmetry, relative convexity, relative area, closure, and so on,

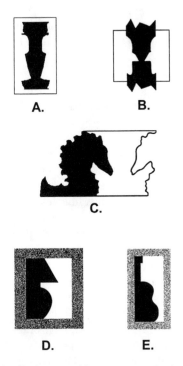

FIG. 3.2.   Sample displays used in our research. A and B were used by Peterson et al (1991). Gestalt configural cues and monocular depth cues favor the interpretation that the black center region is the figure. The white surround regions portray two standing women (in A) and two profile faces (in B). C is a schematic of a stimulus used by Peterson and Gibson (1994a). "Must shape recognition follow figure-ground organization? An assumption in peril." *Psychological Science*, Blackwell Publishing Co. Reprinted with permission. The white region is symmetric around a vertical axis, whereas the black asymmetric region portrays a portion of a seahorse. Thus, for purposes of figure assignment at the edge shared by the black and white regions, the Gestalt configural cue of symmetry competes with an object memory cue. D and E were used by Peterson and Gibson (1993). In these displays, the black and white regions are approximately equated for area and convexity, but the black region is high in denotivity, portraying a portion of a table lamp in D and a portion of a guitar in E.

before figure assignment is complete. Given that a substantial amount of configural processing has taken place on both sides of the contour, it remains to be explained why the region adjacent to the figure is perceived to be shapeless when one-sided contour assignment does occur. The question regarding apparent shapelessness applies regardless of whether the apparently shapeless region would be a familiar or a novel shape if it were seen as the figure (e.g., compare the white regions of Fig. 3.2, parts A and E).

A third unanswered question concerning figure-ground segregation is whether regions adjacent to figures are necessarily completed behind the figure. Can they be completed in front of the figure? Must they be completed at all? The answer will ultimately depend on the extent to which the factors that influence figure-ground segregation determine depth segregation.

A fourth question, related to the third, is whether or not two-dimensional displays are good surrogates for three-dimensional displays. The terms figure and ground, introduced by Rubin and used by the Gestalt psychologists, were originally used to describe the perception of two-dimensional displays. The Gestalt psychologists explicitly assumed that two-dimensional displays were good surrogates for three-dimensional displays (e.g., Rubin, 1915/1958); more recently, others have argued that they are not (e.g., Marr, 1982). In fact, two-dimensional displays may be good surrogates for three-dimensional displays for investigating some questions but not others.

A fifth question concerning figure-ground segregation is whether or not it should be considered a stage of processing. Many investigators consider figure-ground segregation to be a stage of processing that serves to separate the wheat of candidate objects from the chaff of shapeless grounds. Following figure-ground segregation, the former can be matched to object memories, and can serve as targets for action, whereas the latter can be safely eliminated from further processing. It is easy to conceptualize figure-ground segregation as a stage of processing if one accepts the assumption that figure-ground assignment precedes access to object memories. Hence, the answer to the fifth question is likely to be related to the answer to the first question.

CHAPTER OUTLINE

In the remainder of this chapter, I will address the five questions raised previously. In the second section, I review evidence indicating that, contrary to traditional assumptions, memories of object structure (at least) are accessed before figural status is determined (Question 1). Next, I discuss a model that accounts for these effects and provides a mechanism for the apparent shapelessness of grounds (Question 2). Recent evidence supporting the model is reviewed. At the end of the third section, I begin to consider whether regions adjacent to a figure are necessarily amodally completed behind the figure (Question 3). Then, I show that in some ways two-dimensional displays are good surrogates for three-dimensional displays, whereas in other ways they are not (Question 4). Consideration of three-dimensional displays has led me to conclude that figure-ground segregation is not a stage of processing (Question 5) and to propose that it is simply one possible outcome of the interactions among cues to shape and depth. Other outcomes are possible, some of which will be discussed in this chapter. Conceiving of figure-ground segregation as an outcome rather than as a stage opens up new questions about how various visual properties interact to produce the perception of shape and distance. Some of these questions are raised at the end of the chapter.

TWO-DIMENSIONAL DISPLAYS

Object Memory Effects on Figural Status

My colleagues and I found that, contrary to the figure-ground first assumption, memories of the structure of known objects are accessed sufficiently early in perceptual processing to affect figure assignment (Peterson & Gibson, 1994a, 1994b; Peterson, Harvey, & Weidenbacher, 1991). These results were obtained in experiments using both two-dimensional and three-dimensional displays. The research conducted with two-dimensional displays will be discussed in this section; research using three-dimensional displays will be discussed in the third section.

In our stimuli, the edge between two regions sketches an identifiable portion of a known object along one side only. The side of the edge on which the portion of the known object is sketched is called the high-denotative side. The term high-denotative reflects the fact that a large percentage of pilot observers viewing the high-denotative regions agreed on which shape was portrayed along the high-denotative side; in other words, the high-denotative side of the border reliably elicited the same basic level shape perception in pilot observers. The opposite side of the border, called the low-denotative side, did not elicit high agreement about which object, if any, it portrayed. We found it impossible to create articulated regions that were meaningless to all observers, although we could create regions that elicited agreement from less than 25% of our pilot observers. We interpret the denotivity of a stimulus as an index of its goodness of fit to an object memory, with higher levels of denotivity indicating better matches.

Sample two-dimensional stimuli are shown in Fig. 3.2, parts A–E, where the high-denotative regions portray portions of a standing woman in white on the left and right sides of the black central shape (Fig. 3.2, part A), profiles of two identical faces in white (Fig. 3.2, part B), a portion of a seahorse in black (Fig. 3.2, part C), a portion of a table lamp in black (Fig. 3.2, part D), and a portion of a guitar in black (Fig. 3.2, part E). In many of the displays we used (e.g., Fig. 3.2, parts A–C), Gestalt configural cues (e.g., symmetry, smallness of relative area, enclosure) or the monocular depth cue of interposition, or both, favored the interpretation that the low-denotative region was the figure. In other two-dimensional displays, the high- and low-denotative regions were equated for the Gestalt configural cues (and the monocular depth cues were absent; e.g., Fig. 3.2, parts D and E). In this second type of display (but not the first), the only known cue to figural status that distinguished between the two regions was the object memory cue.

We presented our two-dimensional displays in both upright and inverted orientations and sometimes in orientations in between (e.g., Peterson & Gibson, 1994a, 1994b; Peterson et al., 1991). (The term upright refers to the orientation of the display in which the known object was portrayed in its typical upright orientation. Inverted displays were rotated 180° around the z axis.) We manipulated stimulus orientation because the object recognition literature had shown that it takes less time to identify objects when they are seen in their typical upright orientation than when they are rotated away from their upright (e.g., Jolicœur, 1988; Tarr & Pinker, 1989). These identification results could be taken to indicate that some critical threshold necessary for identification is reached earlier in time for upright displays than for displays misoriented from upright. (See Perrett, Oram, & Ashbridge, 1998, for a recent articulation of this view.)

We related these orientation-dependent identification effects to figure assignment as follows. It is generally accepted that figure assignment occurs quite early in the course of perceptual organization. Therefore, it seemed reasonable to argue that only those variables assessed within some critical time frame can affect figure assignment. Thus, if memories of object structure do affect figure assignment, their influence might be evident when displays with a high-denotative region are shown in an upright orientation but not when they are shown in an inverted orientation. For inverted displays, figural status might be determined before memories of object structure reach some critical threshold necessary to affect figure assignment. Changing the orientation of our displays from upright to inverted left unchanged the other cues that were present and known to affect figural status (e.g., overlap, symmetry, enclosure, smallness of relative area, convexity). Therefore, any increased likelihood of seeing the high-denotative regions of our displays as figures when the stimuli were upright versus inverted could be attributed to object memory cues that were present in the upright condition and diminished or absent in the inverted condition.

Consistent with the idea that memories of object structure can affect figure assignment (provided they are accessed quickly), we found that high-denotative regions were more likely to be seen as figures when the displays were upright rather than inverted. The same pattern of results was found both under brief masked exposure conditions in which observers reported which region first appeared to be the figure (Gibson & Peterson, 1994; Peterson & Gibson, 1994a) and under long exposure conditions in which observers reported perceived reversals of figure and ground (Peterson et al., 1991; Peterson & Gibson, 1994b). These results led us to propose that memories of object structure can be accessed sufficiently early in the course of perceptual organization to influence figure assignment. Inverting the displays slowed access to the critical object memories, thereby diminishing, or removing, their contributions to perceived organization.

On the basis of these experiments, we proposed that edges, detected early in the course of perceptual processing (and not just edges assigned to regions already partially or wholly determined to be figures) are the substrate for accessing memories of object structure. In our view, edge-based access to memories of object structure occurs in parallel with assessments of the configural cues and the depth cues, rather than afterwards (the parallel hypothesis). Our results can also be understood within an hierarchical interactive model in which regions (rather than edges) are matched to object memories following initial assessments of the configural cues (Vecera & O'Reilly, 1998, 2000). Presently, it is difficult to distinguish the hierarchical interactive model from our parallel model (Peterson, 1999b; Vecera & O'Reilly, 2000, but see Peterson, 2003). Both models account for our data indicating that object memories are accessed before figure assignment is complete and for converging evidence provided by others (e.g., Vecera & Farah, 1997). The critical difference is whether initial access to object memories is considered to be edge based or region based.

Cue Competition

Our experiments conducted with two-dimensional displays indicated that the object memory cue does not necessarily dominate putatively lower level cues to figure status, such as interposition, symmetry, and smallness of relative area. Nor do low-level cues necessarily dominate the putatively higher level object memory cue. We investigated this question directly in experiments using the displays shown in Fig. 3.3 (Peterson & Gibson, 1994a). In each display, a high-denotative region and a low-denotative region shared a central edge. The horizontal symmetry (i.e., reflectional symmetry around a vertical axis) of the high- and low-denotative regions was manipulated orthogonally. The stimuli were exposed briefly (14 ms to 100 ms) and masked immediately. Observers reported whether the region lying on the left or the right side of the central edge appeared to have a definite shape by pressing a key to their left or their right. They were given an option to press neither key if both regions appeared to be shaped by the central border or if neither region did.

The data from an unpublished experiment ($N = 24$ participants; 100-ms stimulus exposure) are shown in Table 3.1. The results clearly indicate that both memories of object structure and the configural cues of symmetry affect perceived figural status. Averaging over symmetry conditions, high-denotative regions were more likely to be seen as figures when the displays were upright (74.5%) rather than inverted (58%). And, considering only inverted displays with one symmetric and one asymmetric region (regardless of denotivity), symmetric regions (72%) were

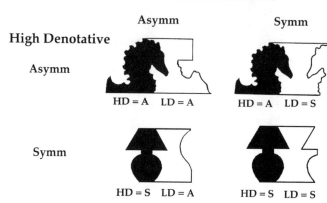

Low Denotative

FIG. 3.3. The four types of stimuli used by Peterson and Gibson (1994a). "Most shape recognition follow figure-ground organization? An assumption in peril." *Psychological Science,* Blackwell Publishing Company. Reprinted with permission. In all stimuli, a high-denotative and a low-denotative region shared a central edge. In this figure, high-denotative regions are shown on the left in black, and low-denotative regions are shown on the right in white. In the experiment, the high-denotative regions appeared equally often on the left and the right and in black and in white. Also in this figure, the white regions are outlined in black on the top, bottom, and outer sides. This black outline is necessary to delimit the white regions of the stimuli from the white background. In the experiment, the black and white stimuli were shown on a gray background; no black outline surrounded the white regions. Symm = Symmetric around a vertical axis drawn through the center of the region. Asymm = Asymmetric.

more likely than adjacent asymmetric regions to be seen as figures. This percentage is consistent with recent estimates of the strength of the symmetry cue reported by others (e.g., Driver, Baylis, & Rafal, 1992).

The condition that permits an assessment of how the Gestalt cue of symmetry and the object memory cue fare when they are placed in conflict is the condition in which the low-denotative region was symmetric (LD$_S$) and the high-denotative region was asymmetric (HD$_A$). For inverted versions of these LD$_S$/HD$_A$ displays, the high-denotative region was seen as the figure in only 29% of the trials (i.e., the symmetric low-denotative region was seen as the figure in 71% of the trials). This percentage reflects the strength of the symmetry cue when the object memory cue is absent or diminished by virtue of stimulus inversion. When competition from memories of object structure was present in the upright condition, however, the high-denotative regions were twice as likely to be seen as figures as they were in the inverted condition (59% vs. 29%). In other words, the percentage of figure reports consistent with the symmetry cue decreased markedly, to 41%. The comparison of

TABLE 3.1

Percentage of Trials on Which the High-Denotative
Region Was Seen as the Figure as a Function of the
Symmetry and the Orientation of the Adjacent High-
and Low-Denotative Regions

High Denotative	Low Denotative	
	ASYMM	SYMM
ASYMM		
Upright	72%	59%
Inverted	64%	29%
SYMM		
Upright	87%	80%
Inverted	72%	67%

Note. ASYMM = asymmetric; SYMM = symmetric.

performance obtained with upright and inverted displays revealed that memories of object structure do affect figural status when they are placed in competition with the Gestalt configural cue of symmetry.

Despite the substantial and significant increase in the likelihood of seeing HD_A regions as figures in upright compared with inverted LD_S/HD_A displays, the high-denotative regions were not seen as figures in the upright displays much more often than half the time. This finding suggests that the object memory cue does not necessarily dominate the putatively lower level cue of symmetry; each cue seemed to determine figure assignment approximately half the time. Thus, it is not the case that the high-level cue necessarily dominates the low-level cues, as many others have assumed (e.g., Göttschaldt, 1926/1938; Köhler, 1929/1947), nor is it the case that the low-level cues necessarily dominate the high-level cue, as others have claimed (e.g., Pylyshyn, 1999). The data in Table 1, along with the previous observations published by Peterson and Gibson (1994a), suggest that the object memory cue is simply one more cue to figural status; it is not given substantially more weight than the configural cue of symmetry.

In the experiment just described and others like it, observers were given the option to report that both regions appeared shaped by the central border or that neither region did. Observers rarely used this third response option. This finding implies that one-sided contour (or edge) assignment occurred in these experiments. In other words, when a cue did not determine figural status, the region carrying that cue appeared to be shapeless near the central edge. Consider LD_S/HD_A displays: When symmetry did not determine figure assignment, the symmetric low-denotative region appeared shapeless near the edge it shared with the high-denotative region. (Hence, its symmetry could not be seen.) Likewise, when memories of object structure did not determine figural status, the high-denotative region appeared to be shapeless near the border it shared with the low-denotative figure. (Hence, it could not be identified.)

The local apparent shapelessness of a high-denotative region adjacent to a low-denotative figure can easily be accounted for by a theory in which object memories are accessed for figures and not for grounds. On a theory in which memories of object structure are accessed before figural status is determined, how can one account for the apparent shapelessness of a high-denotative region seen as a ground? And on either theory, how can one account for the apparent shapelessness of a symmetric region seen as a ground? The parallel interactive model of configural analyses (PIMOCA), described in the next section, explains apparent shapelessness by positing competition between configural cues on opposite sides of an edge. PIMOCA explains the apparent shapelessness of the relatively weakly cued side of an edge, regardless of its denotivity.

Accounting for the Apparent Shapelessness of Grounds in Two-Dimensional Displays

PIMOCA (Peterson, 2000; Peterson, de Gelder, Rapcsak, Gerhardstein, & Bachoud-Lévi, 2000) integrates the parallel hypothesis (Peterson, 1994b, 1999b; Peterson & Gibson, 1994a) with inhibitory cross-border connections, a feature commonly employed in interactive hierarchical models (see Kienker, Sejnowski, Hinton, & Schumacher, 1986; Vecera & O'Reilly, 1998). According to PIMOCA, illustrated in Fig. 3.4, configural cues on the same side of an edge cooperate, whereas configural cues on opposite sides of an edge compete.

In PIMOCA, memories of object structure are considered to be configural cues, as are the traditional Gestalt configural cues. This is because, for effects of object memories on figure assignment to be observed, the parts of known objects must be

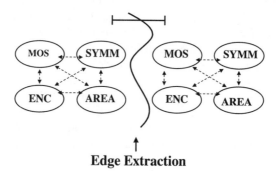

Edge Extraction

FIG. 3.4. The parallel interactive model of configural analysis (PI-MOCA). MOS = memories of object structure. SYMM = symmetry. ENC = enclosure. The double-headed arrows indicate cooperative interactions; the horizontal bar with two end stops indicates a competitive interaction. Adapted from *Vision Research, 40*, Peterson et al., Object memory effects on figure assignment, p. 1565. Copyright 2000, with permission from Elsevier Science.

in the proper configuration, and the known object must be portrayed in its typical orientation. Effects of object memories on figure assignment were not found when high-denotative regions were reconfigured by rearranging the parts, a change that rendered them low in denotivity (Gibson & Peterson, 1994; Peterson, et al., 2000; Peterson, Gerhardstein, Mennemeier, & Rapcsak, 1998; Peterson et al., 1991). Showing observers the known object from which the reconfigured version was created and pointing out the correspondence between the parts did not restore the object memory effects on figure assignment (Peterson et al., 1991). Thus, it is the configuration itself that is important for the object memory effects, not higher level knowledge regarding the object. Furthermore, the memories of object structure relevant to figure assignment are not holistic (Peterson, 2002). Instead, the relevant remembered configurations appear to be spatially limited (i.e., smaller than the whole object).

According to PIMOCA, the perception of shape in two-dimensional displays consisting only of configural cues is only the perception of shape attributes, such as symmetry versus asymmetry, convexity versus concavity, closure, area, part configuration, familiarity, and so on. When these configural attributes are suppressed in such two-dimensional displays, shape cannot be seen. Thus, the cross-edge competition in PIMOCA accounts for a weakly cued region adjacent to a relatively strongly cued region being perceived as locally shapeless, regardless of whether it is high or low in denotivity. Processing of configural properties continues on the strongly cued side of the shared edge, and a shape is ultimately perceived there.

Tests of PIMOCA's Predictions

We recently tested PIMOCA's predictions regarding cross-edge inhibition using the stimuli shown in Fig. 3.5–3.7 (Peterson & Kim, 2001). On each trial, two shapes were shown sequentially—a black silhouette followed by a line drawing. All of the black silhouettes were novel shapes; hence, their edges were low in denotivity on the black side. As well, they were all symmetric, enclosed, and substantially smaller in area than the white screen on which they were displayed. The black silhouettes appeared centered on fixation, and a new one appeared on every trial. Thus, for all silhouettes a number of configural factors cued the black regions to be figures, as did the cues of expectation and fixation location (Peterson & Gibson, 1994b). Most (75%) of the silhouettes were low in denotivity (LD) along the white (W) side of their left and right borders as well as along the black (B) side. Samples of these $B_{LD}W_{LD}$ silhouettes are shown in Fig. 3.5.

The remaining 25% of the silhouettes were high in denotivity (HD) on the white side of their left and right borders. Samples of these $B_{LD}W_{HD}$ silhouettes are shown in Fig. 3.6. For the $B_{LD}W_{HD}$ silhouettes, one configural factor—memory for object structure—cued the white side of the black-white border as the figure. Because the black side of the border was strongly cued to be the figure by many configural factors (see previous listing), we expected observers to perceive the black regions as the shaped figures and the white regions as shapeless grounds in these $B_{LD}W_{HD}$.

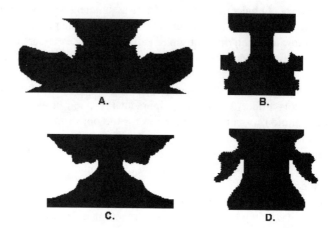

FIG. 3.5. Four sample $B_{LD}W_{LD}$ silhouettes used by Peterson and Kim (2001). B is from *Visual Cognition, 8* (3/4/5), Peterson & Kim, pp. 329–348. Copyright 2001, reprinted with permission of Psychology Press, Ltd., Hove, UK.

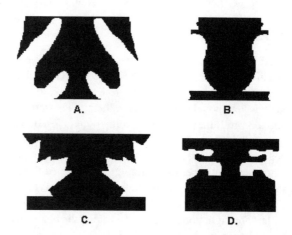

FIG. 3.6. Four sample B_{LD} W_{HD} silhouettes used by Peterson and Kim (2001). The white sides of the left and right borders of the black regions are high in denotivity. The object sketched in part on the white side is a hand in A, a bell in B, a leaf in C, and a faucet in D. B is from *Visual Cognition, 8* (3/4/5), Peterson & Kim, pp. 329–348. Copyright 2001, reprinted with permission of Psychology Press, Ltd., Hove, UK.

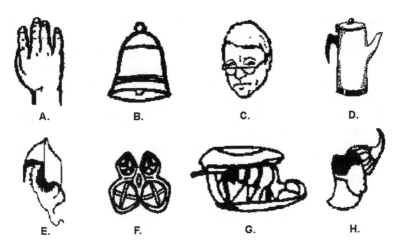

FIG. 3.7. Sample line drawings used by Peterson and Kim (2001). A–D are line drawings of known objects; E–H are line drawings of novel objects. Line drawings of novel objects were always preceded by B_{LD} W_{LD} silhouettes like those in Fig. 3.5. Half of the line drawings of known objects were also preceded by B_{LD} W_{LD} silhouettes like those in Fig. 5; these were control trials. The other half of the line drawings of known objects were preceded by B_{LD} W_{HD} silhouettes in which the HD region, perceived as ground, sketched a portion of the same basic level object. Examples of these experimental trials would be Fig. 3.7, parts A and B, preceded by Fig. 3.6, parts A and B, respectively. B and F are from *Visual Cognition, 8* (3/4/5), Peterson & Kim, pp. 329–348. Copyright 2001, reprinted with permission of Psychology Press, Ltd., Hove UK. E–H are from *Journal of Verbal Learning and Verbal Behavior, 23,* Kroll & Potter, pp. 39–66. Copyright 1984, reprinted with permission from Academic Press.

silhouettes as well as in the $B_{LD}W_{LD}$ silhouettes. Indeed, that is what observers typically reported seeing when they looked at these displays within the context of the experiment (and for the brief durations used in the experiment). According to PIMOCA, the apparent shapelessness of the white regions near the border of the black figure is mediated in part by inhibition of object memories that were accessed on the relatively weakly cued side of the edge.

We tested for the proposed inhibition using a priming paradigm. Silhouettes like those in Fig. 3.5 or 3.6 were presented for 50 ms as primes before line drawings like those in Fig. 3.7. Participants categorized the line drawings as known or as novel objects by pressing one of two buttons as quickly and as accurately as they could. Line drawings were exposed until a response was made.

A different silhouette was shown before each of the line drawings. $B_{LD}W_{LD}$ silhouettes (Fig. 3.5) were shown before all of the line drawings of novel objects.

The novel line drawings and their paired silhouette primes were included only so the observers had to make a decision before responding to the real line drawings; none of the novel line drawings was preceded by a silhouette with a matching shape in either the figure or the ground. The responses to the novel line drawings will not be considered further in this chapter. $B_{LD}W_{LD}$ silhouettes were also shown before half of the line drawings of known objects (these were control prime trials). $B_{LD}W_{HD}$ silhouettes were shown before the remaining half of the line drawings of known objects. On these experimental prime trials, a portion of the same basic level object portrayed by the line drawing was sketched along the white side of the borders of the silhouette prime (cf. Fig. 3.6, parts A and B, with Fig. 3.7, parts A and B). The borders of the silhouette and the line drawing were different (i.e., a different version of the same basic level object was portrayed by each) to increase the likelihood that any priming we observed would be mediated by memories of object structure rather than by edge descriptions alone.

We were primarily interested in the participants' latency to correctly categorize the known line drawings, depending on the nature of the preceding prime silhouette

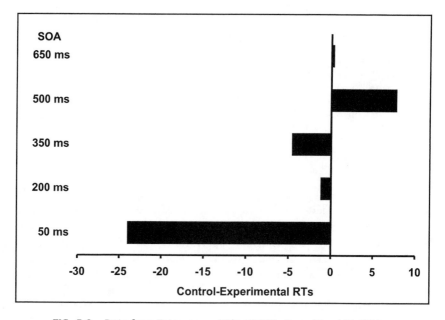

FIG. 3.8. Data from Peterson and Kim (2001, Experiment 2). SOA = stimulus onset asynchrony between the silhouette and the line drawing. In this experiment, the silhouette was exposed for the entire SOA. At the shortest SOA, observers were significantly slower to correctly classify known objects in the experimental condition than in the control condition. This difference may reflect the inhibition of object memories accessed for regions adjacent to strongly cued figures (i.e., the black silhouettes).

(control vs. experimental). If the memories of object structure matching the ground side of $B_{LD}W_{HD}$ silhouettes were inhibited, as predicted by PIMOCA, then the latency to correctly classify line drawings of objects from the same basic level category should be longer on experimental prime trials than on control prime trials. Peterson and Kim (2001) obtained evidence for the predicted inhibition. As shown in Fig. 3.8, observers' mean latency to accurately categorize line drawings as known was longer on experimental than on control prime trials. This pattern was obtained when the stimulus onset asynchrony (SOA) between the silhouette prime and the line drawing target was short—50 ms (Exp. 2) or 83 ms (Exp. 1).

We took these results to reflect the inhibition of object memories matching the white side of the border of the $B_{LD}W_{HD}$ experimental prime silhouettes. We investigated the longevity of the inhibition by testing for priming at longer SOA conditions. Our results suggested that the object memories were inhibited for a brief time only. These results have been replicated with masked primes and a different control condition (e.g., using control prime silhouettes that portrayed portions of objects from a different superordinate class than their paired line drawings; Skow Grant, Lampignano, Kim, & Peterson, 2002). These results are consistent with the proposal that memories of object structure matched by the relatively weakly cued side of a border are inhibited.

According to PIMOCA, cooperation between configural cues on the same side of an edge and competition between configural cues on opposite sides of an edge produces the perception of definite shape on one side and shapelessness on the other side—one-sided edge assignment. PIMOCA's predictions regarding inhibition extend to all configural cues on the relatively weakly cued side of an edge. Therefore, PIMOCA can account for the perceived shapelessness of symmetric regions, and convex regions, seen as grounds. Tests of whether these inhibitory effects extend to the other configural cues are currently underway.

Possible Neural Substrates of PIMOCA

Suppression arising from competitive mechanisms has been observed in ventral area V4 of the monkey (e.g., Jagadeesh, Chelazzi, Mishkin, & Desimone, 2001; Reynolds, Chelazzi, & Desimone, 1999). Consistent evidence in humans was obtained using functional magnetic resonance imaging (fMRI; Kastner, De Weerd, Desimone, & Ungerleider, 1998). The suppression in those experiments arose from competition between two objects present in the same receptive field rather than from competition between configural cues on opposite sides of an edge. However, other evidence indicates that area V4 might be critical for figure-ground perception. For instance, Pasupathy and Connor (1999) found that V4 neurons respond to local convexity, one of the Gestalt configural cues. Peterson (2003) proposed that the spatially limited configurations mediating the object memory effects on figure assignment might be coded in V4 as well. In addition, Kastner, de Weerd, and Ungerleider (2000) observed neural correlates of texture segregation in V4 and TEO. Hence, it would not be unreasonable to investigate whether evidence of

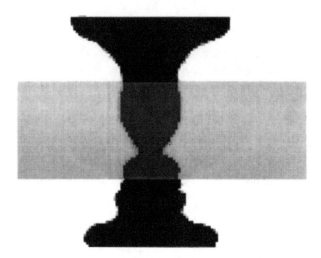

FIG. 3.9.   A Rubin vase-faces stimulus in which the gray portion of
the region adjacent to the black figure appears to complete in front
of, rather than behind, the figure.

the competitive interactions between configural cues on opposite sides of a border
can be observed in V4.

Apparent Shapelessness and Completion

In two-dimensional displays, where no other depth cues or transparency cues are
present, the perception of shapelessness on one side of a border may just be relative
depth perception. It is thought that the ground, lacking a border near the figure,
appears to complete amodally behind the figure. Must shapeless regions adjacent to
figures appear to continue behind the figure? The illustration in Fig. 3.9 shows that
when transparency cues are added, portions of the region adjacent to the figure can
separate into two surfaces—one completes in front of the figure (the transparent
gray surface); the other completes amodally behind the figure (the white surface).
Fig. 3.9 demonstrates that the two figural properties of being shaped by a border
and being in front of adjacent regions at that border can be uncoupled; the figure
appears to lie behind the gray transparency (although it does appear to lie in front
of the white ground).

Another demonstration that the figural properties of shape and relative nearness
can be uncoupled is discussed in the next section. In addition, question 4 (whether
two-dimensional displays are good surrogates for three-dimensional displays) and
question 5 (whether figure-ground segregation should be considered a stage of
processing) will be considered in the next section.

THREE-DIMENSIONAL DISPLAYS

To investigate whether or not object memories affect the assignment of figural status in three-dimensional displays, Peterson and Gibson (1993) created black and white stereograms by adding binocular disparity to the two vertical edges of either the high-denotative or the low-denotative region of stimuli like those shown in Fig. 3.2, parts D and E. (Fig. 3.10 shows sample stereograms.)

These stereograms were presented on a large random dot background. Each display was shown in two conditions. In one condition, binocular disparity specified that the high-denotative region was in front of the projection plane and that the low-denotative region lay on the projection plane. This condition was called the cooperation condition because the object memory cue and the binocular disparity cue cooperate to specify that the high-denotative region is the figure. In the other condition, binocular disparity specified that the low-denotative region was in front of the projection plane and that the high-denotative region lay on the projection plane. This condition was called the competition condition because the object memory cue and the binocular disparity cue specify that the figure lies on opposite sides of the central edge.[1]

The critical condition was the competition condition. We predicted that if the object memory cue affects the perceived organization of three-dimensional displays, then observers should be less likely to see the disparity-consistent organization in competitive stereograms than in cooperative stereograms. That is, observers should be less likely to see the low-denotative region as the shaped entity lying in front of the high-denotative region in competitive stereograms than they are to see the high-denotative region as the shaped entity lying in front of the low-denotative region in cooperative stereograms. If observers were equally likely to see the disparity-consistent interpretation in both cooperative and competitive stereograms, that would indicate that memories of object structure do not affect the perceived organization of three-dimensional displays.

We showed these displays to observers for long durations (30–40-s) and asked them to report whether the region lying on the right or the left of the central edge appeared to have a definite shape and to lie in front of the adjacent region at the central border. Observers indicated what they saw throughout the viewing period by pressing one of two horizontally oriented keys. As in previous experiments, they were given the option to press neither key if both regions appeared to have a definite shape, or if neither region appeared to be in front at the central edge.

Before each trial, observers were instructed to view the stereograms under one of two intentional sets (Peterson & Hochberg, 1983). On half of the trials, they were asked to try to perceive the region on the right of the central edge

---

[1] Peterson and Gibson (1993) used the terms *cooperative* and *competitive*. Strictly, these terms apply only on the assumption that figural regions (i.e., shaped regions) are necessarily perceived nearer to the viewer than adjacent regions.

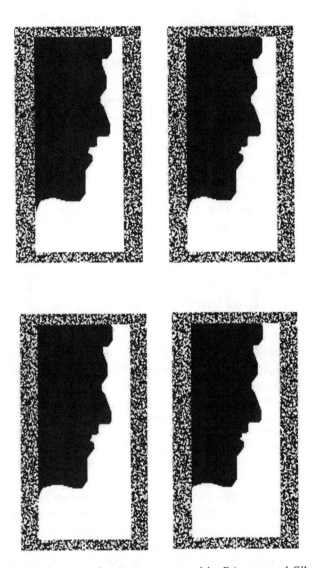

FIG. 3.10. Two sample stereograms used by Peterson and Gibson (1993). If fusion is achieved by diverging the eyes, the stereogram pair in the top of the figure is a cooperative pair, and the stereogram pair in the bottom of the figure is a competitive pair. In cooperative stereograms, binocular disparity and object memories both specify that the high-denotative region (shown in black here) is the figure (shaped and in front). In competitive stereograms, binocular disparity specifies that the low-denotative region (shown in white here) is in front, whereas object memories specify that the high-denotative region is the shaped entity; the shaped entity is typically perceived to lie in front of the adjacent region. Hence, the object memory cue competes with binocular disparity. The stereograms in Peterson and Gibson's (1993) experiments were shown on a random-dot background, only a portion of which is reproduced here.

FIG. 3.10. (continued) From *Cognitive Psychology, 25,* Peterson & Gibson, pp. 383–429. Copyright 1993, reprinted with permission from Academic Press.

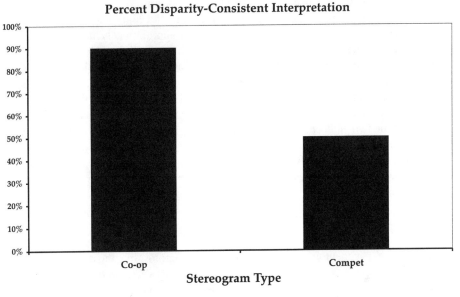

FIG. 3.11. A schematic of the typical results obtained by Peterson and Gibson (1993) on trials on which observers tried to perceive the disparity-consistent interpretation of the two types of stereograms. Co-op = cooperation condition. Compet = competition condition. In the Co-op condition, the high-denotative region was the figure in the disparity-consistent interpretation. In the Compet condition, the low-denotative region was the figure in the disparity-consistent interpretation.

as satisfying the two criteria listed previously. On the other half of the trials, they were asked to try to perceive the region on the left of the central edge as satisfying those two criteria. (Across the four stimuli used in this experiment, the right-left location of the high- and low-denotative regions was balanced within and counterbalanced across observers.) The data were summarized as the mean durations that the region specified to be in front by binocular disparity (i.e., the disparity-consistent interpretation) was perceived as the shaped, near figure at the central edge on trials on which observers followed instructions to try to perceive that region as the figure (see Fig. 3.11).[2]

In cooperative stereograms, the high-denotative region was more likely than the low-denotative region to be perceived as the shaped occluding figure at the central

---

[2]Results were very similar when expressed as the mean duration of the first percept reported on each trial.

edge (i.e., the disparity-consistent interpretation). These results were expected regardless of whether disparity alone determined the perception of three-dimensional displays or whether object memories contributed as well. The contributions of these two cues cannot be separated unless one compares performance in the cooperation condition with performance in the competition condition.

Critically, in competitive stereograms, the low- and high-denotative regions were each perceived as the figure at the central edge approximately half of the time. In these stereograms, binocular disparity specified that the low-denotative region was the occluding object at the central border, but memories of object structure specified that the high-denotative region was the shaped entity there. The results suggest that, in these particular three-dimensional displays, neither the binocular disparity cue nor the object memory cue was necessarily dominant in determining which of the two adjacent regions was the shaped, near region at the central edge.

In summary, these results showed that memories of object structure can affect figure assignment in three-dimensional displays, even when the depth cue of binocular disparity specifies that the edge shared by a high- and a low-denotative region should be assigned to the low-denotative region.

Perceived Distance

In another experiment using black and white stereograms, like those in Fig. 3.10, we asked observers to report the apparent distance between the projection plane and the black and white surfaces at each of their sides. That is, observers estimated the perceived distance between the white region and the projection plane near its outer edge and near the central edge; they also estimated the perceived distance between the black region and the projection plane near its outer edge and near the central edge. Magnitude estimations of perceived distance were elicited for each type of stereogram under each of the two intentional sets (i.e., "try to perceive the black region as the figure" and "try to perceive the white region as the figure"). These magnitude estimations can reveal whether or not the disparity cue is necessarily suppressed when observers see the disparity-inconsistent interpretation of competitive stereograms.

As can be seen in Fig. 3.12, part A, when observers saw the disparity-consistent interpretation of cooperative stereograms, they saw a sharp, deep depth discontinuity between the high- and low-denotative regions at the central edge. The high-denotative region appeared to be located at the same distance from the projection plane as a standard stereogram with the same disparity (magnitude = 100), whereas the low-denotative ground appeared to lie far behind the figure (and close to the projection plane) at both the central edge and at its outer edge.

When observers saw the disparity-inconsistent interpretation of the cooperative stereograms, however, they perceived much less depth in the displays (Fig. 3.12, part C). Both the high- and low-denotative regions appeared to lie close to the projection plane, and a much smaller difference in depth was seen at the central

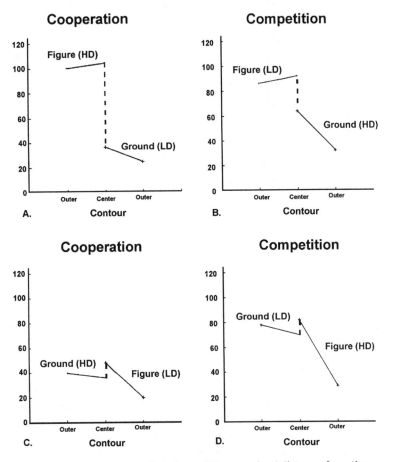

FIG. 3.12. Magnitude estimations of the perceived distance from the projection screen at both the center and the outer edges of regions perceived to be figures and grounds in both the cooperation (A) and (C) and the competition conditions (B) and (D). Magnitude estimations for disparity-consistent interpretations are shown in (A) and (B); magnitude estimations for disparity-inconsistent interpretations are shown in (C) and (D). The solid lines connect judgments made for a single region. The dashed line simply portrays graphically the inferred depth edge between the two regions. From *Cognitive Psychology*, 25, Peterson & Gibson, pp. 383–429. Copyright 1993, reprinted with permission from Academic Press.

border. The magnitude estimations suggest that observers may have been suppressing the binocular disparity cue to follow the instructions to try to see the low-denotative region as the figure in the cooperative stereograms. If so, the small percentage of time they succeeded in seeing this interpretation (see Fig. 3.11) suggests that this strategy was not very successful. I next consider the distance estimations obtained for competitive stereograms to investigate whether disparity was always suppressed when observers saw the disparity-inconsistent interpretation of a three-dimensional display.

Consider first the magnitude estimations obtained when observers perceived the disparity-consistent interpretation of competitive stereograms (i.e., the low-denotative region appeared to be the shaped region and to lie in front of the shapeless high-denotative region). Observers' magnitude estimations indicated that, when the disparity consistent interpretation was perceived, the low-denotative region of competitive stereograms appeared to be approximately as far in front of the projection plane as did the high-denotative region of cooperative stereograms (cf. magnitude estimations for the perceived figures in Fig. 3.12, parts A and B). A shallower depth step was perceived between the high- and low-denotative regions near the central edge of the competitive stereograms, however. Indeed, as can be seen in Fig. 3.12B, the high-denotative ground of competitive stereograms appeared to slant in depth across its spatial extent. It seemed to lie farther from the projection plane near the central edge than near its outer edge, although it still appeared to lie behind the low-denotative region there. Reasons for the perception of this slant will be considered later. For now, I leave the issue of slant aside and continue to explore the question of whether binocular disparity is necessarily suppressed when the disparity-inconsistent interpretation of competitive stereograms was perceived.

The magnitude estimations obtained when the disparity-inconsistent interpretation of competitive stereograms was perceived are not consistent with the suppression hypothesis (Fig. 3.12, part D). When, contrary to the disparity cue, the high-denotative region was seen as the figure in competitive stereograms, the low-denotative region did not appear to lie on or near the projection plane, as would be expected were the disparity cue suppressed. Rather, the low-denotative region appeared to lie much farther in front of the projection plane than the high-denotative region did when it was perceived as the ground in cooperative stereograms (cf. Fig. 12, parts C and D).

Thus, perception of the disparity-inconsistent interpretation of competitive stereograms does not necessarily entail the suppression of the binocular disparity signal. In contrast, recall that when the configural cue of object memory does not determine figure assignment, it is suppressed (Peterson & Kim, 2001; Skow Grant et al., 2002). It appears that the interactions between binocular disparity and the configural cues are different from the interactions among the configural cues themselves. This finding may not be surprising inasmuch as configural cues are shape cues, whereas binocular disparity is predominantly a depth cue. The object memory cues and binocular disparity are processed in separate neural pathways (i.e.,

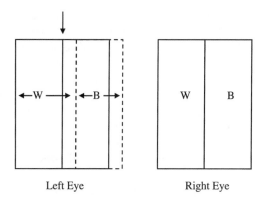

Left Eye   Right Eye

FIG. 3.13. A schematic of how a black and white stereogram was constructed such that binocular disparity indicated that the black region on the right was in front of the projection plane. Following standard procedure, the black region was shifted to the right in the left eye's view relative to its location in the right eye's view. Its shifted location is indicated by the dashed line contours in the left eye's view. This shift creates a space between the original edge of the white region and the new location of the edge of the black region. This space was filled with the color of the unshifted region (white in this example). Therefore, the white region was wider in the left eye's view than in the right eye's view. Thus, the slant of the white region was ambiguous: It could either be a flat plane located at the distance of the projection plane or a slanted plane rising up from its outer edge toward it's inner edge (the edge it shares with the black region).

dorsal and ventral pathways, respectively; Ungerleider & Mishkin, 1982; Young, 1995). The interactions within the ventral pathway that determine perceived shape (e.g., the interactions modeled by PIMOCA) might be quite different from the interactions between the ventral and the dorsal pathways.

I return now to the fact that the high-denotative regions of competitive stereograms appeared to slant upwards in depth from their outer border toward the central border both when they were seen as figures and when they were seen as grounds (Fig. 3.12, parts D and B, respectively). Note that a much smaller degree of slant was perceived in low-denotative regions of cooperative stereograms (Fig. 3.12, parts A and C). This originally puzzling result (see Peterson & Gibson, 1993) ultimately led me to understand that the slant of the region specified to lie behind in the black and white stereograms was ambiguous. The ambiguity was an unintentional consequence of the manner in which we made the stereograms, described next and illustrated in Fig. 3.13.

To portray, say, a black region on the right side of the central edge as lying farther in front of the projection plane than a white region on the left side of the central edge, we shifted the location of the entire black region to the right in the left eye's view relative to its location in the right eye's view. (This is the standard method for creating crossed disparity.) Shifting a region lying on the right of the central edge farther to the right necessarily left a space between the black and white regions in the left eye's view. In random-dot stereograms, this space is typically filled with random dots uncorrelated with those already filling the two regions. In the black and white stereograms used by Peterson and Gibson (1993), this space was filled with the lightness of the unshifted region (white, in the sample case discussed). As a consequence, the region specified to be behind in the black and white stereograms was wider in the left eye's view than in the right eye's view. A display with these properties specifies either a flat surface lying on the projection plane and extending behind the front surface or a surface contacting the projection plane at its outer edge and slanting upwards in depth toward the central edge. (For discussion, see Howard & Rogers, 1995.) Thus, the slant of the region specified to lie behind by disparity was ambiguous in both the cooperative and the competitive black and white stereograms. It is noteworthy that the slanted interpretation was fitted to the back region predominantly in competitive stereograms (see Fig. 3.12, parts B and D); it was not perceived in the cooperative stereograms (see Fig. 3.12, parts A and C).

Might the fact that our black and white stereograms ambiguously specified a slanting far surface account for our finding that memories of object structure affected the perceived organization of competitive stereograms? The slant of the ground can be rendered unambiguously in random-dot stereograms. Gibson and I (Peterson & Gibson, 1993, Experiment 1) failed to find object memory effects on figure assignment using random-dot stereograms. However, I did not then and I do not now take those results as evidence that object memory effects are present only when three-dimensional displays are ambiguous, for a number of reasons.

First, Gibson and I predicted that memories of object structure would not affect figure assignment in random-dot stereograms because it takes longer to detect the edge between the high- and low-denotative regions in random-dot stereograms than in black and white stereograms. (Luminance edges can be detected early in processing, whereas disparity edges can be detected only after the solution to the correspondence problem has begun to emerge.) As a consequence, edge-based access to object memories might not occur quickly enough in random-dot stereograms to affect figure assignment (Peterson & Gibson, 1993).

Second, even if the central edge is detected sufficiently quickly in random-dot stereograms, the dots comprising the stereograms may have added too much noise to the edge to support good edge-based matches to object memories. Evidence consistent with this latter hypothesis was obtained in an experiment in which observers viewed 300-ms masked exposures of stereograms in which binocular disparity indicated that a high-denotative region lay in front of the projection plane and an adjacent low-denotative region lay on the projection plane. Their task was to identify the object portrayed by the high-denotative region. For random-dot stereograms, observers identified only 29% of the objects portrayed by high-denotative regions. In contrast, for black and white stereograms, they identified 75% of the objects portrayed by high-denotative regions (Peterson & Gibson, 1991,

1993). To the extent that identification responses under these conditions can be taken as an index of the goodness of the edge-based match to object memories, these data suggest that matches to object memories mediated by edges in random-dot stereograms are poor compared with matches mediated by edges in black and white stereograms.

Furthermore, as discussed in the next section, that shaped apertures can be perceived demonstrates that object memories affect the perceived organization of unambiguous three-dimensional displays. Therefore, although the ambiguous slant of the background of the black and white stereograms used by Peterson and Gibson (1993) may have affected their perceived organization, it does not appear to be a necessary condition for the observation of object memory effects on figure assignment in three-dimensional displays.

Shaped Apertures

Consider a hand-shaped aperture cut into a surface mounted on a pole outdoors, as illustrated in Fig. 3.14. When this display is viewed from nearby, the binocular disparity cues are strong; each eye has different information about distant regions seen through the aperture. Other depth cues including linear perspective, relative size, texture density gradient, and interposition specify the layout of the scene beyond the surface into which the aperture has been cut. In addition, a few edges in the scene are good candidates for completion behind the mounted surface. These are all cues that the edge of the hand-shaped aperture belongs to the mounted surface. However, configural cues (including enclosure, convexity, and memories of object structure) specify that a shaped entity lies on the aperture side of the edge. What is perceived? The mounted surface with the aperture cut in it appears to be the near surface. The edge shared by the aperture and the near surface is seen as one of the occluding edges of the near surface. Nevertheless, the aperture appears to have a definite shape—that of a hand.

That a hand-shaped aperture can be perceived in the real three-dimensional scene illustrated in Fig. 3.14 indicates that object memory effects do extend to three-dimensional displays (as do the effects of the Gestalt configural cues). Therefore, for testing the role of configural cues in perception, two-dimensional displays are good surrogates for three-dimensional displays. In the three-dimensional version of Fig. 3.14, the distance to the objects seen through the aperture is specified unambiguously; nevertheless, object memory effects on perception are clearly evident. Hochberg (1998) and Palmer (1999) have also discussed cases in which shaped apertures can be seen. The case of a keyhole discussed by Hochberg is particularly telling because in that case we have a name for a shape that has primarily been seen in aperture form.

Remarkably, in the shaped aperture example, the two properties of a figure's border have been uncoupled (or at least, these properties have been assigned with differential strength to these two regions). The shaping property of the border has been assigned to the aperture, yet the occluding property of the border has been

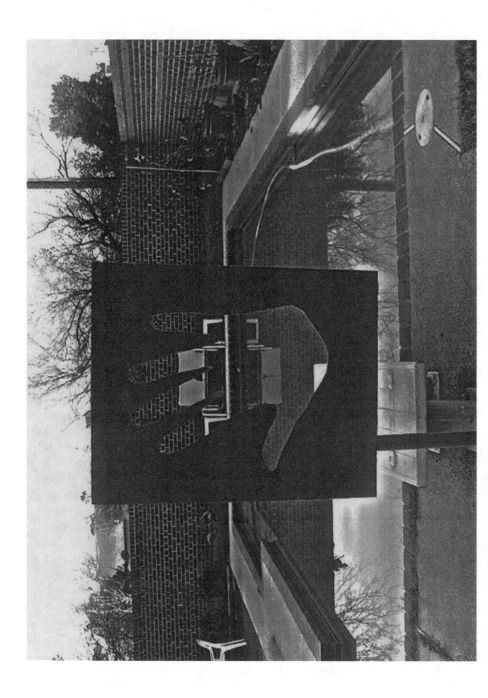

assigned to the near surface. The demonstration that the two properties of a figure's border can be uncoupled in three-dimensional displays lends further support to the idea that the interactions between depth cues and configural cues are different from the interactions among configural cues. The three-dimensional cues specify which of two adjacent regions is the near surface (and they may also specify shape), whereas the configural cues specify where a shaped entity lies relative to a border shared by two regions. It seems that these two properties of near and shaped are perceptually coupled only (1) when the two types of cues specify the same region as the shaped near surface or (2) when there is a null signal in one type of cue. Most two-dimensional displays used to investigate figure assignment meet Criterion (2): Configural cues are present, but depth cues tend to be absent. In such displays, the shaped entity appears to be the near entity. Accordingly, at first glance, two-dimensional displays may seem to be good surrogates for three-dimensional displays because, for three-dimensional displays, the near surface is likely to be the shaped surface. However, the shaped aperture case demonstrates that two-dimensional displays cannot stand in for three-dimensional displays for the purposes of investigating whether the shaping and occluding properties of a border are necessarily assigned to the same side.[3] In other words, two-dimensional displays can sometimes but not always serve as surrogates for three-dimensional displays.

OLD AND NEW QUESTIONS

The five questions raised at the beginning of this chapter have been addressed, and partial answers have been provided to some of them. My colleagues and I have shown that memories of object structure affect figure assignment. Therefore, the traditional answer to the first question—Why can figures be identified if they are familiar, whereas grounds cannot?—is wrong. It is not the case that object memories are accessed for figures and not for grounds. Rather, the solution implemented by the visual system appears to be more complex. I discussed PIMOCA, which

---

[3]Recall that in the black and white competitive stereograms tested by Peterson and Gibson (1993), the shaping and occluding properties of the figure border were perceptually coupled. Perhaps the ambiguous slant of the back surface allowed the coupling to be maintained. This hypothesis requires further investigation.

←——

FIG. 3.14. A photograph of a real three-dimensional display in which a hand-shaped hole was cut into a surface and mounted on a pole outdoors. The shape of the hand is clearly perceived, despite (1) the hand appearing to be surface-free and (2) the edge it shares with the surface into which the hole was cut appearing to be an occluding border of that surface. Of course, this picture can only provide a two-dimensional depiction of an actual three-dimensional display.

uses cross-edge inhibition to account in part for why regions adjacent to strongly cued figures cannot be identified and appear shapeless (Questions 1 and 2). PI-MOCA is a model of the interactions between and among the configural cues, which constitute a subset of the cues that determine shape and occlusion. Additional research must investigate the form of the interactions among the configural cues and between the configural cues and the depth cues.

On the basis of examples discussed in this chapter, it is clear that regions adjacent to figures are not necessarily completed behind them (Question 3). When the region sharing an edge with a figure can be separated into two surfaces, a transparent overlay and an opaque ground, the transparent overlay completes in front of the figure, and the other surface appears to complete amodally behind the figure (Fig. 3.9). Under these conditions, scission has occurred for the region that is not shaped by the shared edge. The edge still appears to be an occluding contour of the figure. In the shaped aperture case, illustrated in Fig. 3.14, however, the edge shared by two regions appears to shape one region (the aperture) and to be the occluding contour of the region lying on the opposite side (and perhaps also to shape that region). The shaped aperture case demonstrates that two-dimensional displays can serve only a limited role as surrogates for three-dimensional displays.

The present chapter raises new questions, including the following: What is the ontological status of the shaped aperture? Is it a figure? It has a definite shape but it may not have a surface. It certainly does not appear to be a surface lying at the farthest distance visible through the aperture, nor does it appear to be a surface lying closer to the viewer than the surface into which the aperture has been cut. Physically, the shaped aperture has no surface, but can the visual system perceive a surfaceless shape? Or, in the absence of cues to transparency, does the visual system fit a transparent surface within the boundary of the shaped aperture? If so, then shaped apertures constitute a new case of amodal completion—a completed surface is present but is not perceived. Regardless of whether or not amodal completion occurs, the shaped aperture outcome is not a case of figure-ground segregation, which entails one-sided contour assignment. Instead, it is a special case of figure-figure segregation, the properties of which remain to be determined experimentally.

A second question raised by the shaped aperture case is whether the shaping property of figures has been assigned to one side only (the aperture side) or whether the near surface appears to be shaped by its occluding contours as well. The configural cues are not balanced in the shaped aperture example. Therefore, PIMOCA predicts that shape will not be seen on the side of the border across from the hand-shaped aperture. However, PIMOCA models the interactions among configural cues only. A critical aspect of the shaped aperture case is that depth cues are present, in addition to configural cues. Investigations of the extent to which the near surface appears to be shaped by the edge it shares with the shaped aperture will provide critical evidence regarding the interactions among configural cues and depth cues in determining both shape and relative depth.

In conclusion, on the basis of the research summarized here, it is clear that figure-ground segregation is not a stage of processing that simply provides the substrate for higher level visual processes. Rather it is one possible outcome of interactions among image segregation cues (including configural cues, depth cues, motion, texture, shading, etc.) cues that jointly determine perceived shape, perceived surface properties, and perceived relative depth. These attributes need not be coupled, although they often are, in particular when figure-ground segregation occurs.

REFERENCES

Driver, J., & Baylis, G. C. (1996). Edge-assignment and figure-ground segmentation in short term visual matching. *Cognitive Psychology, 31,* 248–306.

Driver, J., Baylis, G. C., & Rafal, R. D. (1992). Preserved figure-ground segregation and symmetry perception in visual neglect. *Nature, 360,* 73–75.

Gibson, B. S., & Peterson, M. A. (1994). Does orientation-independent object recognition precede orientation-dependent recognition? Evidence from a cueing paradigm. *Journal of Experimental Psychology: Human Perception and Performance, 20,* 299–316.

Göttschaldt, K. (1938). Gestalt factors and repetition (continued). In W. D. Ellis (Ed.), *A sourcebook of Gestalt psychology.* London: Kegan Paul, Trech, Tubner. (Original work published 1938).

Hochberg, J. (1998). Gestalt theory and its legacy. In J. Hochberg (Ed.), *Perception and cognition at century's end* (pp. 253–306). New YorK: Academic Press.

Howard, I. P., & Rogers, B, J, (1995). *Binocular vision and stereopsis.* New YorK: Oxford University Press.

Jagadeesh, B., Chelazzi, L., Mishkin, M., & Desimone, R. (2001). Learning increases stimulus salience in anterior inferior temporal cortex of monkey. *Journal of Neurophysiology, 86,* 290–303.

Jolicœur, P. (1988). Mental rotation and the identification of disoriented objects. *Canadian Journal of Psychology, 42,* 461–478.

Kastner, S., De Weerd, P., Desimone, R., & Ungerleider, L. G. (1998). Mechanisms of directed attention in the human extrastriate cortex as revealed by functional MRI. *Science, 282,* 108–111.

Kastner, S., De Weerd, P., & Ungerleider, L. G. (2000). Texture segregation in the human visual cortex: A functional MRI study. *Journal of Neurophysiology, 83,* 2453–2457.

Kennedy, J. M. (1974). *A psychology of picture perception.* San Francisco: Jossey-Bass.

Kienker, P. K., Sejnowski, T. J., Hinton, G. E., & Schumacher, L. E. (1986). Separating figure from ground in a parallel network. *Perception, 15,* 197–216.

Köhler, W. (1947) *Gestalt psychology.* New YorK: New American Library. (Original work published 1929)

Kroll, J. K., & Potter, M. C. (1984). Recognizing words, pictures, and concepts: A comparison of lexical, object, and reality decisions. *Journal of Verbal Learning and Verbal Behavior, 23,* 39–66.

Marr, D. (1982). *Vision.* SanFrancisco: W. H. Freeman.

Palmer, S. E. (1999). *Vision science: Photons to phenomenology.* Cambridge, MA: MIT Press.

Pasupathy, A., & Connor, C. E. (1999). Responses to contour features in macaque area V4. *Journal of Neurophysiology, 82,* 2490–2502.

Perrett, D., Oram, M. W., & Ashbridge, E. (1998). Evidence accumulation in cell populations responsive to faces: An account of generalization of recognition without mental transformations. *Cognition, 67,* 111–145.

Peterson, M. A. (1994a). The proper placement of uniform connectedness. *Psychonomic Bulletin and Review, 1,* 509–514.

Peterson, M. A. (1994b). Shape recognition can and does occur before figure-ground organization. *Current Directions in Psychological Science, 3,* 105–111.

Peterson, M. A. (1999a). On the role of meaning in organization. *Intellectica, 28,* 37–51.

Peterson, M. A. (1999b). What's in a stage name? *Journal of Experimental Psychology: Human Perception and Performance, 25,* 276–286.

Peterson, M. A. (2000). Object perception. In E. B. Goldstein (Ed.), *Blackwell handbook of perception* (pp. 168–203). Oxford Blackwell Publishers, Ltd.

Peterson, M. A. (2003). Overlapping partial configurations in object memory: An alternative solution to classic problems in perception and recognition. In M. A. Peterson & G. Rhodes (Eds.), *Perception of faces, objects, and scenes: Analytic and holistic processes.* (pp. 269–294) New York: Oxford University Press.

Peterson, M. A., de Gelder, B., Rapcsak, S. Z., Gerhardstein, P. C., & Bachoud-Lévi, A.-C. (2000). Object memory effects on figure assignment: Conscious object recognition is not necessary or sufficient. *Vision Research, 40,* 1549–1567.

Peterson, M. A., Gerhardstein, P. C., Mennemeier, M., & Rapcsak, S. Z. (1998). Object-centered attentional biases and object recognition contributions to scene segmentation in right hemisphere- and left hemisphere-damaged patients. *Psychobiology, 26,* 557–570.

Peterson, M. A., & Gibson, B. S. (1991, November). *Shape representation contributions to the organization of 3-D displays.* Paper presented at the Psychonomic Society Meeting, San Francisco, CA.

Peterson, M. A., & Gibson, B. S. (1993). Shape recognition contributions to figure-ground organization in three-dimensional displays. *Cognitive Psychology, 25,* 383–429.

Peterson, M. A., & Gibson, B. S. (1994a). Must shape recognition follow figure-ground organization? An assumption in peril. *Psychological Science, 5,* 253–259.

Peterson, M. A., & Gibson, B. S. (1994b). Object recognition contributions to figure-ground organization: Operations on outlines and subjective contours. *Perception & Psychophysics, 56,* 551–564.

Peterson, M. A., Harvey, E. H., & Weidenbacher, H. L. (1991). Shape recognition inputs to figure-ground organization: Which route counts? *Journal of Experimental Psychology: Human Perception and Performance, 17,* 1075–1089.

Peterson, M. A., & Hochberg, J. (1983). Opposed-set measurement procedure: A quantitative analysis of the role of local cues and intention in form perception. *Journal of Experimental Psychology: Human Perception and Performance, 9,* 183–193.

Peterson, M. A., & Kim, J. H. (2001). On what is bound in figures and grounds [special issue]. *Visual Cognition. Neural Binding of Space and Time. 8,* 329–348.

Pylyshyn, Z. (1999). Is vision continuous with cognition? The case of impenetrability of visual perception. *Behavioral and Brain Sciences, 22,* 341–423.

Reynolds, J. H., Chelazzi, L., & Desimone, R. (1999). Competitive mechanisms subserve attention in macaque areas V2 and V4. *Journal of Neuroscience, 19,* 1736–1753.

Rubin, E. (1958). Figure and ground. In D. Beardslee & M. Wertheimer (Ed. & Trans.), *Readings in perception* (pp. 35–101). Princeton, NJ: Van Nostrand. (Original work published 1915)

Skow Grant, E., Lampignano, D. L., Kim, J. H., & Peterson, M. A. (2002). *Tests of a competitive interactive model of figure assignment. Journal of Vision, 2,* 472.

Tarr, M. J., & Pinker, S. (1989). Mental rotation and orientation-dependence in shape recognition. *Cognitive Psychology, 21,* 233–282.

Ungerleider, L. G., & Mishkin, M. (1982). Two cortical visual systems. In D.G. Ingle, M. A. Goodale, & R. J. Q. Mansfield (Eds.), *Analysis of visual behavior* (pp. 549–586) Cambridge, MA: MIT Press.

Vecera, S. P., & Farah, M. J. (1997). Is visual image segmentation a bottom-up or an interactive process? *Perception & Psychophysics, 59,* 1280–1296.

Vecera, S. P., & O'Reilly, R. C. (1998). Figure-ground organization and object recognition processes: An interactive account. *Journal of Experimental Psychology: Human Perception and Performance, 24,* 441–462.

Vecera, S. P., & O'Reilly, R. C. (2000). Graded effects in hierarchical figure-ground organization: Reply to Peterson (1999). *Journal of Experimental Psychology: Human Perception and Performance, 26,* 1221–1231.

Young, M. P. (1995). Open questions about the neural mechanisms of visual pattern recognition. In M. I. Gazzaniga (Ed.), *The cognitive neurosciences* (pp. 463–474). Cambridge, MA: MIT Press.

4 Visual Perceptual Organization: A Microgenetic Analysis

Ruth Kimchi
University of Haifa

INTRODUCTION

The visual world consciously perceived is very different from the retinal mosaic of intensities and colors that arises from external objects. We perceive an organized visual world consisting of discrete objects, such as people, houses, and trees, that are coherently arranged in space. Some internal processes of organization must be responsible for this achievement.

The Gestalt school of psychology was the first to study the problem of perceptual organization. According to the Gestaltists, organization is composed of grouping and segregation processes (Koffka, 1935; Kohler, 1929/1947). The well-known principles of grouping proposed by Max Wertheimer (1923/1955) identify certain stimulus factors that determine organization. These factors include proximity, similarity, good continuation, common fate, and closure.

Although the Gestalt work on perceptual organization has been widely accepted as identifying crucial phenomena of perception and their demonstrations of grouping appear in almost every textbook on perception, there has been, until the last decade or so, little theoretical and empirical emphasis on perceptual organization. This may be, in part, because perceptual organization is so deeply ingrained in visual experience that it is often hard to appreciate the difficulties involved in achieving it.

117

Another reason for the paucity of attention to the problem of perceptual organization is that cognitive psychology has been dominated for several decades by the "early feature-analysis" view, according to which early perceptual processes analyze simple features and elements (e.g., sloped line segments) that are integrated later, presumably by attention demanding processes, into coherent objects (e.g., Marr, 1982; Treisman, 1986; Treisman & Gormican, 1988). A major contributor to the popularity of the "early feature-analysis" view has been earlier work on the physiology of vision, most notably the work of Hubel and Wiesel (e.g., 1959, 1968), that has fostered the idea of a hierarchical system that proceeds from extracting simple properties to extracting more complex stimulus configurations in a strictly feedforward way.

Thus, traditional theories of perception have treated organization only briefly. To the extent that they did address organization, they assumed that it occurs early, preattentively, and in a bottom-up fashion to represent units to which attention is deployed for later, more elaborated processing (e.g., Treisman, 1986).

In the last decade or so, there has been a growing body of research on perceptual organization. Clear progress has been made, but there still remain many open questions and controversial issues. In this chapter, I review recent work by my colleagues and I, using mainly (but not exclusively) a microgenetic approach in an attempt to shed light on several of these open issues.

One issue concerns the structures provided by early perceptual processing. The question is whether early perceptual processing provides only simple properties or elements, as assumed by traditional theories of perception, or complex stimulus configurations as implied by the Gestaltists' notion of perceptual organization.

A second issue concerns the order of organizational processing and its time course. First, there is the question of where in visual processing grouping occurs. Some researchers have argued that Gestalt grouping does not occur at such an early stage of vision as has been widely assumed (Palmer, this volume; Palmer & Rock 1994a; Palmer, Neff, & Beck, 1996; Rock & Brosgole, 1964; Rock, Nijhawan, Plamer, & Tudor, 1992). Palmer and Rock (1994a, 1994b; Palmer, this volume) have further argued for a more basic organizational principle, the principle of uniform connectedness, that precedes all other forms of grouping and according to which a connected region of uniform visual property (such as color, texture, and motion) is perceived initially as a single perceptual unit. Other investigators, however, have argued that uniform connectedness does not have a privileged status in perceptual organization (e.g., Han, Humphreys, & Chen, 1999; Kimchi, 1998; Peterson, 1994). A second question concerns the time course of grouping. Several studies have suggested that various grouping processes may vary in their time course, showing, for example, an earlier impact of grouping by proximity than grouping by good continuation or by similarity of shape (e.g., Ben-Av & Sagi, 1995; Han & Humphreys, 1999; Han et al., 1999; Kurylo, 1997).

A third issue concerns the stimulus factors that engage the mechanism of organization. New grouping factors have been added to the list of classical principles of grouping (Palmer, 1992, this volume; Palmer & Rock, 1994a), and others are yet to be determined. There are also the questions of how several grouping factors are integrated and what the strength of their combined influence is. The Gestalt grouping principles, as well as the new ones, can predict the outcome of grouping with certainty only when there is no other grouping factor influencing the outcome, but they cannot predict the outcome of a combination of factors. The visual system, however, clearly integrates over many grouping factors.

A fourth issue concerns the role of past experience in perceptual organization. The question is whether past experience influences the products of organization, as assumed by the traditional view, or whether it has a direct influence on organization, as suggested by recent findings demonstrating that knowledge of specific object shapes affects figure-ground segregation (e.g., Peterson, this volume; Peterson & Gibson, 1994), image segmentation (Vecera & Farah, 1997), and grouping (Kimchi & Hadad, 2002).

Finally, a fifth issue concerns the role of attention in organization. The question is whether organization occurs preattentively, as has been widely assumed, or whether it involves focused attention. Some studies have suggested that grouping requires attention (Mack, Tang, Tuma, Kahn, & Rock, 1992; Rock, Linnet, Grant, & Mack, 1992), though other findings have demonstrated that certain grouping occurs under conditions of inattention (e.g., Moore & Egeth, 1997).

In the remainder of this chapter, I present findings that address these issues. I begin with a general description of the major approach we have taken to study perceptual organization—the microgenetic approach—and the paradigm we have used to study microgenesis—the primed matching paradigm. I then present studies that have examined the microgenesis of the perceptual organization of hierarchical stimuli and line configurations, demonstrating relative dominance of global structures or elements at different times along the progressive development of organization, depending on certain stimulus factors and their combinations. Next, I describe evidence for the role of past experience in perceptual grouping. Then, I describe recent experiments that we have done to examine the role of attention in different types of organization and the time course of these organizations. I present preliminary results suggesting that not all groupings are created equal in terms of time course and attentional demands. I close by considering the implications of all these findings to the five issues raised above.

MICROGENETIC ANALYSIS AND THE PRIMED MATCHING PARADIGM

One of the major ways we have used to address issues of perceptual organization has been to study the microgenesis of organization, namely, the time course of the development of the representation of visual objects. This microgenetic analysis is important for understanding the processes underlying organization, rather than just the final product of these processes.

To study the microgenesis of organization we used the primed matching paradigm. The basic procedure (Beller, 1971) is as follows: Participants view a priming stimulus followed immediately by a pair of test figures, and they must judge, as rapidly as possible, whether the two test figures are the same as each other or different from one another. The speed of "same" responses to the test figures depends on the representational similarity between the prime and the test figures: Responses are faster when the test figures are similar to the prime than when they are dissimilar to it. Thus, primed matching enables us to assess implicitly the participant's perceptual representations.

This paradigm also enables us to explore the time course of organization (e.g., Kimchi, 1998, 2000; Sekuler & Palmer, 1992). If we assume that the internal representation of a visual stimulus develops over time, then only the early representation of the priming stimulus would be available for priming at short prime duration. Therefore, responses to test figures that are similar to the early representation of the prime should be facilitated. Later representations are available only at longer prime durations, facilitating positive responses to test figures that are similar to these representations. Thus, if we vary the duration of the prime, and construct test figures that are similar to different aspects of the prime (e.g., components or global configuration), then responses to such test pairs at different prime durations would reveal which structures are available in earlier and later representations of the priming stimulus. Note that both findings of representational change and findings of no representational change during the microgenesis of the percept would be informative.

PERCEPTUAL ORGANIZATION OF HIERARCHICAL STIMULI: MICROGENESIS AND STIMULUS FACTORS

Hierarchical Stimuli and the Global Advantage Effect

Since the seminal work of Navon (1977), hierarchical stimuli, in which larger figures are constructed by suitable arrangement of smaller figures, have been extensively used in investigations of global versus local perception. In a typical experiment in the global/local paradigm, the stimuli consist of a set of large letters constructed from the same set of smaller letters having either the same or different identity as the larger letter. The observers are presented with one hierarchical stimulus at a time and are required to identify the larger (global) or the smaller (local) letter in separate blocks of trials. All else being equal, a global advantage is observed: The global letter is identified faster than is the local letter, and conflicting information between the global and the local levels exerts asymmetrical global-to-local interference (e.g., Navon, 1977).

Although the phenomenon seems to be robust (to the limits of visibility and visual acuity) and has been observed under various exposure durations, including short ones (e.g., Navon, 1977; Paquet & Merikle, 1988), the mechanisms underlying the global advantage effect or its locus are still disputed (see Kimchi, 1992, in press, for a review). Whereas several investigators interpreted the global advantage as reflecting the priority of global structures at early perceptual processing (e.g., Broadbent, 1977; Han, Fan, Chen, & Zhuo, 1997; Navon, 1977, 1991; Paquet & Merikle, 1988), other investigators suggested that the global advantage arises in some postperceptual process (e.g., Boer & Keuss, 1982; Miller, 1981a, 1981b; Ward, 1982).

A more direct way to examine whether early perceptual processing provides global structures is to study the microgenesis of the organization of hierarchical stimuli. In addition, previous work by Goldmeier (1972) and Kimchi (1988, 1990; Kimchi & Palmer, 1982, 1985) suggests that the relative dominance of the global and local structures of hierarchical stimuli may depend on the number and relative size of the elements. They found that patterns composed of a few, relatively large elements are perceived in terms of global form and figural parts. The elements are perceptually salient and interact with the global form. On the other hand, patterns composed of many, relatively small elements (like the ones typically used in the global/local paradigm) are perceived in terms of global form and texture, and the two are perceptually separable.

Microgenesis of the Perceptual Organization of Hierarchical Stimuli

To examine the relative dominance of the global configuration versus the local elements during the evolution of the percept, I studied the microgenesis of the perceptual organization of hierarchical stimuli that vary in number and relative size of their elements (Kimchi, 1998, Experiment 1). The priming stimuli were few- and many-element patterns presented for various durations (40, 90, 190, 390, or 690 ms). Each trial included a prime followed immediately by a pair of test figures. There were two types of same-response test pairs defined by the similarity relation between the test figures and the prime. In the element-similarity test pair, the figures were similar to the prime in their elements but differed in their global configurations. In the configuration-similarity test pair, the test figures were similar to the prime in their global configurations but differed in their elements. In addition, an X was presented as a neutral prime and served as a baseline condition for the two types of test pairs. An example of priming stimuli and their respective same- and different-response test pairs is presented in Fig. 4.1, part A.

If the local elements are represented early and the global configuration is constructed only later, then at short prime durations correct same responses to the element-similarity test figures would be faster than responses to the configuration-similarity test figures. The opposite pattern of results is expected if the global configuration is initially represented. In that case, at short prime durations, correct same responses to the configuration-similarity test figures would be faster than

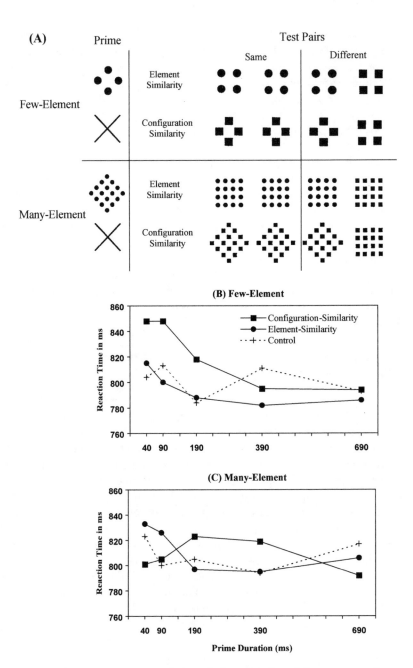

FIG. 4.1. (A) Examples of the priming stimuli and the same- and different-response test pairs for few-element and many-element patterns in Kimchi's (1998) primed-matching experiment with

responses to the test figures having the same elements as the prime. Given that prime-test similarity in elements entails dissimilarity in configuration, and vice versa (see Fig. 4.1, part A), two possible effects may contribute to differences between configuration-similarity and element-similarity test pairs: a facilitation due to prime-test similarity and an interference due to prime-test dissimilarity. Facilitation and inhibition are assessed in comparison with the neutral condition. At longer prime durations, the differences between the two types of test pairs are expected to disappear because presumably both the global configuration and the elements are represented by then.

The results are presented in Fig. 4.1, parts B and C. The results for the few-element stimuli (Fig. 4.1B) showed an early representation of the local elements: Prime-test similarity in elements produced faster responses than similarity in con-figuration at the shorter prime durations (40, 90, and 190 ms). A comparison with the control condition reveals that this difference was mainly due to inter-ference produced by dissimilarity in elements. The absence of facilitation for the element-similarity condition under the earlier prime durations suggests an early representation of the configuration, albeit a weak one. The early representation of the configuration was not strong enough to cancel interference due to dissim-ilarity in elements. No significant difference between element and configuration similarity and no significant facilitation or inhibition were observed at the longer prime durations of 390 and 690 ms, suggesting that, by that point, elements and configuration were equally available for priming.

The results for the many-element stimuli (Fig. 4.1C) showed an early rep-resentation of the configuration: Prime-test similarity in configuration produced faster responses than similarity in elements at the shorter prime durations (40 and 90 ms). Both facilitation due to similarity in configuration and inhibition due to dissimilarity in configuration contributed to this difference. The pattern of reac-tion time (RT) seemed to reverse at the longer prime duration of 190 and 390 ms: Similarity in elements actually produced significantly faster responses than similarity in configuration. No priming effects were observed at the 690-ms prime duration.

These results indicate that the relative dominance of global configuration and elements in the course of the organization of hierarchical stimuli depends on the number and relative size of the elements. A pattern composed of a few, relatively large elements is represented initially both in terms of its individual elements

---

FIG. 4.1. (*continued*) hierarchical stimuli. (B) Mean correct same RTs for each prime-test similarity (element similarity, configuration similarity, and neutral) as a function of prime duration, for the few-element primes, and (C) for the many-element primes. From "Uniform Connectedness and Grouping in the Perceptual Organiza-tion of Hierarchical Patterns," by R. Kimchi, 1998, *Journal of Ex-perimental Psychology: Human Perception and Performance, 24,* p. 1107, 1108. Copyright 1998 by APA. Reprinted with permission.

and its global configuration, but the representation of the global configuration is weaker than that of the elements. The global configuration consolidates with time and becomes equally available for priming as the elements at around 400 ms. On the other hand, the initial representation of a pattern composed of many, relatively small elements is its global configuration, without individuation of the elements. The individuation of the elements occurs later in time: The elements are available for priming at about 200 ms, and for a while they seem to be somewhat more readily available for priming than the global configuration. By around 700 ms, the global configuration and the elements of the many-element patterns seem to be equally available for priming.

Accessibility of Global Configurations and Local Elements to Rapid Search

Further support for the difference in the early representations of few- and many-element patterns (elements for the former and global configuration for the latter) has come from visual search, which is another way to address the question regarding the structures that are provided by early perceptual processing.

In visual search, the task is to detect as quickly and as accurately as possible the presence or absence of a target among other items (distractors) in the display. The number of distractors varies. Correct reaction times to the target are examined as a function of the total number of items (target and distractors) in the display, and the slope of the RT function over number of items indicates search rate. If the time to detect the target is independent or nearly independent of the number of items in the display and the target seems to pop out, then target search is considered fast and efficient, and target detection occurs under widely spread attention. If the time to detect a target increases as the number of other items in the display increases, then search is considered difficult and inefficient, and target detection requires focused attention (e.g., Duncan & Humphreys, 1989; Enns & Kingstone, 1995; Treisman & Gormican, 1988).

Given the widespread view that early perceptual processes are rapid and effortless—whereas later processes are more effortful, time-consuming and attention demanding (e.g., Neisser, 1967; Treisman & Schmidt, 1982)—visual pop-out for a given property has been interpreted as evidence that it is extracted by early perceptual processes (e.g., Enns & Rensink, 1990; Treisman & Schmidt, 1982).

To examine whether the global configuration or the local elements of few- and many-element stimuli are accessible to rapid search, participants were required, in separate blocks, to detect the presence or absence of a global target or a local target (Kimchi, 1998, Experiment 3). In the global search, the target differed from the distractors only in the global shape; in the local search, the target differed from the distractors only in the local elements. The number of items in the display was 2, 6, or 10. An example of the stimulus displays for the two types of search in few- and many-element conditions is presented in Fig. 4.2, for a display size of 6.

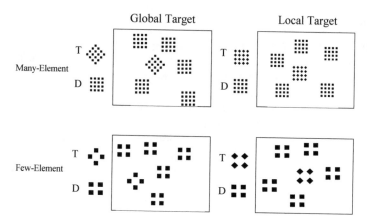

FIG. 4.2. The targets (T) and distractors (D) in Kimchi's (1998) visual search experiment (see text for details).

The microgenetic analysis for hierarchical stimuli predicts that the global configuration of many-element stimuli is more likely to be accessible to rapid search than the local elements because the global configuration is represented prior to the individuation of the elements. For the few-element patterns, on the other hand, the local elements are more likely to be accessible to rapid search than is the global configuration because the microgenetic findings indicate that the local elements of few-element patterns are represented prior to the full consolidation of the global configuration.

The results of the visual search converged with the microgenetic findings. When target and distractors were many-element patterns, the results showed high-speed pop-out search for the global targets (mean search rate 1.29 ms/item for target-present trials and 5.97 ms/item for target-absent trials), indicating the accessibility of the global configuration to rapid search. Search for the local targets of many-element patterns was slow and inefficient (mean search rates 33.88 ms/item for the target-present and 78.06 ms/item for target-absent trials), suggesting that the detection of the local targets involved focused attention. For the few-element patterns, on the other hand, a high-speed pop-out search was observed for local targets (mean search rates 2.90 ms/item for target-present and 14.26 ms/item for target-absent trials), indicating the accessibility of the local elements to rapid search. Search for global targets of the few-element patterns was slower (mean search rates 13.27 ms/item for the target-present and 28.76 ms/item for target-absent trials), suggesting the involvement of focused attention. Note that although search for the global target in the few-element condition was slower than search for the local targets, it was not as slow as search for the local elements in the many-element condition. These results provide further evidence for some early representation of the global configuration of the few-element patterns and for no early individuation of the local elements of the many-element patterns.

Summary

Taken together, the microgenetic and the visual search results suggest that the elements of few-element stimuli are represented early along with a weak representation of the global configuration. The grouping of few, relatively large elements into global configuration consumes time and requires focused attention. On the other hand, the global configuration of many-element stimuli is represented early, and the individuation of the local elements occurs later in time and requires focused attention. The early, rapid organization of many, relatively small elements into global configurations seems to be mandatory because search for local targets appeared inefficient despite the local search and global search being administered in separate blocks.

PERCEPTUAL ORGANIZATION OF LINE CONFIGURATIONS: MICROGENESIS AND STIMULUS FACTORS

To obtain further insights into the processes of perceptual organization and the stimulus factors that engage the mechanism of organization, I have studied the time course of the organization of line segments into configurations. Previous work with line configurations demonstrated configural dominance in discrimination and classification tasks both for connected line configurations (e.g., Kimchi & Bloch, 1998; Lasaga, 1989) and for disconnected ones (e.g., Kimchi, 1994; Pomerantz, Sager, & Stoever, 1977). These findings, however, do not necessarily imply that the global configuration of line segments is available in early perceptual processing because discrimination and classification performance can be based on later rather than earlier representations.

In a series of experiments I examined the relative dominance of configuration and components during the microgenesis of the organization of line configurations, using primed matching once again. The priming stimuli varied in the grouping factors present in the image (connectedness, proximity, collinearity, closure, and collinearity and closure combined).

Grouping Line Segments by Connectedness, Collinearity, and Closure

In the first experiment (Kimchi, 2000, Experiment 1), the priming stimuli were a diamond and a cross configurations that varied in the connectedness between their line components (no gap, small gap, and large gap) and were presented for various durations (40, 90, 190, and 390 ms). Connectedness was manipulated between subjects. The gaps between the component lines subtended $0.29°$ each in the small gap condition, and $1°$ each in the large gap condition. There were two types of same-response test pairs. The figures in the configuration-similarity test pair were similar to the prime in both configuration and line components, whereas the figures in the component-similarity test pair were similar to the prime in lines but dissimilar in configuration. A random array of dots was used as a neutral prime and served as a control condition for the assessment of facilitation and inhibition effects. The priming stimuli and the same- and different-response test pairs are presented in Fig. 4.3. The line segments of the cross are likely to be grouped by collinearity, whereas the line segments of the diamond are more likely to be grouped by closure. The relatability theory (Kellman, this volume; Kellman & Shipley, 1991; Shipley & Kellman, 1992), which formalizes the Gestalt principle of good continuation, suggests that the visual system connects two noncontiguous edges that are relatable so that the likelihood of seeing a completed figure increases systematically with the size of the angle that must be interpolated, with the 50% threshold occurring at around 90°. According to this criterion, the cross configuration is characterized by high relatability (an angle of 180°—collinearity), and diamond configuration is characterized by low relatability (an angle of 90°). The diamond configuration, however, possesses closure, whereas the cross does not.

For this set of stimuli, priming effects of the configuration would manifest in facilitation for the configuration-similarity condition and possibly interference for the component-similarity condition (due to dissimilarity in configuration). Priming effects of the line components would manifest in facilitation for both similarity conditions (because both types of test pairs are similar to the prime in components).

The results (see Fig. 4.4) showed early availability of the configuration that was manifested in facilitation for the configuration-similarity test pairs and inhibition for the component-similarity test pairs. These priming effects were observed under the shortest exposure duration of 40 ms and did not vary with prime duration. These effects were more pronounced for the no-gap (Fig. 4.4, part A) and the small-gap (Fig. 4.4, part B) conditions than for the large-gap condition (Fig. 4.4, part C), suggesting that proximity between the line segments has an effect on the early availability of global configuration. Note, however, that no facilitation due to component similarity alone was observed, even for the large-gap condition.

The early availability of configural organization observed in this experiment may have been overestimated for three reasons. One, there was an asymmetry between the two same-response test pairs with respect to their similarity relation to the prime: The configuration-similarity test pair was similar to the prime in both lines and configuration, whereas the component-similarity test pair was similar in lines but dissimilar in configuration. This asymmetry could have biased the participants in overreacting to configuration dissimilarity in the component-similarity condition. Two, the participants may have been biased toward complete configurations because all the test figures were connected configurations. Three, the figures in each of the two different-response test pairs differed from one another in both components and configuration so that participants could adopt a strategy of relying only on configural information in making their same/different judgments, thus

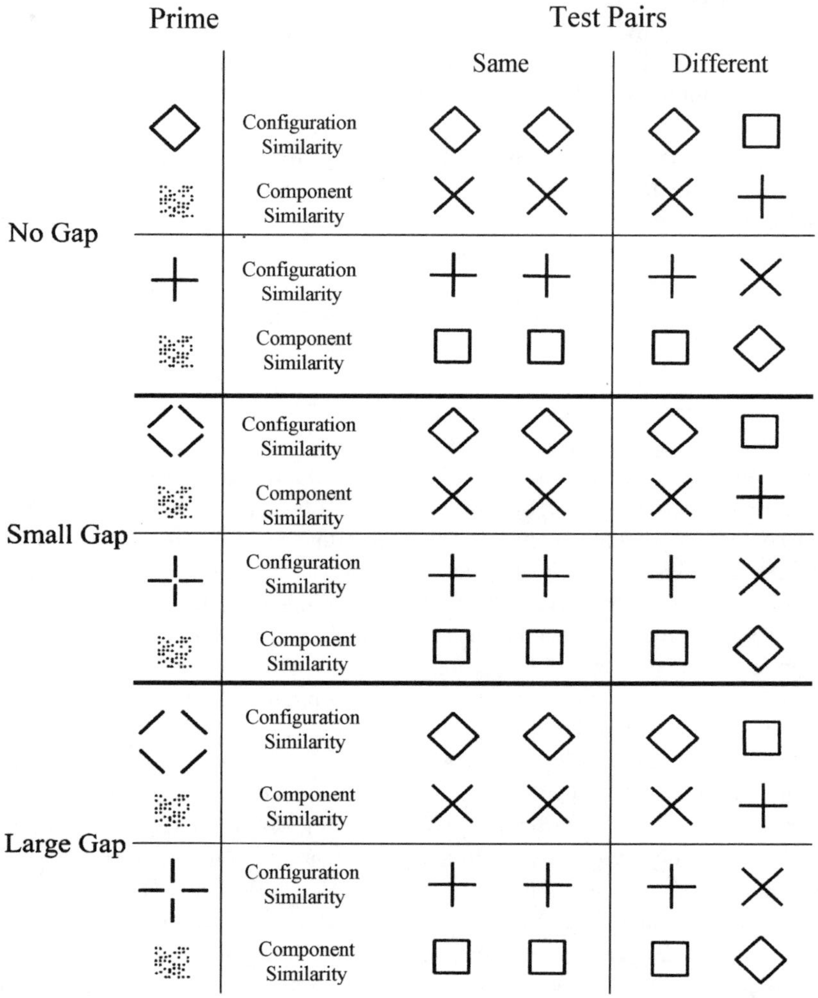

FIG. 4.3. The priming stimuli and the same- and different-response test pairs for the no-gap, small-gap, and large-gap conditions in Kimchi's (2000, Experiment 1) primed-matching experiment with line configurations. From "The Perceptual Organization of Visual Objects: A Microgenetic Analysis," by R. Kimchi, 2000, *Vision Research, 40*, p. 1336. Copyright 2000 by Elsevier Science Ltd. Reprinted with permission.

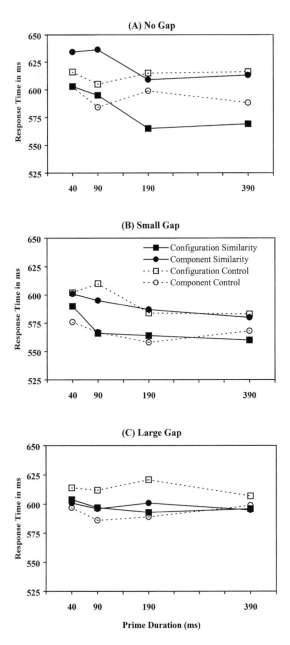

FIG. 4.4. Mean correct same RTs for each prime-test similarity as a function of prime duration (collapsed across prime type) for each gap condition in Kimchi's (2000, Experiment 1) primed-matching experiment with line configurations. From "The Perceptual Organization of Visual Objects: A Microgenetic Analysis," by R. Kimchi, 2000, *Vision Research, 40*, p. 1338. Copyright 2000 by Elsevier Science Ltd. Reprinted with permission.

biasing them toward the configuration.[1] These potential biases are controlled for in the experiment described next, which was conducted with the stimuli presented in Fig. 4.5, part A.

Collinearity and Closure Combined

In this experiment (Kimchi, 2000, Experiment 2) the primes were square configu- rations that varied in proximity between the components (small gap, large gap). For these stimuli, the components are likely to be grouped into a configuration by the combination of collinearity and closure. The figures in the configuration-similarity test pair were similar to the prime in configuration but dissimilar in components, whereas the figures in the component-similarity test pair were similar to the prime in components but dissimilar in configuration (see Fig. 4.5, part A). For this set of stimuli, priming effects of the configuration would manifest in facilitation for the configuration similarity condition and possibly interference for the component similarity condition (due to dissimilarity in configuration). Priming effects of the line components would manifest in facilitation for the component similarity con- ditions and possibly interference for the configuration similarity condition (due to dissimilarity in components).

The results (see Fig. 4.5, parts B and C) showed clear priming effects of the configuration, namely, facilitation for configuration similarity and inhibition for component similarity. These priming effects were observed under the earliest prime duration of 40 ms and did not vary significantly with prime duration. These results converged with the previous ones, indicating an early representation of the global configuration. Because there was no bias toward the configuration in this exper- iment, this convergence indicates that the early availability of the configuration observed in the previous experiment is not likely to be due to any bias.

With this set of stimuli, however, no effect of proximity was observed: The priming effects of the configuration were equally strong and equally early (ob- served under 40-ms prime duration) for strong proximity/small gap (Fig. 4.5, part B) and for weak proximity/large gap (Fig. 4.5, part C). This difference in the effect of proximity suggests that proximity between components has a larger effect on the early availability of the global configuration when only closure (as in the diamond prime, Fig. 4.3) or only collinearity (as in the cross prime, Fig. 4.3) is present in the stimulus than when closure and collinearity are combined (as in the square prime,

---

[1]The results of this experiment were completely replicated in an experiment in which the figures in the component-similarity test pairs were single lines rather than a connected configuration. This replica- tion weakens the arguments concerning potential biases due to connected test figures for a configuration- based same/different judgment. But this experiment introduced another problem, namely, that the test figures in the component similarity condition differed from the prime also in number of lines (whereas each of the test figures in the configuration-similarity condition included four lines as did the prime).

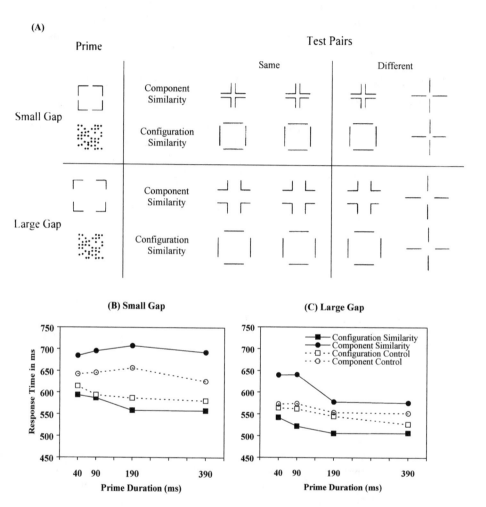

FIG. 4.5. (A) The priming stimuli and the same- and different-response test pairs for the small-gap and large-gap conditions in Kimchi's (2000, Experiment 2) primed-matching experiment with square configurations. (B) Mean correct same RTs for each prime-test similarity as a function of prime duration for the small-gap condition, and (C) for the large-gap condition. From "The Perceptual Organization of Visual Objects: A Microgenetic Analysis," by R. Kimchi, 2000, *Vision Research, 40,* p. 1340, 1341. Copyright 2000 by Elsevier Science Ltd. Reprinted with permission.

Fig. 4.5). Some evidence for the potential power of the combination of closure and collinearity comes also from the work of Donnelly, Humphreys and Riddoch (1991), which demonstrated that the combination of closure and collinearity results in an efficient visual search, much more so than in the presence of closure alone.

Open-Ended Line Segments Versus Closed Figural Elements

A comparison of the microgenetic findings for the line configurations and those for the hierarchical stimuli raises an interesting discrepancy. The findings for the hierarchical stimuli showed an early representation of the components for stimuli composed of four relatively large elements, whereas the findings for stimuli composed of four line segments showed an early representation of the configuration. This apparent discrepancy might be due to a difference in the salience of the components (greater for the solid circles and squares in the hierarchical stimuli than for the line segments) or, alternatively, to a difference in the nature of the components (open-ended lines vs. closed shapes). To rule out a simple salience account, I studied the microgenesis of organization for patterns composed of four outline shapes (see Fig. 4.6) for which the difference in salience in comparison to the line segments was minimized (Kimchi, 2000, Experiment 3). The results converged with the results for the few-element hierarchical stimuli, showing an early relative dominance of the elements. This finding rules out a simple salience account; rather, the early grouping of the local elements, or, alternatively, the early individuation of the local elements, seems to depend not only on the number and the relative size of the elements but also on their properties, with closure at the local level presumably being important for element individuation.

Summary

Taken together, these microgenetic findings demonstrate that open-ended line segments are rapidly organized into configurations provided the presence of collinearity, closure, or both. These results also yield information about the relationship between the grouping factors of closure, collinearity, and proximity. Proximity between line components facilitates grouping by either closure (as in the diamond prime) or collinearity (as in the cross prime), but the combination of closure and collinearity (as in the square primes) dominates proximity in early perceptual grouping. In contrast to open-ended line segments, closed figural elements are individuated early and are grouped into configurations over time.

In addition, the finding that the configural organization of disconnected line segments was available under the same short duration (i.e., 40 ms) as the configuration of the connected line segments suggests that uniform connectedness (UC) may not have a privileged role in perceptual organization, as claimed by Palmer

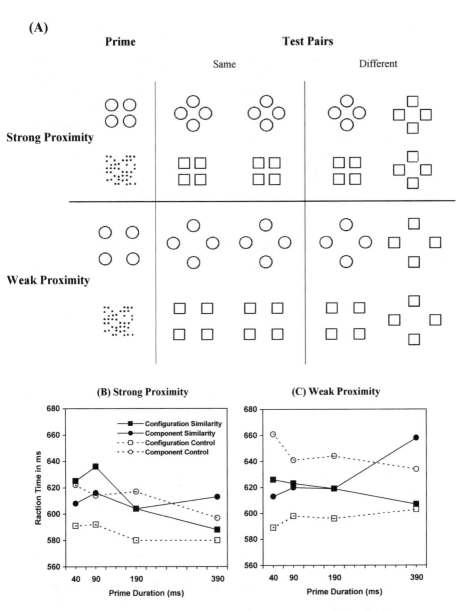

(A)

Prime · Test Pairs

Same · Different

Strong Proximity

Weak Proximity

(B) Strong Proximity · **(C) Weak Proximity**

Raction Time in ms

- ■— Configuration Similarity
- ●— Component Similarity
- □ - - Configuration Control
- ◇ - - Component Control

Prime Duration (ms)

FIG. 4.6. (A) The priming stimuli and the same- and different-response test pairs for the two proximity conditions in Kimchi's (2000, Experiment 3) primed-matching experiment with the few-element stimuli. (B) Mean correct "same" RTs for each prime-test similarity as a function of prime duration for strong proximity, and (C) for weak proximity among the elements. From "The Perceptual Organization of Visual Objects: A Microgenetic Analysis," by R. Kimchi, 2000, *Vision Research, 40,* p. 1340, 1341. Copyright 2000 by Elsevier Science Ltd. Reprinted with permission.

133

and Rock (1994a, 1994b). Palmer and Rock's theory predicts that the early representation of the primes in Fig. 4.3 in the no-gap condition would be the complete diamond and cross configurations, by virtue of UC. Parsing processes can then divide the uniformly connected diamond or cross into four component lines at the interior concave discontinuities. On the other hand, the theory predicts that the early representations of the primes in the small-gap and large-gap conditions are the component lines because each of the lines forms a UC region. Grouping processes can then group the four lines into a diamond or a cross configuration. The results, however, showed early priming of the configuration for both connected and disconnected configurations.

THE ROLE OF PAST EXPERIENCE IN PERCEPTUAL ORGANIZATION

Phenomenologically, a very fragmented image is perceived initially as a random array of pieces, but, once recognized, it is perceived as an organized picture. The question is whether past experience (in particular, object memories) has a direct influence on perceptual organization, or only on the output of organizational processes. The traditional and widely held view has been that organization must precede object recognition because it requires a candidate object on which to work (e.g., Marr, 1982; Neisser, 1967; Treisman, 1986). In this view, perceptual organization is accomplished on the basis of low-level, bottom-up cues, without access to object representations in memory.

To examine whether past experience exerts an influence on perceptual grouping, Hadad and I used primed matching and manipulated the familiarity of the prime and its connectedness (Kimchi & Hadad, 2002). To manipulate familiarity we used as primes Hebrew letters, presented upright (familiar) or inverted (unfamiliar). This manipulation of familiarity allowed us to equate the familiar and the unfamiliar stimuli in their bottom-up grouping factors (e.g., connectedness, collinearity, proximity). The disconnected primes were formed by dividing each letter into four line segments at the interior concave discontinuities (Hoffman & Richards, 1984) and introducing small or large gaps between the line segments. A neutral prime, consisted of a random array of dots, served as a baseline condition. The primes were presented for various durations (40, 90, 190, 390, and 690 ms). The priming stimulus was followed immediately by a pair of test figures. We used two types of same-response test pairs: The figures in the similarity test pair were similar to the prime, and the figures in the orientation-dissimilarity test pair were 180° rotational transforms of the prime. An example of upright and inverted primes and their respective same- and different-response test pairs in the three gap conditions (no gap, small gap, and large gap) is presented in Fig. 4.7. Familiarity was manipulated within subjects and connectedness between subjects. For the sake of simplicity, I refer hereafter only to the similarity test pairs. For

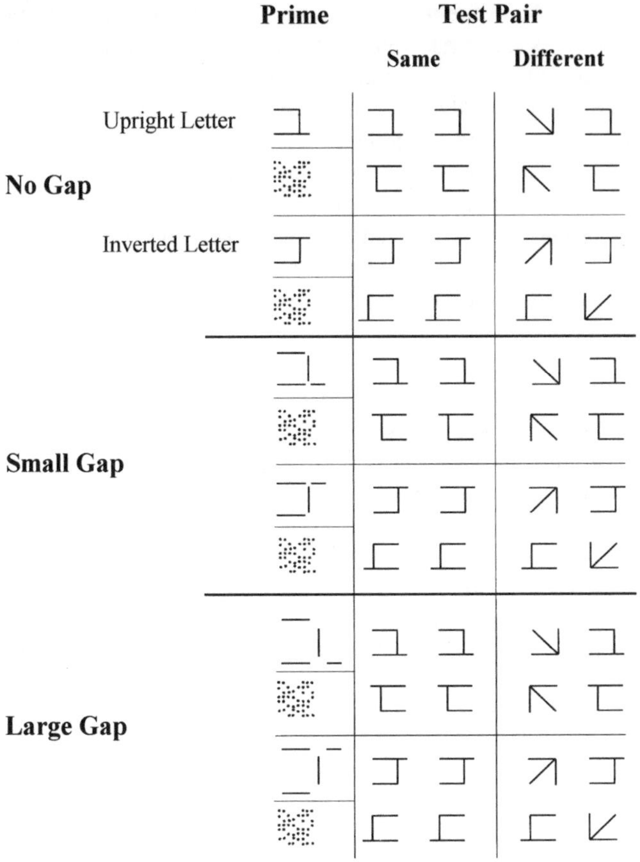

FIG. 4.7. Examples of upright and inverted primes and the *same*- and *different*-response test pairs in the no-gap, small-gap, and large-gap conditions. For each prime, the similarity test pair is the upper pair and the orientation-dissimilarity test pair is the lower pair. The random array of dots serves as a neutral prime, providing a baseline (control) for each of the test-pair types. From "Influence of Past Experience on Perceptual Grouping," by R. Kimchi and B. Hadad, 2002, *Psychological Science, 13*, p. 44. Copyright 2002 by APS. Reprinted with permission from Blackwell Publishers.

these test pairs, priming effects of the configuration would manifest themselves in facilitation.

The traditional view predicts additive effects of connectedness and familiarity on priming. According to this view, the primes (whether upright or inverted) get organized only on the basis of bottom-up cues, without any influence from object memories. Consequently, connectedness would affect the organization of the primes. Upright primes are then recognized faster than inverted primes because they are more likely to activate object representations and thereby speed responses to similar figures. This would result in additive effects of connectedness and familiarity on priming. An advantage of familiar relative to unfamiliar primes would indicate an influence of past experience on the output of organization rather than on organization itself. However, if familiarity interacts with connectedness so that the effect of disconnectedness on priming is more detrimental for unfamiliar than for familiar primes, this would indicate that object memories contribute to the grouping of the line segments into a configuration. The microgenetic analysis enables us to determine how early in time the effect of familiarity is exerted relative to that of connectedness.

The results for the similarity condition are presented in Fig. 4.8, parts A (upright primes) and B (inverted primes). These results show that familiarity interacted with connectedness in their effect on priming: Connectedness had no effect on the priming of familiar primes, whereas the priming effects of unfamiliar primes varied as a function of connectedness. For the upright primes, both connected and disconnected primes produced equal amounts of facilitation that was observed under the earliest duration of 40 ms and did not vary with prime duration (Fig. 4.8, part A). The results for inverted primes were quite different, showing that priming effects were affected by connectedness and by prime duration (Fig. 4.8, part B). Inverted connected primes produced facilitation that was as strong and as early as the facilitation produced by upright primes. Disconnectedness, however, had a detrimental effect on priming. The facilitation observed in the small-gap condition was significantly smaller than the one in the no-gap condition, and for the large-gap condition facilitation was observed only later in time.

These findings suggest an influence of past experience on the rapid grouping of line segments into a configuration. The effect of past experience manifested itself at the same time as the effect of connectedness, as indicated by the finding that the configuration of connected upright letter, the configuration of disconnected upright letter, and the configuration of connected inverted letter all were available under exposure duration of 40 ms. In the absence of familiarity and connectedness (as with the disconnected inverted primes), the grouping of the disconnected line segments into a configuration occurred later in time.

An alternative account for the observed priming effects of the configuration for the upright letters may be similarity in identity between the prime and the test figures, without any prior organization, rather than effects of familiarity on grouping. According to this alternative account the upright primes activate object representations, get identified, and facilitate responses to test figures with the same identity. Previous findings, however, indicate that partial information or stimulus degradation affects identification speed (e.g., Everett, Hochhaus, & Brown, 1985; Snodgrass & Corwin, 1988). Therefore, an effect of connectedness would be expected for the upright primes, but no such effect was found (see Fig. 4.8, upright primes). Thus, although we cannot rule out completely some effect of identity, the results are more compatible with the grouping account.

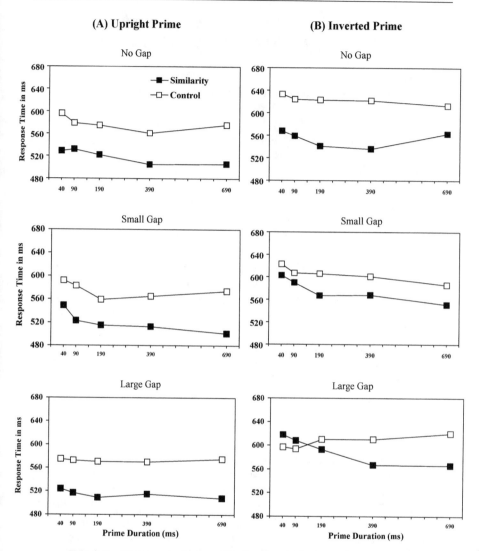

FIG. 4.8. Mean correct same RTs for the similarity and the control conditions as a function of prime duration for each gap condition for (A) upright primes and (B) inverted primes.

These results converge with the previous ones in demonstrating that uniform connectedness does not have a special role in perceptual organization. This is not to say that connectedness does not play a role in organization. The strength of connectedness manifested itself with the connected inverted primes. But connectedness is one of a number of cues that determine perceptual organization. We have shown that input from object memories is also among these cues.

SIMPLE SPATIAL FILTERING MECHANISMS OR
SOPHISTICATED GROUPING PROCESSES?

One may argue that the results concerning the early representations of the hierarchical stimuli and the line configurations are due to spatial filters based on spatial-frequency channels operating at early visual processing (e.g., Ginsburg, 1986). Several investigators have already suggested that the global advantage observed with many-element hierarchical stimuli is mediated by low-spatial-frequency channels (e.g., Badcock, Whitworth, Badcock, & Lovegrove, 1990; Hughes, Fendrich, & Reuter-Lorenz, 1990; Lamb & Yund, 1993; Shulman, Sullivan, Gish, & Sakoda, 1986; Shulman & Wilson, 1987). Thus, blurring by large-scale, low-resolution filters at early stages of visual processing may account for the early representation of the global structures of the many-element patterns. Such blurring may also account for the early representation of the large elements of the few-element patterns due to their large absolute size.

Similarly, it can be argued that due to blurring by low-spatial-frequency channels, the existence of small gaps between line segments should not greatly affect priming, thus yielding a similar priming effect of the global configuration for connected and disconnected line segments.

Several findings, however, are not compatible with this account. First, it has been found that relative size of the elements (i.e., the size of the elements relative to the configuration in which they are embedded) rather than their absolute size is critical for the early organization of hierarchical stimuli. For example, Peled and I (Kimchi & Peled, 1999) examined whether absolute or relative size of elements governs priming effects for few-element patterns by using patterns in which the element number was held constant at four and the elements size varied in three conditions: (1) absolutely large, relatively large elements; (2) absolutely small, relatively large elements; and (3) absolutely small, relatively small elements. The first two conditions produced a similar pattern of results, indicating early priming effects of the elements. A different pattern of results was observed for the third condition. These results suggest that relative rather than absolute size of the elements is critical for determining early organization. Enns and Kingstone (1995) used visual search with few-element stimuli that varied in the absolute size of the elements (small vs. large), but the small and large elements had similar, large relative size. Search slopes for the local elements were shallow and did not differ for the small and large elements. Their results, then, demonstrate that few, relatively large elements, regardless of whether their absolute size is large or small, are accessible to rapid search.

The critical role of relative size suggests that simple spatial filtering mechanisms cannot fully account for the early organization of hierarchical stimuli. Ivry and Robertson's (1998) view that focuses on relative rather than absolute spatial frequencies in the image also cannot easily account for the early organization of hierarchical stimuli. According to Ivry and Robertson, the difference between global and local information is a difference along a continuum of spatial frequency. Therefore, the difference in the processing of few- and many-element stimuli is not compatible with their approach because the spatial frequency of the elements is relatively higher than that of the configuration for both types of stimuli (see also Behrmann & Kimchi, this volume).

Second, blurring by low spatial frequency channels cannot account for the finding, observed with the line configurations, that the effect of proximity on priming depended on the presence (or absence) of other grouping factors in the image (i.e., that proximity among the line segments facilitated grouping when either closure or collinearity was present but had no effect when closure and collinearity were combined). Nor can it account for the differential effect of connectedness on priming for familiar and unfamiliar stimuli, namely, that connectedness had no effect for familiar primes, but the priming effects for the unfamiliar primes varied as a function of connectedness. If the early priming of the global configuration of disconnected line segments were due to blurring by low-resolution filters, then connected and disconnected primes would have similar priming effects, regardless of whether other grouping factors are present or absent or whether the stimuli are familiar or unfamiliar.

Taken together, these findings suggest that early organization is unlikely to be due to simple spatial filtering at early perceptual processing. Rather, more sophisticated processes of grouping and individuation are likely to be involved in early organization. These processes rely on a host of cues, such as number and relative size of the elements, connectedness, collinearity, proximity, and familiarity.

THE ROLE OF ATTENTION IN PERCEPTUAL ORGANIZATION

Contrary to the assumptions of traditional theories of visual perception that perceptual organization occurs preattentively, Mack, Rock and their colleagues have claimed that no organization occurs without attention (Mack et al., 1992; Rock, Linnet et al., 1992). In their inattention paradigm, they used a relatively difficult primary task in which subjects had to determine whether the horizontal or vertical line of a briefly presented cross is longer. The display contained elements in the background of the cross for all of the initial trials. On the fourth, inattention trial the background elements were organized into rows (or columns) according to lightness or proximity, and the subjects were asked, after reporting which line of the cross was longer, about the background organization. Subjects could not report whether the background organization was vertical or horizontal. These kinds of findings led Rock and Mack to the conclusion that no Gestalt grouping takes place without attention. However, the poor knowledge of the subjects may reflect poor explicit memory rather than an indication of no organizational processing.

To circumvent the issue of explicit memory, Moore and Egeth (1997) used the inattention paradigm but devised indirect online measures of unattended processing. Their primary task was to determine which of two horizontal lines was longer. On the inattention trial the elements in the background were grouped by luminance into inducers biasing the horizontal line length by creating the Muller-Lyer or Ponzo illusion. Subjects were unable to report the background organization, but their line-length judgments were influenced by the illusions. These findings suggest that grouping by similarity in luminance does occur under conditions of inattention, albeit without subjects' awareness.

In addition, it has been suggested that grouping is not the unitary phenomenon referred to in much of the literature but rather involves two distinct processes: Clustering, or unit formation, which determines which elements belong together, and configuring, or shape formation, which determines how the grouped elements appear as a whole based on the interrelations of the elements (Koffka, 1935; Rock, 1986; Trick & Enns, 1997). This suggestion raises the possibility that different groupings may vary in their attentional demands, depending on the processes involved, with configuring being more demanding than just clustering.

Organization Without Attention

To examine whether organization can take place without attention, and whether different groupings vary in their attentional demands, Razpurker-Apfeld and I (Kimchi & Razpurker-Apfeld, 2001) used the method developed by Driver and his colleagues (cited in Driver, Davis, Russell, Turatto, & Freeman, 2001) to obtain online measures of unattended processing, and manipulated the grouping of the unattended elements. On each trial, subjects were presented with two successive displays, each appeared for 200 ms, and separated by 150 ms. Each display consisted of a central square matrix surrounded by background elements (see Fig. 4.9). The subject's task was to judge whether the two successive central target squares were same or different. The organization of the background elements stayed the same or changed across successive displays, independently of whether the successive target squares were same or different. The colors of the elements always changed between the two successive displays to disentangle a change in color per se from a change in organization.

We employed three different background organizations (between subjects), examples of which are presented in Fig. 4.9 (in grayscale). One organization was the classical Gestalt grouping of elements into columns or rows by color similarity (Fig. 4.9, part A), similar to the one used by Driver et al. (2001). The second organization was grouping elements into a square or a cross by color similarity (Fig. 4.9, part B). These two types of organization involve grouping elements together into units on the basis of common color. We conjectured, however, that configuring is less demanding in the former, which requires determination of the orientation (vertical or horizontal) of the units, than in the latter, which requires

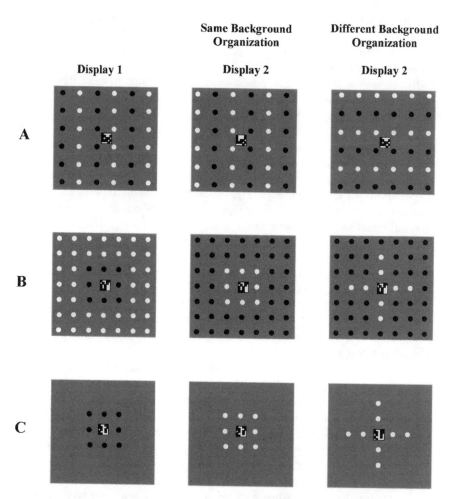

Display 1   Display 2   Display 2

A

B

C

FIG. 4.9. Examples (in grayscale) of the displays for a single trial
in the study of Kimchi and Razpurker-Apfeld (2001). The central target squares in Display 1 and Display 2 can be the same or different. The background elements can be grouped into columns/rows by
color similarity (A), into square/cross by color similarity (B), or into
square/cross (C). The background organization either stays the same
across Display 1 and Display 2 or changes (independently of whether
the central square changes or not). The colors of background elements always change between Display 1 and Display 2.

the formation of a distinctive shape. The third type of organization also required grouping elements into a square or a cross (Fig. 4.9, part C), but because this grouping is supported by several gestalt factors including proximity, similarity of color, similarity of luminance, and similarity of shape, and it does not involve segregation from other elements, it may be less demanding than the grouping into square/cross by color similarity.

If organization of the background elements occurs without attention, then target-same judgments would be faster and more accurate when the background organization stays the same than when it changes, and target-different judgments would be faster and more accurate when the background organization changes than when it stays the same.

The results are presented in Fig. 4.10. An influence of the background organization on the same-different judgments was observed for grouping elements into columns/rows by color similarity (Fig. 4.10, part A): Subjects were faster with their target-same judgments if the background organization stayed the same, and target-different judgments were faster if the background organization changed. In contrast, no effect of the background organization on subjects' performance was found for grouping elements into square/cross by color similarity (Fig. 4.10, part B). Yet, background organization clearly influenced subjects' judgments when grouping into a square or a cross did not involve segregation from other elements (Fig. 4.10, part C). For all three conditions, we found that the surprise questions at the end of the experiment replicated the results of Mack et al. (1992): Subjects were unable to report the background organization of the immediately preceding background displays.

We hypothesized that grouping elements into columns/rows by color similarity would be more attention demanding than grouping elements into square/cross by color similarity because configuring is simpler in the former than in the latter. We found, however, that under certain conditions (i.e., when no segregation from other elements is required), grouping into a shape can occur under inattention, suggesting that the process of shape formation per se cannot account for the difference between grouping into columns/rows and grouping into a shape by color similarity. Presumably, grouping that requires segregation from other elements is more attention demanding when it involves configuring into a shape than into a vertical or horizontal pattern because segregation in the former case also requires resolving figure-ground relations for the segregated units, whereas all units in the latter are designated as "figures."

Time Course of Organization

Interestingly, we found that differences in the time course of grouping parallel these differences in attentional demands. We used primed matching to explore the time course of three types of organization, similar to the ones manipulated in our inattention experiment. The priming stimuli and their respective same and different test pairs are presented in Fig. 4.11 (in grayscale; the actual elements in

(A) Columns/Rows by Color Similarity

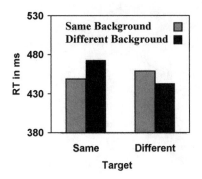

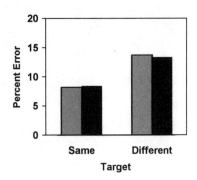

(B) Square/Cross by Color Similarity

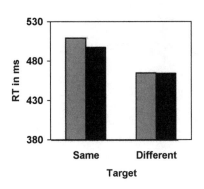

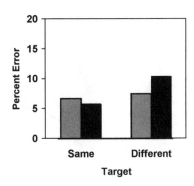

(C) Square/Cross

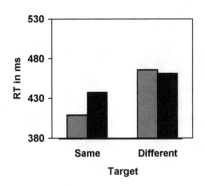

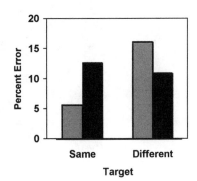

FIG. 4.10. Mean correct target-same and target-different RTs and percent error as a function of background (same or different) for the three background groupings in Kimchi and Razpurker-Apfeld's experiment (2001).

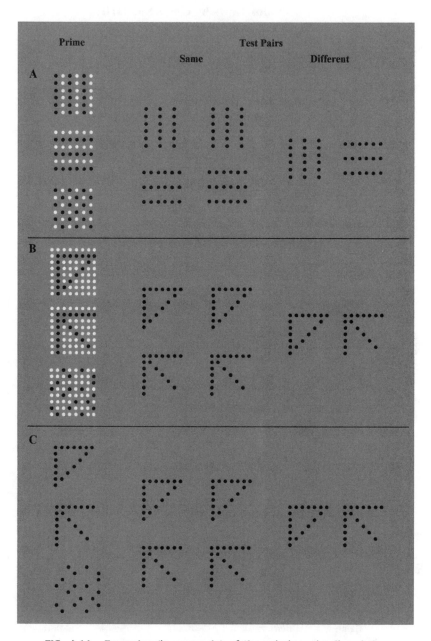

FIG. 4.11. Examples (in grayscale) of the priming stimuli and the same- and different-response test pairs in Kimchi and Razpurker-Apfeld's (2001) primed-matching experiment. The primes can be organized into columns/rows by color similarity (A), into triangle/arrow by color similarity (B), or into triangle/arrow (C). The color of the circle elements always changed between the prime and the test figures.

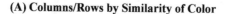

(A) Columns/Rows by Similarity of Color

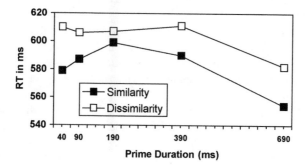

(B) Triangle/Arrow by Similarity of Color

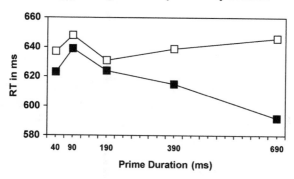

(C) Triangle/Arrow Configuration

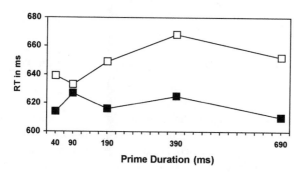

FIG. 4.12. Mean correct same RTs for the similarity and dissimilarity conditions as a function of prime duration (collapsed across prime type) for each of the three types of organization in Kimchi and Razpurker-Apfeld's (2001) primed-matching experiment.

145

the experiment were colored). In one condition the priming stimuli were colored elements that grouped into columns/rows by similarity of color (Fig. 4.11, part A). In a second condition the priming stimuli were colored elements grouped into a triangle or an arrow by color similarity (Fig. 4.11, part B). In the third condition, the priming stimuli were colored elements grouped into a triangle or an arrow, and no segregation from other elements was involved (Fig. 4.11, part C). Each of the test pairs was similar to one prime and dissimilar to the other. The color of the elements of the test figures was always different from that of the elements of the priming stimuli.

The results are presented in Fig. 4.12. Similarity between the prime and the test figures produced faster responses than dissimilarity under all prime durations, including the shortest duration of 40 ms, for organization into columns/rows by common color (Fig. 4.12, part A) and for organization into triangle/arrow when no segregation from other elements was required (Fig. 4.12, part C). For organization into triangle/arrow by common color, significant priming due to prime-test similarity was observed only under longer prime durations (Fig. 4.12, part B).

Summary

These results show that grouping elements into a vertical or a horizontal pattern by color similarity, and grouping elements into a shape (when no segregation from other elements is involved) occur rapidly and under conditions of inattention. Grouping elements into a shape by color similarity demands attention and consumes time. These findings suggest that quite an elaborated form of grouping can take place rapidly and without attention, albeit without subjects' awareness. Grouping into a shape that requires resolving figure-ground relations for segregated units appears to be time consuming and attention demanding. Further research is required to better understand the differences between attentional and inattentional grouping.

IMPLICATIONS TO ISSUES OF PERCEPTUAL ORGANIZATION

The findings reviewed in this chapter show that configural organization and global structures can be available early, presumably as a result of early rapid grouping, or can emerge later in time, as a result of late or slower attention demanding grouping, depending on the grouping operations, stimulus factors, and past experience. I turn now to the implications of these findings for the issues raised in the beginning of the chapter.

A first important implication is that early perceptual processing provides more complex structures than has been assumed by traditional theories of perception. The traditional theories, dominated by the early feature-analysis view, have assumed that early perceptual processes analyze only simple elements and properties. Contrary to this assumption, we found that global configurations, based on the interrelation among simple elements and line segments, are available for priming even under exposure durations as short as 40 ms, and are accessible to rapid search. Other investigators have reported similar results. Early levels of perceptual processing have been found to be sensitive to scene-based properties (e.g., Enns & Rensink, 1990; He & Nakayama, 1992; Kleffner & Ramachandran, 1992), to complete configurations rather than to components (e.g., Rensink & Enns, 1995), and to part-whole information (e.g., Wolfe, Friedman-Hill, & Bilsky, 1994). These findings provide converging evidence for early representation of complex configurations. In light of this evidence, a view that holds that only simple properties are available in early perceptual processing is hardly tenable.

A second implication is that both stimulus factors and past experience have an effect on perceptual organization. Some of the stimulus factors found to engage the mechanisms of early organization include number and relative size of elements, collinearity, proximity, connectedness, and closure (see also, for example, Kellman, this volume; Kovács & Julesz, 1994). Uniform connectedness (Palmer, this volume; Palmer & Rock, 1994a, 1994b), however, does not seem to have a privileged status in organization (see also Han et al., 1999; Peterson, 1994).

The importance of stimulus factors has been demonstrated in several of our findings. Thus, we have found that the priming effects of equally familiar stimuli depend on the grouping factors present in the image. For example, the priming effects of the global configuration of disconnected line segments with relatively weak proximity (large gap) between the line segments were stronger when both collinearity and closure were present in the image than when only collinearity or closure were present. In addition, familiar and unfamiliar primes produced similar priming effects of the configuration when connectedness was present in the image.

The influence of past experience on organization has been demonstrated in the findings of differential effects of priming of the global configuration for disconnected stimuli that were equated for the grouping factors present in the image but differed in familiarity (upright and inverted letters). The global configurations of upright letters were available for priming early, regardless of connectedness, whereas the configurations of disconnected inverted letters were not available until later. Our findings converge with other findings that have demonstrated the contribution of input from higher level object representations to figure assignment (e.g., Peterson, this volume; Peterson & Gibson, 1994) and image segmentation (Vecera & Farah, 1997).

These findings are incompatible with the traditional feedforward view that assumes perceptual organization is accomplished solely on the basis of bottom-up cues and is immune to influence from past experience (e.g., Marr, 1982). Rather, these findings are consistent with a hierarchical interactive model with temporally cascaded processing that includes feedforward and feedback mechanisms (e.g., McClelland & Rumelhart, 1981; Vecera & O'Reilly, 1998). They can also be accounted for by the parallel model proposed by Peterson (e.g., this volume) in which object recognition processes influence organization in parallel with lower level cues. Our finding that the effect of familiarity on the integration of the line segments manifested at the same time as the effect of connectedness suggests that at least some aspects of object representations in memory may be accessed in parallel with image-based cues. Presently, however, it is difficult to distinguish between the models (Peterson, 1999; Vecera & O'Reilly, 2000), and further research is needed to evaluate the relative adequacy of these models for perceptual organization.

A third implication is that not all groupings are created equal in terms of time course and attentional demands: Certain forms of grouping take place early, rapidly, and without attention, whereas other forms of grouping occur later, consume time, and require attention. Thus, for example, we found that grouping of elements into columns/rows by common color occurs rapidly and without attention. Grouping of many small elements into a shape also occurs rapidly and without focused attention, provided that no segregation from other elements is involved. On the other hand, grouping a few, relatively large closed elements into a configuration consumes time and requires focused attention. We also found that if the grouping of many elements into a configuration involves segregation of grouped elements into figure and ground, then it consumes time and cannot take place without attention.

Other studies reported in the literature also have demonstrated that different groupings vary in time course and attentional demands (e.g., Ben-Av & Sagi, 1995; Han & Humphreys, 1999; Han et al., 1999; Kurylo, 1997). Further support for the suggestion that not all groupings are created equal comes from the work Behrmann and I did with two agnosic patients (Behrmann & Kimchi, this volume). The patients had no problem grouping elements into columns/rows by proximity or by luminance, and grouping by collinearity. Nonetheless, they exhibited difficulties (and to different degrees) in grouping elements into configuration, even in the simpler case that does not involve segregation from other elements and in grouping by closure.

Clearly, our findings, along with other findings reported in the literature (e.g., Moore & Egeth, 1997), do not support the radical claim made by Mack and Rock (e.g., Mack et al., 1992) that no Gestalt grouping takes place without attention. Further research is required, however, to elucidate the different perceptual-organizational processes that differ in time course and attentional demands.

Recent neurophysiological findings are consistent with the behavioral findings reviewed in this chapter, indicating that grouping and segregation take place as early as the primary visual cortex, presumably as a result of horizontal interactions and back projections from higher to lower centers of the visual system (e.g., Lamme, Super, & Spekreijse, 1998; Spillmann, 1999; Westheimer, 1999). For example, responses of neurons in the primary visual cortex (V1) to stimuli inside the classical receptive fields can be modulated by contextual stimuli outside the receptive field (e.g., Lamme et al., 1998; Sugita, 1999; Zipser, Lamme, & Schiller,

1996), suggesting that even the earliest stage of visual cortical processing is involved in complex visual perception such as grouping of image fragments. There is also evidence for mutual bottom-up and top-down reciprocity (e.g., Bullier & Nowak, 1995; Lee & Nguyen, 2001; Zhou, Friedman, & von der Heydt, 2000), suggesting that input from higher level representations can contribute to early organization.

CONCLUSIONS

The findings reviewed in this chapter indicate that early perceptual processing involves organizational processes of grouping and individuation, providing more complex structures than has been assumed by the traditional view. These processes rely on a host of cues, including lower level cues, such as connectedness and collinearity, and higher level cues, such as input from object representations. We have further shown that these organizational processes vary in their time course and attentional demands. These findings are part of recent developments in the psychological and physiological research on visual perception that provide converging evidence for a highly interactive perceptual system in which both image-based and object-based properties contribute to the early organization of visual objects.

ACKNOWLEDGMENTS

Preparation of this chapter was supported in part by the Max Wertheimer Minerva Center for Cognitive Processes and Human Performance, University of Haifa. I thank Marlene Behrmann for useful comments on an earlier draft and Irene Razpurker-Apfeld and Aliza Cohen for general assistance. Correspondence should be addressed to Ruth Kimchi, Department of Psychology, University of Haifa, Haifa 31905, Israel. Electronic mail: rkimchi@research.haifa.ac.il.

REFERENCES

Badcock, C. J., Whitworth, F. A., Badcock, D. R., & Lovegrove, W. J. (1990). Low-frequency filtering and processing of local-global stimuli. *Perception, 19,* 617–629.
Beller, H. K. (1971). Priming: Effects of advance information on matching. *Journal of Experimental Psychology, 87,* 176–182.
Ben-Av, M. B., & Sagi, D. (1995). Perceptual grouping by similarity and proximity: Experimental results can be predicted by intensity auto-correlations. *Vision Research, 35,* 853–866.
Boer, L. C., & Keuss, P. J. G. (1982). Global precedence as a postperceptual effect: An analysis of speed-accuracy tradeoff functions. *Perception & Psychophysics, 13,* 358–366.
Broadbent, D. E. (1977). The hidden preattentive process. *American Psychologist,* 109–118.

Bullier, J., & Nowak, L. G. (1995). Parallel versus serial processing: New vistas on the distributed organization of the visual system. *Current Opinion in Neurobiology, 5,* 497–503.

Donnelly, N., Humphreys, G. W., & Riddoch, M. J. (1991). Parallel computations of primitive shape descriptions. *Journal of Experimental Psychology: Human Perception and Performance, 17,* 561–570.

Driver, J., Davis, G., Russell, C., Turatto, M., & Freeman, E. (2001). Segmentation, attention and phenomenal visual objects. *Cognition, 80,* 61–95.

Duncan, J., & Humphreys, G. W. (1989). Visual search and stimulus similarity. *Psychological Review, 96,* 433–458.

Enns, J. T., & Kingstone, A. (1995). Access to global and local properties in visual search for compound stimuli. *Psychological Science, 6,* 283–291.

Enns, J. T., & Rensink, R. A. (1990). Influence of scene-based properties on visual search. *Science, 24,* 721–723.

Everett, B. L., Hochhaus, L., & Brown, J. R. (1985). Letter-naming as a function of intensity, degradation, S-R compatibility, and practice. *Perception & Psychophysics, 27,* 467–470.

Ginsburg, A. P. (1986). Spatial filtering and visual form information. In K. R. Boff, L. Kaufman, & J. P. Thomas (Eds.), *Handbook of human perception and performance* (pp. 1–41). New York: Wiley.

Goldmeier, E. (1972). Similarity in visually perceived forms. *Psychological Issues, 8,* (1, Whole No. 29). (Original work published 1936)

Han, S., Fan, S., Chen, L., & Zhuo, Y. (1997). On the different processing of wholes and parts: A psychophyiological analysis. *Journal of Cognitive Neuroscience, 9,* 687–698.

Han, S., & Humphreys, G. W. (1999). Interactions between perceptual organization based on Gestalt laws and those based on hierarchical processing. *Perception and Psychophysics, 61,* 1287–1298.

Han, S., Humphreys, G. W., & Chen, L. (1999). Uniform connectedness and classical Gestalt principles of perceptual grouping. *Perception and Psychophysics, 61,* 661–674.

He, Z. J., & Nakayama, K. (1992). Surfaces versus features in visual search. *Nature, 359,* 231–233.

Hoffman, D. D., & Richards, W. A. (1984). Parts of recognition. *Cognition, 18,* 65–96.

Hubel, D. H., & Wiesel, T. N. (1959). Receptive fields of single neurones in the cat's striate cortex. *Journal of Physiology, 148,* 574–591.

Hubel, D. H., & Wiesel, T. N. (1968). Receptive fields and functional architecture of monkey striate cortex. *Journal of Physiology, 195,* 215–243.

Hughes, H. C., Fendrich, R., & Reuter-Lorenz, P. (1990). Global versus local processing in the absence of low spatial frequencies. *Journal of Cognitive Neuroscience, 2,* 272–282.

Ivry, R., & Robertson, L. C. (1998). *The two sides of perception.* Cambridge, MA: MIT Press.

Kellman, P. J., & Shipley, T. F. (1991). A theory of visual interpolation in object perception. *Cognitive Psychology, 23,* 141–221.

Kimchi, R. (1988). Selective attention to global and local levels in the comparison of hierarchical patterns. *Perception and Psychophysics, 43,* 189–198.

Kimchi, R. (1990). Children's perceptual organization of hierarchical patterns. *European Journal of Cognitive Psychology, 2,* 133–149.

Kimchi, R. (1992). Primacy of wholistic processing and global/local paradigm: A critical review. *Psychological Bulletin, 112,* 24–38.

Kimchi, R. (1994). The role of wholistic/configural properties versus global properties in visual form perception. *Perception, 23,* 489–504.

Kimchi, R. (1998). Uniform connectedness and grouping in the perceptual organization of hierarchical patterns. *Journal of Experimental Psychology: Human Perception and Performance, 24,* 1105–1118.

Kimchi, R. (2000). The perceptual organization of visual objects: A microgenetic analysis. *Vision Research, 40,* 1333–1347.

Kimchi, R. (in press). Relative dominance of holistic and component properties in the perceptual organization of visual objects. In M. A. Peterson & G. Rhodes (Eds.), *Perception of faces, objects, and scenes: Analytic and holistic processes*. Oxford University Press.

Kimchi, R., & Bloch, B. (1998). Dominance of configural properties in visual form perception. *Psychonomic Bulletin and Review, 5,* 135–139.

Kimchi, R., & Hadad, B. (2002). Influence of past experience on perceptual grouping. *Psychological Science, 13,* 41–47.

Kimchi, R., & Palmer, S. E. (1982). Form and texture in hierarchically constructed patterns. *Journal of Experimental Psychology: Human Perception and Performance, 8,* 521–535.

Kimchi, R., & Palmer, S. E. (1985). Separability and integrality of global and local levels of hierarchical patterns. *Journal of Experimental Psychology: Human Perception and Performance, 11,* 673–688.

Kimchi, R., & Razpurker-Apfeld, I. (November, 2001). *Perceptual organization and attention.* Paper presented at the 42nd Annual Meeting of the Psychonomic Society, Orlando, FL.

Kimchi, R., & Peled A. (1999). The role of element size in the early organization of hierarchical stimuli. Unpublished manuscript.

Kleffner, D. A., & Ramachandran, V. S. (1992). On the perception of shape from shading. *Perception & Psychophysics, 52,* 18–36.

Koffka, K. (1935). *Principles of Gestalt psychology.* New York: Harcourt Brace Jovanovich.

Kohler, W. (1947). *Gestalt psychology.* New York: Liveright. (Original work published 1929)

Kovács, I., & Julesz, B. (1994). Perceptual sensitivity maps within globally defined visual shapes. *Nature, 370,* 644–646.

Kurylo, D. D. (1997). Time course of perceptual grouping. *Perception and Psychophysics, 59,* 142–147.

Lamb, M., & Yund, E. W. (1993). The role of spatial frequency in the processing of hierarchically organized structure. *Perception and Psychophysics, 54,* 773–784.

Lamme, V. A., Super, H., & Spekreijse, H. (1998). Feedforward, horizontal, and feedback processing in the visual cortex. *Current Opinions in Neurobiology, 8,* 529–535.

Lasaga, M. I. (1989). Gestalts and their components: Nature of information-precedence. In B. S. S. Ballesteros (Ed.), *Object perception: Structure and process* (pp. 165–202). Hillsdale, NJ: Erlbaum.

Lee, T. S., & Nguyen, M. (2001). Dynamics of subjective contour formation in the early visual cortex. *Proceedings of the National Academy of Sciences, 98,* 1907–1911.

Mack, A., Tang, B., Tuma, R., Kahn, S., & Rock, I. (1992). Perceptual organization and attention. *Cognitive Psychology, 24,* 475–501.

Marr, D. (1982). *Vision.* San Francisco: W. H. Freeman.

McClelland, J. L., & Rumelhart, D. E. (1981). An interactive activation model of context effects in letter perception: Part 1. An account of basic findings. *Psychological Review, 88,* 375–407.

Miller, J. (1981a). Global precedence in attention and decision. *Journal of Experimental Psychology: Human Perception and Performance, 7,* 1161–1174.

Miller, J. (1981b). Global precedence: Information availability or use: Reply to Navon. *Journal of Experimental Psychology: Human Perception and Performance, 7,* 1183–1185.

Moore, C. M., & Egeth, H. (1997). Perception without attention: Evidence of grouping under conditions of inattention. *Journal of Experimental Psychology: Human Perception and Performance, 23,* 339–352.

Navon, D. (1977). Forest before trees: The precedence of global features in visual perception. *Cognitive Psychology, 9,* 353–383.

Navon, D. (1991). Testing a queue hypothesis for th eprocessing of global and local information. *Journal of Experimental Psychology: General, 120,* 173–189.

Neisser, U. (1967). *Cognitive psychology.* New York: Appleton Century Crofts.

Palmer, S. E. (1992). Common region: A new principe of perceptual grouping. *Cognitive Psychology, 24,* 436–447.

Palmer, S. E., Neff, J., & Beck, D. (1996). Late influences on perceptual grouping: Amodal completion. *Psychonomic Bulletin and Review, 3,* 75–80.

Palmer, S. E., & Rock, I. (1994a). Rethinking perceptual organization: The role of uniform connect-edness. *Psychonomic Bulletin and Review, 1*, 29–55.

Palmer, S. E., & Rock, I. (1994b). On the nature and order of organizational processing: A reply to Peterson. *Psychonomic Bulletin and Review, 1*, 515–519.

Paquet, L., & Merikle, P. M. (1988). Global precedence in attended and nonattended objects. *Journal of Experimental Psychology: Human Perception and Performance, 14*, 89–100.

Peterson, M. A. (1994). The proper placement of uniform connectedness. *Psychonomic Bulletin & Review, 1*, 509–514.

Peterson, M. A. (1999). What's in a stage name? *Journal of Experimental Psychology: Human Perception and Performance, 25*, 276–286.

Peterson, M. A., & Gibson, B. S. (1994). Must shape recognition follow figure-ground organization: An assumption in peril. *Psychological Science, 9*, 253–259.

Pomerantz, J. R., Sager, L. C., & Stoever, R. J. (1977). Perception of wholes and their component parts: Some configural superiority effects. *Journal of Experimental Psychology: Human Perception and Performance, 3*, 422–435.

Rensink, R. A., & Enns, J. T. (1995). Preemption effects in visual search: evidence for low-level grouping. *Psychological Review, 102*, 101–130.

Rock, I. (1986). The description and analysis of object and event perception. In K. R. Boff, & L. Kaufman, & J. P. Thomas (Eds.), *Handbook of perception and human performance* (Vol. 33, pp. 1–71). New York: Wiley.

Rock, I., & Brosgole, L. (1964). Grouping based on phenomenal proximity. *Journal of Experimental Psychology, 67*, 531–538.

Rock, I., Linnet, C. M., Grant, P., & Mack, A. (1992). Perception without attention: Results of a new method. *Cognitive Psychology, 5*, 504–534.

Rock, I., Nijhawan, R., Plamer, S. E., & Tudor, L. (1992). Grouping based on phenomenal similarity of achromatic color. *Perception, 21*, 779–789.

Sekuler, A. B., & Palmer, S. E. (1992). Perception of partly occluded objects: A microgenetic analysis. *Journal of Experimental Psychology: General, 121*, 95–111.

Shipley, T. F., & Kellman, P. (1992). Perception of occluded objects and illusory figures: Evidence for an identity hypothesis. *Journal of Experimental Psychology: Human Perception and Performance, 18*, 106–120.

Shulman, G. L., Sullivan, M. A., Gish, K., & Sakoda, W. J. (1986). The role of spatial-frequency channels in the perception of local and global structure. *Perception, 15*, 259–273.

Shulman, G. L., & Wilson, J. (1987). Spatial frequency and selective attention to local and global information. *Neuropsychologia, 18*, 89–101.

Snodgrass, J. G., & Corwin, J. V. (1988). Perceptual identification thresholds for 150 fragmented pictures from the Snodgrass and Vanderwart picture set. *Perceptual and Motor Skills, 67*, 3–36.

Spillmann, L. (1999). From elements to perception: Local and global processing in visual neurons. *Perception, 28*, 1461–1492.

Sugita, Y. (1999). Grouping of image fragments in primary visual cortex. *Nature, 401*, 269–272.

Treisman, A. (1986). Properties, parts and objects. In K. R. Boff, L. Kaufman, & J. P. Thomas (Eds.), *Handbook of perception and human performance* (Vol. 35, pp. 1–70). New York: Wiley.

Treisman, A., & Gormican, S. (1988). Feature analysis in early vision: Evidence from search asymmetries. *Psychological Review, 95*, 15–48.

Treisman, A., & Schmidt, H. (1982). Illusory conjunctions in the perception of objects. *Cognitive Psychology, 14*, 107–141.

Trick, L. M., & Enns, J. T. (1997). Clusters precede shapes in perceptual organization. *Psychological Science, 8*, 124–129.

Vecera, S. P., & Farah, M. J. (1997). Is visual image segmentation a bottom-up or an interactive process? *Perception and Psychophysics, 59*, 1280–1296.

Vecera, S. P., & O'Reilly, R. (1998). Figure-ground organization and object recognition processes: An interactive account. *Journal of Experimental Psychology: Human Perception and Performance, 24*, 441–462.

Vecera, S. P., & O'Reilly, R. C. (2000). Graded effects in hierarchical figure-ground organization: Reply to Peterson (1999). *Journal of Experimental Psychology: Human Perception and Performance, 26*, 1221–1231.

Ward, L. M. (1982). Determinants of attention to local and global features of visual forms. *Journal of Experimental Psychology: Human Perception and Performance, 8*, 562–581.

Wertheimer, M. (1955). Gestalt theory. In W. D. Ellis (Ed.), *A source book of Gestalt psychology* (pp. 1–16). London: Routhedge & Kegan Paul. (Original work published 1923)

Westheimer, G. (1999). Gestalt theory reconfigured: Max Wertheimer's anticipation of recent developments in visual neuroscience. *Perception, 18*, 5–15.

Wolfe, J. M., Friedman-Hill, S., & Bilsky, A. R. (1994). Parallel processing of part-whole information in visual search tasks. *Perception and Psychophysics, 55*, 537–550.

Zhou, H., Friedman, H. S., & von der Heydt, R. (2000). Coding of border ownership in monkey visual cortex. *Journal of Neuroscience, 20*, 6594–6611.

Zipser, K., Lamme, V. A., & Schiller, P. H. (1996). Contextual modulation in primary visual cortex. *The Journal of Neuroscience, 16*, 7376–7389.

5 Visual Perception of Objects and Boundaries: A Four-Dimensional Approach

Philip J. Kellman
University of California, Los Angeles

To see an object means to detect and represent a bounded volume of matter. To see objects accurately means that our perceptual representations correspond to facts about the physical world: what things cohere and where the world breaks apart. Carving the world into objects links fundamental aspects of physical reality to a primary format of cognitive reality. Our comprehension of scenes and situations is written in the vocabulary of objects, and to objects we assign basic properties important for thought and action, such as shape, size, and substance.

In ordinary situations, object perception is fast and effortless. Some lines of research suggest that we can obtain representations of object unity and shape in a third of a second or perhaps even much less. It is probable that we can do this with more than one object at a time. Perceiving on average several objects a second, in 16 waking hours of a normal day, object perception is something we do perhaps 10^5–10^6 times. We might suspect that something we do so often is important. Of course, the frequency of object perception is not the reason for its importance; rather, we do it so frequently because object perception organizes thought and action, is central to language, is salient in cognitive development, and anchors learning throughout life.

Mapping the world's objects into mental representations does not come easily, however. Despite its introspective ease, the underlying processes of object perception have proved complicated and have resisted satisfactory explanations.

In recent years, researchers' efforts have brought clear progress. The requirements for object perception, the information that makes it possible, and processes and brain mechanisms that carry it out are all beginning to be understood in greater detail. In this chapter, I suggest an overall framework for thinking about object perception. Within that framework, I focus on several important issues at the frontiers and some research efforts that may help to push them back.

The chapter is organized into three sections. In the first, I consider a schematic model of object perception, indicating the particular tasks that need to be accomplished and how they might fit together. In that context, I explore in some detail basic issues in segmentation and grouping, especially the idea of complementary contour and surface interpolation processes and the formal notion of contour relatability as an account of the information underlying contour interpolation.

In the second section, I take up issues that challenge existing models of object perception by falling outside of their scope. Components of object perception, such as edge finding, boundary assignment, and contour and surface interpolation have most often been studied in static, two-dimensional cases. I describe research showing that accounts of segmentation and grouping in object perception will require at least a four-dimensional account, incorporating all three spatial dimensions and time. These phenomena and findings will require major additions to object-perception models, especially existing neural-style models that build on two-dimensional spatial relations of oriented units in early cortical areas. At the same time, recent findings suggest continuity between existing geometric models of segmentation and grouping and object formation from three-dimensional and spatiotemporal (motion-based) information. Specifically, straightforward extensions of the geometry of contour relatability provide a unified formal account of contour interpolation in two- and three-dimensional and spatiotemporal object perception. This unified geometric account may help suggest more general models of neural mechanisms.

In a final section, I take up the question of the general character of object perception. Whereas my discussion emphasizes relatively local, autonomous perceptual mechanisms, other investigations have suggested a role for more global or top-down factors, or both. One line of current research may help to clarify the separate contributions of these different components in the visual processing of objects.

TASKS AND PROCESSES IN OBJECT PERCEPTION

Object perception involves several conceptually distinct information-processing tasks and representations. (These may or may not be realized as separate processes or mechanisms in the brain.) Fig. 5.1 combines current knowledge with some hypotheses about processes, representations, and how they interact. It is

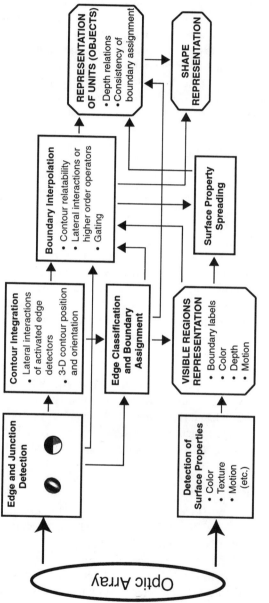

FIG. 5.1. A framework for object perception. Rectangles indicate functions or processes and octagons indicate representations. (See text for details.) From Kellman, Guttman, Wickens "Geometric and Neural Models of Object Perception." In *From Fragments to Objects: Segmentation and Grouping in Vision*, by T. F. Shipley and P. J. Kellman (Eds.). 2001, Amsterdam: Elsevier. Copyright 2001 by Elsevier Science. Reprinted with permission.

perhaps a framework more than a model, intended to provide a context for research discussed later. In the diagram, some components and their connections reflect established findings, whereas others represent newer conjectures. There are significant differences in how much is known about what goes on inside the specific boxes indicating particular representations or processes.

Rectangular boxes indicate functions or processes, and octagonal ones indicate representations. The model has few representations: output representations of shape and unity (specification of regions belonging to a single object) and one intermediate representation—*the visible regions representation*. I discuss the nature of these representations and the reasons for including them later.

General Considerations in the Model

The input to the model is the optic array. Although we will consider first information in momentary, static views of the environment, the true inputs include the time-varying optic array, sampled by two eyes. Later I focus on evidence supporting the idea that object formation is at least a four-dimensional process (i.e., involving three spatial dimensions and time).

Two processing streams handle complementary aspects of object formation. One deals with contours and junctions; the other deals with surface characteristics. The surface-processing stream extracts characteristics of luminance, color, texture, depth, and motion and represents these properties with relation to their surface locations; this information is used later to determine connections among spatially distinct visible regions. The contour stream locates discontinuities in luminance, color, texture, depth, and motion; these are used to locate edges and junctions, and, later, meaningful contours and object shape. This division into edge and contour processes was suggested previously (e.g., Grossberg & Mingolla, 1985), and it was foreshadowed by seminal work by Yarbus (1967). (See also Humphreys, Cinel, Wolfe, Olson, & Klempen, 2000, and Humphreys, this volume.)

The major processes and representations are briefly described later. For a more detailed discussion of the model, see Kellman, Guttman and Wickens (2001).

Edge and Junction Detection

An important early step on the way to object representations is locating significant edges and junctions in the scene. Not only is edge detection a point of entry into scene segmentation, but it is also crucial for defining shapes of perceived objects. For segmentation, the importance of edges is straightforward. For any visual processor to segment the world into objects, differences must exist between different objects or between objects and (projectively) adjacent visible surfaces. Abrupt changes in surface characteristics mark the locations of contours or edges. The changes are of two general types. Receiving most attention in models of edge detection have been discontinuities in luminance, chromatic, or textural properties in a scene. Their importance derives from the ecological fact that objects tend to be relatively homogeneous in composition (and thus relatively homogeneous in the properties of the light they reflect). At object boundaries, the likelihood is high that the luminance, chromatic, or textural information, or all three, will change.

Edge detection would be possible, however, even in a world of objects of homogeneous surfaces and even illumination, if the surfaces had visible texture. It might be argued, in fact, that the most robust sources of information for edges would still be available in such a world. These are discontinuities caused by the spatial arrangements of objects. At object boundaries, there are likely to be depth discontinuities that lead to gradient discontinuities in stereoscopic depth perception (e.g., Gillam, Chambers, & Russo, 1988) and also to accretion and deletion of texture when the scene is viewed by a moving observer. The ecological basis of these information sources derives from the objects being arrayed in three-dimensional space, and only rarely do adjacent objects' surfaces join to form a smooth gradient. In general, discontinuities of depth and motion are available in optical information whenever there are depth differences in the world across a visible contour. We say that these information sources are more robust because they are more highly correlated with object boundaries than are luminance or chromatic discontinuities. The latter arise often within continuous surfaces of a single object.

Computations leading to perception of contours and edges appear to begin in the early cortical areas, V1 and V2. Cells in these areas respond to oriented luminance contrast at particular spatial frequencies in particular retinal locations (Campbell, Cooper, & Enroth-Cugell, 1969; Hubel & Wiesel, 1968). By area V2, and perhaps earlier, many cells respond selectively to particular binocular disparities, providing the basis for stereoscopic depth perception (Fischer & Poggio, 1979). Some cells in the early cortical areas also respond preferentially to motion, although areas upstream, particularly area V5 (the human homologue to macaque area MT), appear to be specialized for motion processing. A number of specific proposals have been advanced regarding how these early cortical responses can be used to detect luminance edges in the optical projection (e.g., Marr & Hildreth, 1980; Morrone & Burr, 1988). The modeling of object perception based on other types of edge inputs, such as discontinuities in stereoscopic depth and motion, is less advanced (Gibson, Kaplan, Reynolds, & Wheeler, 1969; Julesz, 1971; Shipley & Kellman, 1994). Likewise, further research is needed to determine how the visual system integrates edge information arising from these various sources.

Edge Classification

Detected edges originate from several kinds of sources. Some are boundaries of objects or surfaces, whereas others are textural markings on surfaces or illumination edges (shadows). These different origins have markedly different consequences for perception. *Edge classification* refers to the labeling of edges of different kinds (or their differential use in further processing). One important distinction is the difference between *illumination* and *reflectance edges*. Illumination edges arise when surfaces having the same reflectance properties receive different amounts of illumination. Cast and attached shadows are examples of illumination edges. Note that an edge given by a cast shadow across some surface is not particularly helpful for scene segmentation (of that surface, at least) because there is no object boundary at the location of the shadow. Reflectance edges are edges caused by differences in the light-reflecting properties of two surfaces. Often these differences mark an object boundary, but sometimes they do not. A textural marking on a surface is a reflectance edge, yet it is not a boundary of the surface. Most important for object segmentation is a subset of reflectance edges that are also *occluding edges*. Occluding edges mark locations in the optical projection at which one object or surface ends and another passes behind it.

Classification of edges depends on a number of sources of information. Depth and motion information can be decisive because the existence of depth discontinuities (in a stereoscopic depth map, a map of image velocities, or given by accretion and deletion of visible texture) reliably indicates the presence of an occluding edge.

Contour Junctions

Going hand in hand with edge detection and classification are processes for detecting and classifying contour junctions. Whereas edges may be localized in terms of high rates of change in surface properties, junctions may be characterized as locations in which edges have high rates of change (Heitger et al., 1992; Kellman & Shipley, 1991). One indication of the importance of junctions for a variety of tasks in middle and high-level vision is that investigators have suggested numerous names for them. In models of human and artificial object recognition, they are usually called *corners* or *junctions* (e.g., Barrow & Tenenbaum, 1986; Biederman, 1995). In models of segmentation and grouping, they have been referred to as *tangent discontinuities* (Kellman & Shipley, 1991) or as *key points* (Heitger et al., 1992). Contour junctions can be formally defined as points along a contour that have no unique orientation. More intuitively, a junction is an intersection of two or more contours in the optical projection. Contour junctions include the projections of the sharp corners of objects as well as points of contour intersection in the world. Neurally, detecting junctions may be based on operators that use end-stopped cells (e.g., Heitger et al., 1992; Wurtz & Lourens, 2001) or perhaps high rates of curvature.

Classification of contour junctions plays an important role in segmentation and grouping. Among other things, it provides information for edge classification. For example, a *T* junction usually indicates that one of two intersecting edges passes behind the other (i.e., the latter is an occluding edge). An *X* junction is an important cue for transparency. (See Fig. 5.2.) Obviously, to help with edge classification, junctions themselves must be classified (e.g., into *T*s or *X*s). Little is known about the location or operation of neural mechanisms for classifying junctions.

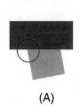 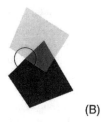

(A)   (B)

FIG. 5.2.   Examples of effects of junction classification on edge classification. (A) A *T* junction indicates an occluding and occluded edge.
(B) An *X* junction indicates transparency.

Boundary Assignment

Closely related to edge classification is boundary assignment. Edges classified as
occluding edges have the property that the Gestalt psychologist Kurt Koffka called
"the one-sided function of contour" (Koffka, 1935). That is, an occluding edge
bounds a surface on only one side. On the other side, the visible surface continues
behind the contour. Said a different way, only one of two visible surfaces meeting at
a contour owns the contour. This assignment of boundary ownership at occluding
edges is what changes in reversible figure-ground displays. Shimojo, Silverman
and Nakayama (1989) proposed the useful terms *intrinsic,* to refer to a contour that
belongs to (bounds) a certain region, and *extrinsic* to refer to a contour that does not.

Boundary assignment is accomplished from information sources similar to edge
classification: Depth and motion discontinuities indicate both that a contour is an
occluding edge and which side is nearer (the nearer side necessarily owns the
contour). Junctions also contribute to boundary assignment. For example, the roof
of a *T* junction is a boundary of the surface opposite the stem of the *T* (see Fig. 5.2,
part A). Another class of boundary assignment cues was identified by Rubin (1915)
in his classic treatment of figure and ground. This class involves relations between
visible areas that influence which area is seen as figure and which as ground. What
is at stake in figure-ground assignment is simply boundary assignment. Rubin's
factors include the following: enclosing areas tend to be seen as grounds, enclosed
as figures; symmetric regions tend to be seen as figures; and convex areas tend to be
seen as figures (see also Peterson, this volume). These cues to boundary assignment
are relatively weak, in that they are readily overridden by depth information given
by stereoscopic or kinematic depth cues or even *T* junctions. Finally, familiarity
of contour shape may influence boundary assignment (Peterson & Gibson, 1991;
von der Heydt, this volume).

The Visible Regions Representation

In the model in Fig. 5.1, there are numerous processes but few representations.
Two are the final outputs of unity and form, and there is one intermediate representation: *the visible regions representation.* This representation explicitly encodes

continuous visible areas; that is, each is a region of visible points that belongs to an uninterrupted surface. It uses inputs from the surface stream, namely spatially contiguous locations possessing homogeneous or smoothly varying surface attributes. In locating continuous surface patches, smoothly changing depth values are primary, but when depth information is minimal (as in the viewing of far away scenes) other properties including lightness, color, and texture can determine visible regions. This grouping complements the edge process: It depends on the *absence* of the surface discontinuities extracted by the edge stream. Information from the contour stream defines the boundaries of tokens in the visible regions representation. In short, the visible regions representation labels connected surface regions and encodes the locations and orientations of their edges and corners. It also labels edges in terms of their boundary assignment (see later discussion).

This representation captures several important properties of representations suggested earlier by other researchers. Consistent with the goals of image segmentation algorithms, it partitions the optic projection into distinct, nonoverlapping regions. Unlike the results of region segmentation processes in machine vision, the visible regions representation should *not* be understood as a set of frontoparallel image fragments. Here the regions have three-dimensional positions and orientations; in this respect, the visible regions representation resembles Marr's (1982) 2.5-dimensional sketch, which assigned to each point an observer-relative depth. Another related proposal is the *uniform connectedness* idea of Palmer and Rock (1994; see also Palmer, this volume): The visual system encodes closed regions with homogeneous surface properties as a single unit. There are important differences from this notion, however. Palmer and Rock treated common surface lightness, color, and texture as the primary determinants of uniform connectedness. By contrast, in the visible regions representation, depth relations, given by stereoscopic and motion parallax cues, take precedence over the commonalty of lightness and color. A surface that is continuous in space but contains discontinuities in surface coloration would be encoded as a single token in the visible regions representation. Conversely, the visible regions representation would encode as *separate* two adjacent, homogeneously textured regions with an abrupt change of depth between them.

What motivates the idea that human perception incorporates an intermediate representation of visible regions? One is the dual nature of human scene perception (c.f. Rock's, 1979, discussion of "dual aspects" in perception). The primary role of perceiving is to produce representations of whole objects and their arrangement in space. Yet we also have an awareness of which parts of objects are occluded and which reflect light to the eyes. These may be considered "distal" and "proximal" modes of perceiving (Rock, 1979). It is the proximal mode that suggests that we have access to a visible regions representation. Artists can hone their awareness to depict only the light reflecting surfaces in their paintings. (Children do much worse, often attempting to put in a drawing the three or four sides of a house in their object representation, despite only two being visible.)

One issue that helps make clear the difference between visible regions and objects, as well as the differences between this proposed representation and other schemes, is the labeling of edges. As noted previously, at each occluding edge the surface on one side of the contour is bounded, whereas the surface on the other side continues behind. A unit in the visible regions representation is labeled as to whether its defining contours are intrinsic or extrinsic to it. Fig. 5.3 shows an example of a display containing two objects and one visible region from that display. The bottom edge is labeled intrinsic, and the two side edges are labeled extrinsic. These are not the only possibilities. The top edge is labeled as a *crease,* a contour that divides two regions that are contiguous and part of the same object (Barrow & Tenenbaum, 1986). Because of edge labeling, units in the visible regions representation are not confusable with bounded entities in the world (e.g., in Fig. 5.3, there are 10 visible regions, but we see only two objects).

As Fig. 5.3 indicates, the visible regions representation also labels tangent discontinuities (contour junctions, shown by circles) as well as the orientation of edges leading into them (shown by arrows). By explicitly labeling these various features of regions, (or implicitly distinguishing their roles in further computations) this representation provides important inputs into further processes, such as contour interpolation and unit formation.

Significant work has been done by the time the visual system obtains a visible regions representation. Yet this representation does not make explicit objects in the physical world (or the objects we perceive). In normal scenes, the chief source of this discrepancy is occlusion. If we define visible to mean "reflects light to the eyes," most objects are only partly visible. Because scenes are three-dimensional, objects are opaque, and light moves in straight lines, most objects are partly occluded. Any three-dimensional object occludes parts of itself when viewed from a particular vantage point. An even greater complication is that most objects are partly occluded by other objects. Visible parts of a single object very often appear in noncontiguous locations on the retina. In a scene partially obscured by foliage (e.g., tree branches), a single object, such as a building, may project to literally hundreds of separate retinal locations. When the observer moves, the problem of spatial fragmentation is exacerbated by the continuously changing projections in which different patches of a partly occluded object are available at different times.

Interpolation Processes: Contours and Surfaces

As mentioned previously, because of occlusion, the relationship between visible regions and the objects in the world is complex. Research suggests that two complementary processes of *interpolation* are used by the visual system to overcome fragmentation (Kellman & Shipley, 1991; Yin, Kellman, & Shipley, 1997).

Contour interpolation connects oriented edges across gaps. It operates on edges satisfying certain geometric relationships. Its products are most often occluded contours, but depending on context and depth relationships in a scene they may also

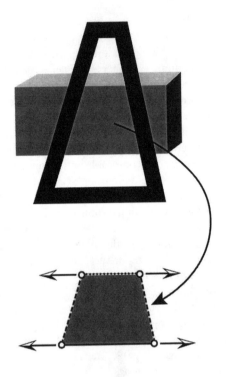

○ Contour junction

────── Intrinsic edge

·------- Extrinsic edge

············ Crease

FIG. 5.3. Example of a visible region and the information encoded in the visible regions representation. A visible region from the center of the upper display is shown in the lower display. Some of the information made explicit in this representation is indicated. Contour junctions are indicated by circles; orientation of edges leading into the junction is indicated by arrows. Solid lines indicate boundaries owned by the region. Straight dotted lines indicate boundaries owned by another region. Dotted lines with circle elements indicate a crease—a contour lying within an object.

be illusory contours. We elaborate significant aspects of the boundary interpolation process later because it forms the focus for much of the rest of this chapter.

The *surface interpolation process* complements the boundary process. It leads to perceived connections among visible regions, even when the object's boundaries are not well specified. Whereas boundary interpolation depends on spatial relations between visible edges, surface interpolation (or spreading under occlusion) depends on similarity of visible surface regions. Although investigation of the surface process is a recent endeavor (Yin, Kellman, & Shipley, 1997, 2000), several aspects are clear. Surface fragments of similar color, luminance, or texture, or all three, can join behind an occluder, despite the absence of contour interpolation. Analogous to phenomena described by Yarbus (1967) in image stabilization experiments, surface quality appears to spread within real contours and also within interpolated contours (Yin et al., 1997). The process can influence boundary assignment and perceived depth (Yin et al., 1997, 2000).

Fig. 5.4 shows an example of the surface spreading process. Because the circles in the display have no tangent discontinuities, they do not participate in contour interpolation processes. Note that the incorporation of the circular areas into the

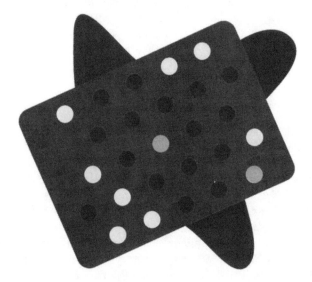

FIG. 5.4. Example of the surface spreading process. The blue circles that fall within relatable edges (or linear extensions of nonrelatable edges) appear as holes, connecting them with the blue surface pieces outside of the gray occluder. In contrast, a blue circle outside of relatable edges is seen as a spot on the gray surface, as are yellow circles. White circles are also seen as holes revealing the white background behind. (See color panel.)

partly occluded figure is selective for areas of matching lightness and color and restricted to operating within the boundaries given by real or interpolated contours (or in some cases, extended tangents of partly occluded contours).

The Units Representation

Regions connected by the interpolation processes feed into two output representations. The *units representation* encodes explicitly the connectedness of visible regions under occlusion. When the surface interpolation process alone has given all or some of these connections, overall shape may be vague. One reason for believing in a units representation separate from a shape representation is that in some circumstances, surface interpolation operates without much support from visible contours. An example would be seeing the sky through numerous branches of a tree. The sky appears to be a connected, but unshaped, unitary surface.

The Shape Representation

More often, boundary interpolation accompanies surface interpolation, and a determinate shape is encoded in the *shape representation*. This representation serves as the primary input to object recognition. This need not be the case, however. As we will consider later, recognition processes may often use shortcuts—activating higher level representations based on even a single feature in a stimulus or, in any case, using far less than a complete and well-defined representation of shape.

Bottom-Up and Top-Down Processes

The model as described is a feedforward or bottom-up view of object perception processes. It does not so far incorporate any feedback from higher levels to earlier ones. Clearly, perception can proceed without such feedback; it must do so in cases in which objects are unfamiliar and asymmetric. Whether there are top-down influences on basic segmentation and grouping processes, as opposed to recognition from partial input, remains controversial (e.g., Kellman, 2000; van Lier, 1999); we take up some of these issues later. One valuable aspect of the current framework is that it allows us to consider explicitly and distinguish possible top-down effects in terms of which higher level processes they come from and which earlier processes they affect. To take one example, Peterson and her colleagues (e.g., Peterson, 1994; Peterson & Gibson, 1991, 1994) found evidence that figure-ground segregation in otherwise ambiguous stimuli can be influenced by the familiarity of a shaped region, such that the familiar shape is preferentially seen as figure. Such an effect could be incorporated into the model, as shown in Fig. 5.5. Boundary assignment is the process that determines figure-ground relationships in the model. If familiar shape influences boundary assignment, the shape of some contour or

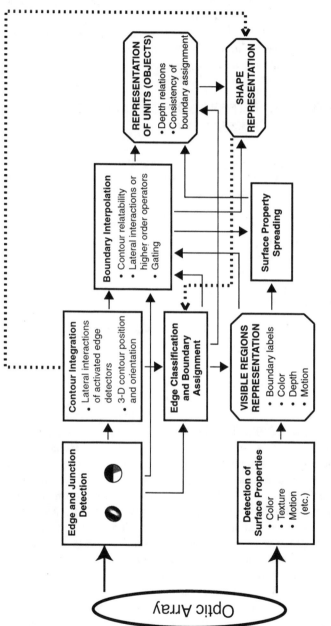

FIG. 5.5. Illustration of top-down effects in the framework of Fig. 5.1. Peterson's effect is shown as an influence of shape on boundary assignment. (See text.) From Kellman, Guttman, and Wickens, "Geometric and Neural Models of Object Perception. In *From Fragments to Objects: Segmentation and Grouping in Vision*. (p. 189), by T. F. Shipley and P. J. Kellman (Eds.). Amsterdam: Elsevier. Copyright 2001 by Elsevier Science. Reprinted with permission.

167

region must be encoded and recognized, that is, matched to some stored memory representation. Finding a match leads to feedback from the shape representation to the computation of boundary assignment.

This example shows how top-down effects can be incorporated into the model. Placing them in this framework may help to sharpen empirical tests. I consider selected ideas and some data about top-down processing later.

CONTOUR INTERPOLATION IN OBJECT PERCEPTION

So far, I have taken a wide-angle view of the processes of object perception. In the remainder of this chapter, I zoom in on the particular problem of *unit formation*—how visible regions get connected—with particular emphasis on the primary process involved in deriving object representations from fragmented input: contour interpolation. I first develop an argument about the generality of contour interpolation processes and then examine the key components of a model of spatial interpolation of contours. These considerations are important in their own right and will provide needed scaffolding for my discussion of three-dimensional and spatiotemporal interpolation.

The Identity Hypothesis in Contour Interpolation

In the model in Fig. 5.1, the boundary interpolation process is intended to apply to several interpolation phenomena that have often been considered distinct. Specifically, it applies to the completion of contours across gaps in partly occluded objects (amodal completion), illusory contours (modal completion), so-called self-splitting figures, and certain transparency phenomena. Specifically, my colleagues and I (Kellman & Loukides, 1987; Kellman & Shipley, 1991) proposed the *identity hypothesis* in contour interpolation: The same underlying process extends contours across gaps in these several different-looking phenomena.

Although this claim is now widely accepted, it is not universally accepted. In this section I elaborate the arguments for the identity hypothesis, indicating its logical and empirical bases, and address some concerns that have been raised about it.

Both empirical evidence and several logical considerations lead to the idea that the contour interpolation process in object formation—the specific process in which visible edges become represented as connected by interpolated contours—is common to occluded contours, illusory contours, and related phenomena. This claim by no means implies that all aspects of the processing of occluded and illusory objects are identical. Indeed, if that were the case, the output representations—that an illusory object is the nearest object to the observer in some visible direction and an occluded object is not—could not differ. Issues of depth relations with surrounding surfaces surely differ for occluded and illusory objects. This difference

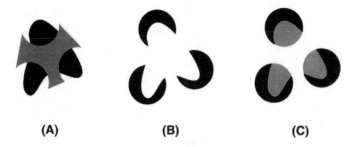

(A)   **(B)**   **(C)**

FIG. 5.6.   Equivalent illusory, occluded, and transparent objects. (A) partly occluded object, (B) illusory object, (C) transparent object. Although they appear quite different, these three images formally are similar in that the same physically specified edges define the central figure in each case. According to the identity hypothesis (see text), the same interpolation process produces contour connections across gaps in these cases.

has sometimes been used to claim that the interpolation process itself differs in these cases (Anderson, Singh, & Fleming, 2002) a claim that does not follow and is almost surely incorrect.

A good beginning is to air out some theory (as some of it is a bit dusty) connected with these central cases of perceptual organization. Consider the displays in Fig. 5.6. These are partly occluded, illusory, and transparent shapes having equivalent physically specified contours and gaps. Phenomenologically, the shapes of the interpolated contours are the same in the three images, yet they differ in appearance. Illusory contours and surfaces appear to cross in front of other surfaces in the scene; they have a robust sensory presence, which led Michotte, Thines and Crabbe (1964) to label their formation as *modal completion* (possessing sensory attributes or modes). Occluded contours pass behind other surfaces. (In the terminology of Michotte et al., they result from *amodal completion,* meaning that they exist perceptually but do not have sensory attributes.) Clearly, occluded contours are out of sight, a fact that leads to perplexities. If a contour or surface is out of sight, in what sense can it be said that we *see* it? If one believes there is a problem here, two resolutions may seem appealing. We could say that we do not really represent hidden contours or surfaces but that our perceptual system simply groups the visible parts that belong to a common object. A second idea is that we do represent the hidden contours, but we cognitively infer, rather than perceive, them.

Both of these ideas, and the line of reasoning that leads to them, need to be reconsidered. The relevant arguments are not new (Gibson, 1966, 1979; Kanizsa, 1979; Koffka, 1935; Michotte et al., 1964) yet they seem to have incompletely penetrated many discussions. The source of the problem is that to see does not necessarily mean to have local sensory responses based on local physical data. Perceptual descriptions are functions of incoming information, but they need not be restricted to some narrow class of functions, such as a one-to-one correspondence between represented properties of objects and local sensations or local stimuli.

The point that seeing is not a summing up of local sensations is a very old one, made convincingly by the Gestalt psychologists, but it is also a tenet of contemporary computational views of perception. Either view can be used to untangle certain perplexities regarding perception of occluded contours. On the computational/representational theory of mind, there is simply no principled difference between representing some contour as going behind another surface and representing some contour in front of another surface. One is not more privileged or real than the other. The argument that one must be a sensory effect and the other a cognitive effect lingers from an epistemology that did not work out. Occluded contours are no more and no less "inferred" than are illusory ones.

Substantial experimental evidence suggests that occluded and illusory contours are processed and represented similarly. They exert similar or identical effects on speed and accuracy in perceptual tasks (Kellman, Yin, & Shipley, 1998; Ringach & Shapley, 1996; Shipley & Kellman, 1992a). Likewise, procedures geared to assessing the precise locations of perceived boundaries lead to the conclusion that interpolated contours in both illusory and occluded cases are represented as being in very specific locations (Kellman, Temesvary, Palmer, & Shipley, 2000).

If there is no theoretical barrier separating represented contours that are occluded or illusory, why do they *look* so different? What is the cause of the robust difference in phenomenology? The answer is that this aspect of our phenomenology—the modal/amodal distinction—appears simply to code whether some surface or contour is nearest to the observer in some visual direction. This piece of information is an important aspect of scene perception that depends on the vantage point of the observer. The parts of an object that are nearest in a visual direction may be reached, grasped, or touched, whereas those equally real edges and surfaces behind some other object may not be reached without going around or through some nearer object.

The understanding of modal/amodal in terms of nearest (or not nearest) in some visual direction (or, equivalently, in terms of a surface area reflecting light directly to the eyes or not) brings up a related theoretical idea. Modern computational analyses as well as many results in perceptual research suggest that it is often advantageous for perceptual systems to represent information in terms that are viewpoint independent. Constancies in perception exemplify this idea. For example, in size constancy, a description of an object's physical size is obtained that does not vary as the observer moves closer or farther from an object. In unit formation, support ratio (Shipley & Kellman, 1992b)—a property that determines strength of contour interpolation—is scale invariant; this has the consequence that the strength of a contour connection does not vary with viewing distance. Representing modal and amodal contours as fundamentally different (or as one being seen and the other inferred) would tend to violate this general tendency in perception. The reason is that what is nearest to the observer from one vantage point may not be from another. Although it may be important to also encode the information about what is nearest in some visual direction, the core representation of contours and surfaces that span gaps in the input should not change as the viewer moves around and experiences changing patterns of occlusion.

The foregoing are rather philosophical arguments. In recent years, more specific logical considerations have emerged, forming essentially a proof that the contour interpolation step in visual processing is shared in common by illusory and occluded contours. I describe these considerations briefly.

Quasimodal Objects.   Kellman, Yin, and Shipley (1998) showed that illusory and occluded edges can join. More accurately, contour interpolation occurs in cases in which the stimulus arrangement fulfills neither the normal conditions for illusory contour nor occluded contour formation. Such contours have been called *hybrid* or *quasimodal* contours. An example is shown in Fig. 5.7. All of the interpolated contours in this display extend between an illusory contour-inducing element on one end and an occluded section on the other. The existence of quasimodal objects highlights the point made previously. The visual system represents interpolated contours and surfaces; sometimes these are in front of other surfaces, and sometimes they are behind. In a quasimodal case, a *single contour* is in front of some surface along part of its length and behind some surface along another part. Although it is a useful piece of information that the edge passes behind and in front of other objects in the scene, the basic representation of contours across gaps seems to incorporate easily segments of both kinds. It is not clear how quasimodal completions could occur from distinct modal and amodal interpolation processes.

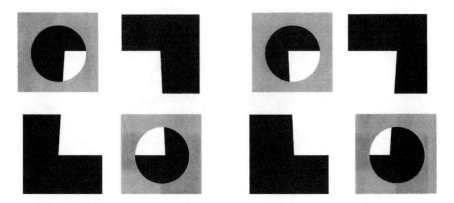

FIG. 5.7. Example of a quasimodal object. The display is a stereo pair that can be free-fused by crossing the eyes. All of the interpolated contours in the central figure are occluded on one end and illusory on the other. (See text.)

Petter's Effect.   The existence of quasimodal contours does not prove the identity hypothesis. After all, it is possible that there are three separate contour completion processes: modal, amodal, and quasimodal. A more conclusive logical argument about the nature of interpolative processes has been implicit in phenomena that have been known since the 1950s. Consider the display in Fig. 5.8, part A, an example of a class of displays studied by Petter (1956). The display has several salient properties. First, although it is a contiguous, homogeneously colored and textured area, it is not seen as a single object. Instead it resolves into two objects, a triangle and a quadrilateral. Second, wherever parts of the two objects lie in the same visual direction, one object is seen as crossing in front of the other. Although all parts of this pictorial display lie in the same depth plane, the visual system appears to obey a constraint that two objects may not occupy the same space.

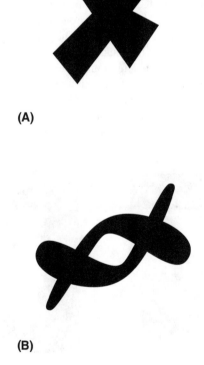

(A)

(B)

FIG. 5.8. (A) Self-splitting object, (B) Example of Petter's effect. Where interpolated contours cross, the one spanning the smaller gap appears in front as an illusory contour, and the one spanning the larger gap appears behind, as an occluded contour.

Where the two objects cross, their physically specified boundaries have gaps, and these gaps are spanned by interpolated edges. In accord with the depth ordering of the two objects, the nearer display has illusory contours, whereas the farther display has occluded contours. In Fig. 5.8A, if the triangle appears in front, it has illusory contours, and the quadrilateral has occluded contours. However, the depth ordering of the two objects is unstable over time; which object appears in front fluctuates. When the triangle switches from being in front to behind, its contours switch from being illusory to being occluded (and vice versa for the quadrilateral).

Self-splitting objects do not always possess this instability of depth order. The display in Fig. 5.8, part B, similar to one devised by Petter (1956), appears more stable. It is seen as containing two interlocking bent objects. The stimulus itself does not have luminance contours defining two objects; the partitioning of the array into two bounded objects is the result of contour interpolation processes.

Implicit in the idea of interlocking, the perceived depth ordering of the two objects in Fig. 5.8B varies across the image; on each side, the thicker object passes in front of the thinner one. Petter (1956) discovered that this perceptual outcome follows a rule, which we can state as follows: *Where interpolated boundaries cross, the boundary that traverses the smaller gap appears to be in front.* Thus, the thicker parts of the objects appear to lay on top of the thinner parts because the former have smaller gaps in their physically-specified contours. Petter's rule also helps us to understand the reversibility of depth order—and of occluded and illusory contours—in Fig. 5.8A: Because the contours of both objects span roughly equal gaps, there is no consistent information about depth order.

The relevance of Petter's (1956) effect to the identity hypothesis may now be apparent. According to Petter's rule, the perception of each interpolated contour as in front or behind—and, in turn, as illusory or occluded (or modal vs. amodal)—depends on its length relative to the interpolated contours that cross it. Logically, this statement implies some sort of comparison or competition involving the crossing interpolations. To accomplish this comparison, the visual system must first register the various sites of interpolation. Comparing the lengths of the crossing interpolations precedes the determination of whether an interpolated contour ultimately will appear as in front of or as behind other contours (and, thus, as illusory or occluded). Therefore, the registration of interpolation sites and lengths must precede the determination of depth ordering. That is, at least in some cases, *contour interpolation processes must operate prior to the processes that determine the final depth ordering of the constructed contours.* This, in turn, implies that there cannot be separate mechanisms for the interpolation of contours in front of and behind other surfaces. At least the steps of locating sites of interpolation and the extents of interpolation must be in common.

Depth Spreading and Object Formation.   Kellman, Yin, and Shipley· (1998) introduced a new type of display that also provides a proof that interpolation cannot be from separate modal or amodal processes because, as in Petter's (1956)

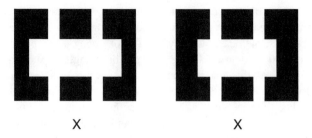

X   X

FIG. 5.9. Display in which interpolation occurs prior to determination of modal or amodal appearance. (See text.)

cases, interpolation must occur before amodal or modal appearance of contours and surfaces can be determined. Fig. 5.9 shows an example of this type of display. It is a stereo pair that may be free-fused by crossing or diverging the eyes. For the analysis here, I assume that the reader has free-fused by crossing the eyes; for diverging, all of the depth relations will be opposite to those in this description.

When fused, the central rectangle appears as the nearest object in the display at its left edge and farthest at its right. With reference to the two white columns in the display, the rectangle appears to pass in front of the one on the left and behind the one on the right. The importance of this simple appearance for the identity hypothesis rests on three elements. First is the mere existence of the rectangle: It is a product of interpolation across two gaps. Second is the notion of depth spreading. Stereoscopic disparity in this display is given only by the positions of the vertical edges of the central rectangle. The middle section of the display (two black squares separated by a white gap) is identical in the images given to the two eyes. There is no information that says the central square is in front or behind either column—this information must come from somewhere else. Depth spreading occurs *within objects* or continuous surfaces. It does not spread unconstrained across the whole scene. Therefore, the rectangle must be a unified object to partake of depth spreading from disparity of the remote vertical edges in the left and right sides of the display.

Now consider the modal or amodal appearances of various contours. The slant in depth of the rectangle's horizontal edges is a consequence of depth spreading. This causes the rectangle to pass in front of the left vertical column; thus, the rectangle here has *illusory* contours and the left column has *occluded* contours where these surfaces cross. On the right, the rectangle passes behind the white column. Opposite to the situation on the left, the rectangle's contours are here occluded and the right column's contours are illusory. Note that not just the modal/amodal appearance of the rectangle's contours but those of the white columns are consequences of depth spreading.

The crucial point is that the amodal or modal appearance of several contours necessarily *follows* from depth spreading, which necessarily requires that interpolation has already occurred. Contour interpolation necessarily precedes determination of the appearance of contours as illusory or occluded in this display. The following reviews the logic:

1. The rectangle as an object is the result of interpolation.
2. Depth spreading presupposes the rectangle as a unified object.
3. Modal or amodal appearance of various contours is the result of depth spreading.

Therefore, interpolation *necessarily* precedes determination of modal or amodal appearance.

In sum, both empirical studies and logical arguments support the idea that contour interpolation relies on a common process that operates without regard to the final determination of illusory or occluded appearance. The phenomenology of an interpolated contour—its appearance as illusory or occluded—relates to the issue of whether it is nearest to the observer in some visual direction or not. Representation of this property depends in turn on mechanisms responsible for assigning relative depth, which lie outside and sometimes operate subsequent to the interpolation process itself.

Some findings have led investigators to suggest that different processes or mechanisms are at work in producing illusory and occluded contours. Peterhans and von der Heydt (1989), for example, reported that single cells in area V2 of the macaque responded to an illusory bar but not to a display that could be interpreted as an occluded bar. This finding can be viewed as evidence for separate mechanisms of illusory and occluded interpolation. There are two specific concerns with connecting the observed data to such a conclusion. First, Peterhans and von der Heydt did find cells in V1 that responded to both their illusory contour and the related occlusion displays, although they suggested that these results may have been artifactual. Another possibility is that the equivalent responses of V1 cells were not artifactual; perhaps the V1 responses indicate a common contour interpolation step in V1, whereas the nonequivalent responses of V2 cells indicate that depth information relevant to the final contour appearance has come into play by that point. Second, as is evident in the foregoing speculation about interpolation in V1 and V2, we currently lack a sufficiently detailed mapping of computations onto cortical layers to use this sort of data to rule out a common interpolation step. Given the logical considerations following from Petter's effect (1956), quasimodal displays and depth spreading displays, as described, putative data suggesting separate visual processes of amodal and modal interpolation must be treated with skepticism. No claim of separate processes can make much sense without giving a new account of the three phenomena and their logical implications. To my knowledge, no such account has been proposed.

The identity hypothesis has several salutary consequences. It has helped in separating the crucial determinants of interpolation from extraneous aspects. It allows convergent evidence about the interpolation processes to be derived from studies of occlusion, illusory contours, and some other contour-connection phenomena. In some cases, one or another of these display types is more convenient. For example, tangent discontinuities may be removed from illusory contour-inducing elements but not from occlusion displays. Both illusory and occluded interpolation displays are used in the research discussed later.

A Model of Contour Interpolation

In this section and the next I present a model of contour interpolation. The model rests on two complementary notions: *tangent discontinuities* and *relatability*. The initiating conditions and geometric relations that govern the connecting of visible fragments across gaps depend on these two kinds of optical information.

Tangent Discontinuities. An important regularity may be observed in Fig. 5.6. In all of the displays, interpolated edges all begin and end at points of tangent discontinuity (TD). In occlusion cases, these are usually T junctions. For illusory contours, they are L junctions. Formation of the illusory contour turns L junctions into what might be called *implicit T junctions,* that is, Ts whose roof is formed by the interpolated edge.

That TDs provide the starting and ending points of interpolation is not a coincidence. Contour interpolation overcomes gaps in the input caused by occlusion. It can be proven that instances of occlusion generically produce TDs in the optical projection (Kellman & Shipley, 1991). This ecological fact underlies the role of TDs in initiating contour interpolation processes: TDs are potential indicators of the loci of occlusion. Not all TDs are points of contour occlusion, but all points of contour occlusion produce TDs.

The fact that occlusion displays always have TDs makes it difficult to test their necessity for interpolation processes; one cannot compare occlusion displays with and without TDs. This situation is one in which the equivalence of interpolation processes in occluded and illusory displays helps the researcher. In illusory contour displays, tangent discontinuities *can* be removed, by rounding off corners, for example. Research shows that this manipulation greatly reduces or eliminates contour interpolation (M. Albert, cited in Hoffman, 1998; Shipley & Kellman, 1990). Likewise, in homogeneous displays that split into multiple objects (sometimes called self-splitting objects or SSOs), rounding the tangent discontinuities eliminates the splitting (Kellman, 2000).

Because only some TDs are loci of occlusion, other information comes into play to determine when interpolation occurs. One influence is the type of contour junction. Some types (e.g., so-called Y junctions) indicate that the boundary has come to an end and does not continue. In other cases, a contour may be seen as passing behind an occluder but does not link up perceptually with any other visible contour.

What determines when contours link up behind occluding surfaces to form objects? In recent years, it has become clear that the visual system uses contour interpolation processes that decide connections between visible areas depending on certain geometric relations of their edges. The most important properties of edges are their positions and orientations leading into tangent discontinuities. The relevant spatial relations bear some close relations to the classic Gestalt notion of *good continuation,* but they also differ from it. These relations have been formally defined as the notion of contour *relatability* (Kellman & Shipley, 1991). The requirements can be summarized intuitively as follows: Two edges separated by a gap or occluder are relatable if they can be connected with a continuous, monotonic (singly inflected) curve. The relatability criterion embodies the constraints that interpolated contours are smooth, monotonic (bending in only one direction), and bend through no more than 90°. Except for the 90° constraint, these conditions can be expressed as the idea that two edges are relatable if their linear extensions meet in their extended regions. Fig. 5.10 shows some examples of relatable and nonrelatable edges in occluded and illusory object displays.

Formally, relatability may be defined with reference to the construction shown in Fig. 5.11. E_1 and E_2 in the drawing represent the edges of surfaces. R and r indicate the perpendiculars to these edges at the point where they lead into a tangent discontinuity, with R defined as the longer of the two. The angle of intersection

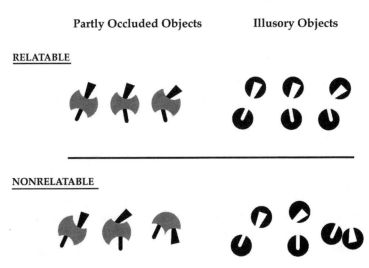

FIG. 5.10.   Examples of relatable and nonrelatable edges in occluded and illusory object displays. From *The Cradle of Knowlege: Development of Perception in Infancy* (p. 143), by P. J. Kellman and M. A. Arterberry, 1998, Cambridge, MA: MIT Press. Copyright 1998 by MIT Press. Reprinted with permission.

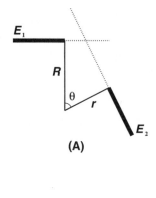

(A)

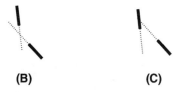

(B)   (C)

FIG. 5.11. Construction used to define relatability. E1 and E2 are edges of surfaces; R and r are perpendiculars to E1 and E2 at points of tangent discontinuity. E1 and E2 are relatable iff $0 \le R\cos\theta \le r$.

between R and r is termed θ. Relatability holds whenever a smooth, monotonic curve can be constructed starting from the endpoint of E_1 (and matching the slope of E_1 at that point) and proceeding through a bend of not more than a 90° to the endpoint of E_2 (and matching the slope of E_2 at that point). More formally, E_1 and E_2 are relatable if and only if

$$0 \le R\cos\theta \le r. \tag{1}$$

This inequality can be explained in two steps. The part on the left side expresses the limitation that the curve constructed to connect $E1$ and $E2$ cannot bend through more than 90°; cos θ is negative for θ greater than 90°. The right-hand side of the inequality states that the projection of R onto r ($R\cos\theta$) must fall within the extent of r. If this inequality is violated (i.e., $R\cos\theta > r$), then any connection between $E1$ and $E2$ would have to be doubly inflected to match the slopes at the TDs or would have to introduce sharp corners where the interpolated edge meets the physically specified edge. According to this model, boundary interpolation does not occur in such cases.

Although the definition gives the limits of relatability, it is not intended as an all-or-none concept. Kellman and Shipley (1992) described contour relatability as decreasing monotonically with deviations from collinearity, falling to 0 at a relative angle of 90°. Singh and Hoffman (1999) proposed a specific measure for this graded decrease.

The notion of contour relatability is often referred to interchangeably with the Gestalt idea of good continuation (Wertheimer, 1923/1958) but differs from it in important ways. For one, the original Gestalt principle has no precise formulation. Wertheimer's original discussion of it contained no definition but gave examples in which the idea was said to be obvious. Nor did later work indicate which of various possible mathematical notions of smoothness or other notions of goodness capture the phenomena. Kellman (2000) argued that most of Wertheimer's examples of good continuation implicate smoothness in the first derivative of functions describing contours, whereas first-derivative discontinuities (tangent discontinuities) indicate possible breakpoints in continuous contours. In the respects in which relatability resembles good continuation, it is a more precise, formal statement of it.

This is not the main issue, however. It appears that a precisely formulated notion of good continuation and relatability are cousins. Although the same principle has been invoked to explain segmentation in visible contiguous lines and figures (Wertheimer, 1923/1958) and in perception of partly occluded objects (Michotte et al., 1964), it is becoming clear that the geometric principles required to explain each of these perceptual tasks are different (Kellman, 2003). Both contexts have in common the notion that tangent discontinuities are significant indicators of segmentation points. The notions of good continuation and relatability are different, however, with the latter being much more restrictive. Two ways in which relatability is a more constrained notion are the monotonicity constraint and the 90° limit on interpolated contours. As mentioned previously, the monotonicity constraint specifies that interpolated edges are singly inflected, (i.e., they bend in only one direction). The 90° constraint specifies that interpolated edges do not bend more than 90°. These theoretical notions have received substantial empirical confirmation (e.g., Field, Hayes, & Hess, 1993; Kellman & Shipley, 1991). They are crucial ingredients in the relatability account of contour interpolation, but neither of these constraints has any counterpart in good continuation. Many excellent demonstrations of good continuation, for example, contain smooth, multiply inflected contours. Likewise, when a continuous contour bends through more than 90°, no break is seen; good continuation has no 90° constraint. These considerations and related research will be described in a forthcoming paper. What is common to both relatability and good continuation is exploitation of contour smoothness, and deviations from it, as information for more than one aspect of visual segmentation and grouping.

Evidence About Contour Relatability.   Results of a number of experiments support relatability as a description of the spatial relationships that support contour interpolation. Some of the best evidence comes from an elegant paradigm introduced by Field et al. (1993) for the study of contour integration. The stimuli in these experiments consisted of arrays of spatially separated, oriented Gabor patches (small elements consisting of a sinusoidal luminance pattern multiplied by a Gaussian window; a Gabor patch closely approximates the ideal stimulus for the oriented receptive fields of V1 simple cells). In some arrays, 12 elements were aligned along a straight or curved path, constructed by having each element in the sequence differ by a constant angle from its neighbors (e.g., 0° for a straight, collinear path; ±15° to create a curved path). The remainder of the array consisted of elements oriented randomly with respect to one another and the path, creating a noisy background. In the experiments, observers judged which of two successively and briefly presented arrays contained a path.

The results of Field et al.'s (1993) experiments strongly supported the geometry of relatability as a description of the conditions under which contour segments connect across gaps. When the positional and angular relations of successive path elements satisfied the relatability criterion, observers detected the stimulus efficiently. Contour detection performance declined gradually as the orientation difference between elements increased, falling to chance at around 90°. Moreover, complete violations of relatability, accomplished by orienting the elements perpendicular to the path rather than end-to-end along it, resulted in drastically reduced task performance. Together, these data suggest that interpolated contour connections require specific edge relationships, the mathematics of which are captured quite well by the notion of relatability. Moreover, interpolated contours become salient, allowing them to play a meaningful role in higher level object perception processes.

I noted previously that relatability expresses a certain notion of contour smoothness. Indeed, its value as a principle of unit formation (connecting separate visible areas into unified objects) may derive from facts about the objects in the world to be perceived. As has been noted in other contexts (e.g., Marr, 1982), objects and surfaces in the world are not random collections of points and attributes but are generally smoothly varying on a number of dimensions, especially spatial position. On the other hand, boundaries between objects may be sites of abrupt change. Relatability intuitively embodies the notion that objects tend to be smooth, such that when gaps are imposed by occlusion, visible edge fragments that can be connected by smooth contours are likely to be parts of the same object.

Recently, Geisler, Perry, Super, and Gallogly (2001) attempted to put these intuitions on a firmer quantitative footing. Their work suggests that relatability captures certain spatial relationships between visible contours that have a high probability of belonging to the same object. Through an analysis of contour relationships in natural images, Geisler et al. found that the statistical regularities governing the probability of two edge elements cooccurring correlate highly with the geometry of relatability. Two visible edge segments associated with the same contour meet the mathematical relatability criterion far more often than not. The success of relatability in describing perceptual interpolation processes appears to derive from ecological regularities in the natural environment.

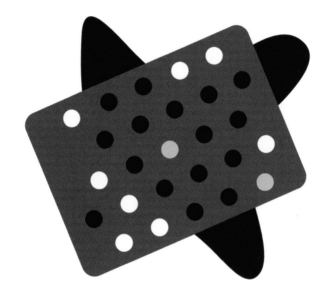

Color Panel for FIG. 5.4

Implementation of the Relatability Geometry.   How are the relationships captured by the geometry of relatability implemented in neural mechanisms of vision? This is an active area of research. Several neural-style models of contour interpolation have been proposed (Grossberg & Mingolla, 1985; Heitger, von der Heydt, Peterhans, Rosenthaler, & Kübler, 1998). None of these fully implements what is known about the geometry of relatability or certain other influences on contour interpolation, such as support ratio (Banton & Levi, 1992; Shipley & Kellman, 1992b) or possible gating effects on interpolation caused by junction types or boundary assignment (Nakayama, Shimojo, & Silverman, 1989).

Nevertheless, existing neural-style models have introduced a number of valuable concepts. Most share the assumption that contour interpolation mechanisms are built on the outputs of orientation-sensitive cells in early cortical visual areas. These cells, sensitive to retinal position, contrast, orientation, and spatial frequency typically provide the inputs into edge and junction detection mechanisms (e.g., Heitger et al., 1992). In turn, contour integration (e.g., Yen & Finkel, 1998) and interpolation processes (e.g., Heitger et al., 1998) may use the outputs of edge and junction analyses. (For a detailed account of the relation of geometric and neural models in object formation, see Kellman, Guttman, & Wickens, 2001.)

THREE-DIMENSIONAL INTERPOLATION IN OBJECT PERCEPTION

The foregoing discussion indicates that, although much remains to be learned, progress has been made in understanding the early and middle vision processes in object perception. From edge detection through interpolation, we know the tasks that visual processes must accomplish, a great deal about the information for the task, and a bit about processes and mechanisms.

Our analysis has been artificially constrained, however. Most of it has addressed object perception in static, two-dimensional displays. This may be an important aspect of the problem, but it is not nearly the whole problem. In ordinary perception, objects are three-dimensional and arranged in three-dimensional space. The inputs to the visual system consist of visible contours oriented not only in frontoparallel planes but also in three-dimensional space. In recent years, these considerations have led us to broaden our investigations of object formation into all three spatial dimensions (as I describe in this section) and to information given over time via motion (as I describe in the next section).

Although the research literature provides some examples of three-dimensional illusory contours (e.g., Gregory & Harris, 1974), there has been little systematic investigation of three-dimensional information in unit formation, its geometry and processes. Over the past few years, my colleagues and I have posed two main

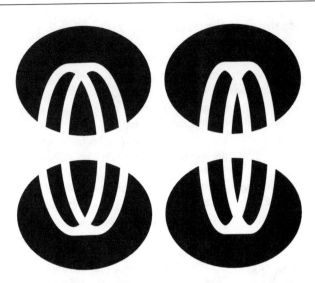

FIG. 5.12. Example of three-dimensional contour interpolation. The
display is a stereo pair, which may be free-fused by crossing the eyes.
When cross-fused, vivid three-dimensional illusory contours are seen
on the left, and occluded contours are seen arcing behind the white
surface on the right. (If the display is fused by diverging the eyes, the
positions of the illusory and occluded contours are reversed.) From
Kellman, P. J. "An Update on Gestalt Psychology." In *Essays in Honor
of Henry and Lila Gleitman*, by B. Landau, J. Jonides, E. Newport,
and J. Sabini (Eds.), 2000, Cambridge, MA: MIT Press. Copyright 2000
by MIT Press. Reprinted with permission.

questions about three-dimensional aspects of interpolation:

1. Do visual interpolation processes use as their inputs three-dimensional relationships of contours and surfaces in the world?
2. Do visual interpolation processes produce as their outputs representations
   of three-dimensional contours and surfaces?

The answers to both questions appear to be yes. As an illustration, consider the demonstration in Fig. 5.12. If this display is viewed stereoscopically
(free-fuse by crossing or diverging the eyes), it gives rise to three-dimensional
illusory contours on one side and three-dimensional occluded contours on
the other. Binocular disparity places the inducing edges at particular three-
dimensional orientations, and contour interpolation processes build the connections, smoothly curving through three dimensions, across the gaps. The demonstration suggests that interpolation processes take three-dimensional positions
and relations as their inputs and build connections across all three spatial
dimensions.

How can these phenomena be studied experimentally and objectively? If the visual system sometimes creates connections of contours and surfaces across gaps, the resulting representations may have important consequences for performance on certain tasks. By discovering such a task, we could use performance measurements on that task to determine the conditions under which such object representations form.

This strategy has been used with two-dimensional displays. Ringach and Shapley (1996), for example, devised the fat-thin method for studying two-dimensional interpolation processes. Illusory squares were created from four partial-circle inducing elements. By rotating the circular inducers around their centers, displays whose width was bulging outward (fat) or compressed inward (thin) were created. The subject's task was to classify displays as fat or thin. Performance on this task turns out to be facilitated by contour interpolation, relative to control displays in which contour interpolation does not occur (Gold, Murray, Bennett, & Sekuler, 2000; Kellman, Yin, & Shipley, 1998; Ringach & Shapley, 1996).

My colleagues and I devised a three-dimensional performance task that is in some ways analogous to the fat-thin task (Kellman, Machado, Shipley & Li, 1996). A full report will appear elsewhere (Kellman, Yin, Garrigan, Shipley, & Machado, 2003); here I note some of the main results.

We used three-dimensional illusory object stimuli such as the one shown in Fig. 5.13, part A. Such displays appear to produce vivid three-dimensional illusory contours and surfaces. We hypothesized that these occur when the physically given contours satisfy a three-dimensional criterion of relatability. The extension from the two-dimensional case is this: Bounding contours are three-dimensional relatable when they can be joined in three dimensions by a smooth, monotonic curve. This turns out to be equivalent to the requirement that, within some small tolerance, the edges lie in a common plane (not necessarily a fronto-parallel plane), and within that plane the two-dimensional relatability criterion applies. Another way of saying the same thing is that the linear extensions of the two edges meet in their extended regions in three-space (and form an angle greater than 90°).

Three-dimensional relatability can be disrupted by shifting one piece in depth, as shown in Fig. 5.13B. Another relatable display and a corresponding shifted, nonrelatable display are shown in Fig. 5.13, parts C and D.

The experimental paradigm used these displays as follows. On each trial, subjects were shown a stereoscopic display. Stereoscopic disparities were produced by outfitting the subject with liquid-crystal-diode (LCD) shutter glasses, in which the left and right eyes' shutters were alternately opened, synchronized with alternating computer images. Subjects made a speeded judgment on each trial about a particular relationship of the upper and lower parts of the display. Displays like those in Fig. 5.13, parts A and B, were said to be in intersecting or *converging* planes. Those in Fig. 5.13, parts C and D, were said to be in *parallel* planes

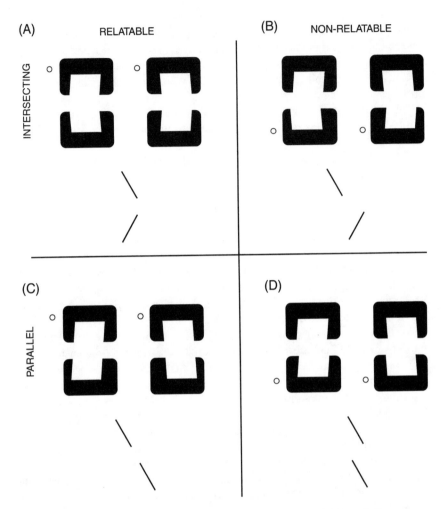

FIG. 5.13. Displays used to study three-dimensional interpolation. Displays are stereo pairs, which may be free-fused by crossing the eyes. (The two small circles in each display can be used as a guide for fusing.) Lines underneath displays indicate side views; orientation is correct for a viewer to the right. (A) three-dimensional relatable display; converging planes; (B) three-dimensional nonrelatable display; converging planes; (C) three-dimensional relatable display; parallel planes; (D) three-dimensional nonrelatable display; parallel planes. (See text.) From Kellman, Guttman & Wickens "Geometric and Neural Models of Object Perception." In *From Fragments to Objects: Segmentation and Grouping in Vision* (p. 236), by T. F. Shipley and P. J. Kellman (Eds.), 2001, Amsterdam: Elsevier. Copyright 2001 by Elsevier Science. Reprinted with permission.

(including coplanar). Note that the classification required from the subject on each trial was orthogonal to the display's status as relatable or nonrelatable. The key predictions were that perception of a unified object would facilitate classification performance, and perceived unity would depend on relatability. The former was expected based on results in two-dimensional displays showing that object completion produces an advantage in detecting boundary orientation. One advantage of this task is that, unlike the two-dimensional analogue, it requires use of a *relation* between the visible parts, which may encourage dependence on interpolation.

Results of one experiment (Kellman, Yin, Garrigan, Shipley, & Machado, 2003) are shown in Fig. 5.14. The graph shows discrimination sensitivity (d') by condition. Two values of depth displacement (used to disrupt relatability) were used, corresponding to about a 5-cm and a 10-cm shift in depth of one of the pieces from

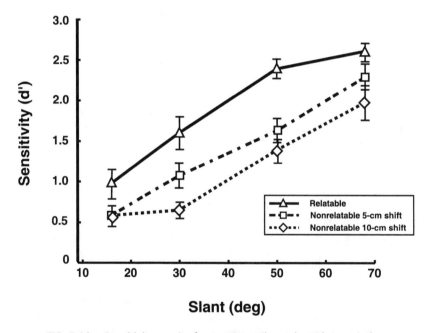

Slant (deg)

FIG. 5.14.   Sensitivity results from a three-dimensional interpolation experiment. Sensitivity is plotted as a function of slant for relatable displays, nonrelatable displays in which one piece was shifted approximately 5 cm in the virtual display, and nonrelatable displays in which the shift was approximately 10 cm. Relatable displays were more accurately and rapidly classified, suggesting that the upper and lower inducing areas were processed as a connected unit. From Kellman, Yin, Garrigan, Shipley, & Machado, 2003.

the observer's viewing distance (100 cm). Participants did the task at four different values of slant; increasing slant made the classification of converging or parallel planes easier. It can be seen that the relatable displays showed a clear superiority over the nonrelatable displays at all slant values. Response times reflected the same advantage: Both parallel and converging relatable displays produced faster, as well as more accurate, responding.

These results suggest that performing the classification of displays as parallel or converging was made easier when the two surface patches were perceived as a single, connected object. Moreover, in most respects a three-dimensional version of contour relatability seems to predict the conditions under which tabs where connected into single objects. Even the smaller value of depth shift disrupted performance markedly.

These data are consistent with the notion that interpolation processes are truly three-dimensional and are described by a notion of three-dimensional relatability. At the same time, there is substantial bootstrapping in this initial set of results. In the same experiment, we validated the paradigm (as being sensitive to object completion) and revealed some determinants of object completion (e.g., it is disrupted by depth shifting of one tab relative to the other).

Accordingly, we must consider alternative explanations for the data. First, it is possible that performance in our task might not really require object completion. Perhaps relatable displays were better processed because their pieces were more nearly equidistant from the observer. Comparing two parts' orientations might be easier when the parts are equidistant. Our design allowed us to check this hypothesis using a subset of the data. As Fig. 5.13 illustrates, a subset of parallel displays used a shift away from the canonical (relatable) stimulus that actually made the two parts more nearly equidistant. We compared these displays (which had roughly 0- or 5-cm depth differences) with relatable parallel displays having parts that differed substantially in depth (10 cm for the largest slant condition). Results showed that relatability, not similarity in depth, produced superior accuracy and speed.

More recently we have used other control groups to test the idea that the effects in this paradigm are due to object completion. Our strategy has been to keep the three-dimensional geometry of the stimulus pieces as similar as possible to that of the original experiment, while using other manipulations that should disrupt object completion. In one control experiment, for example, tangent discontinuities were rounded, a manipulation that disrupts interpolation processes but should have had no effect if comparisons of tabs is coincidentally facilitated by certain geometric arrangements. In this case, the advantage of relatable over nonrelatable displays was completely eliminated. In general, all of the control experiments support the idea that object completion caused the observed performance advantage.

We also examined another important concern. The observed effects appear to be object completion effects, but are they truly *three-dimensional effects*? Introducing binocular depth differences involves monocularly misaligning contours in each eye. Perhaps these monocular effects, not true depth effects, cause the performance decrement. It is known that misalignment of parallel or nearly parallel contours disrupts two-dimensional object completion (Kellman, Yin, & Shipley, 1998; Shipley & Kellman, 1992a).

In designing the original study, we aimed to produce significant depth shifts using misalignments that remained within the tolerances for two-dimensional completion. It has been estimated that contour completion breaks down at about 15 min of misalignment of parallel edges (Shipley & Kellman, 1992a). Our misalignments were on the order of about 10 min in the maximum depth shift condition. To check the effect of monocular misalignment, we carried out a separate experiment. In our binocular, depth-shifted displays, each eye had the same misalignment with opposite sign. In this experiment, we used the same displays but gave misalignment of the same sign in both eyes. Thus, the amount of monocular misalignment was exactly identical in every display as in the original experiment. Because both members of each stereo pair had misalignments of the same sign, shifted displays appeared to be at the same depths as relatable displays but with some lateral misalignment. Results showed no reliable accuracy or speed differences between shifted and relatable displays in this experiment. This outcome is consistent with the idea that the basic experimental effect is a three-dimensional object completion effect. The effects are not explainable by monocular misalignment.

These several experiments make a clear case for contour interpolation as a three-dimensional process. Human visual processing in object formation takes as inputs the positions and orientations of contours in three-dimensional space. Interpolation processes produce as outputs contours and surfaces that extend through all three spatial dimensions. Although this line of research is just beginning, there is considerable support for the notion that a simple piece of geometry—contour relatability—can provide not only an account of two-dimensional spatial interpolation but can be extended to three-dimensional cases.

Even the initial data on three-dimensional interpolation are very challenging for existing models of interpolation. Few if any current models take as their inputs three-dimensional positions and orientations of edges. It is possible that a three-dimensional analogue of the kinds of interactions of oriented units envisioned in neural models of two-dimensional interpolation may offer a plausible route for understanding the neural mechanisms underlying three-dimensional interpolation. Alternatively, it is possible that early interpolation processes are actually done in a two-dimensional substrate, but depth information is used to correct the results somehow. The latter possibility seems unlikely, but it would be more consistent with neural models that depend heavily in their initial stages on two-dimensional orientation information in early visual cortical areas. These possibilities remain to be explored. What is clear is that human perception produces interpolations spanning all three dimensions, whereas current models do not.

SPATIOTEMPORAL INTERPOLATION

Complex perceptual systems are exclusively the property of mobile organisms. Most research on interpolation processes in object formation has emphasized static, two-dimensional displays, but object perception processes must serve the moving observer and may need to use information available over time. When looking through dense foliage, for example, an observer may see bits of light and color from the scene behind but may be unable to detect specific objects or spatial layout. However, if the observer moves parallel to the occluding foliage, the scene behind may suddenly be revealed. This ordinary experience suggests that humans can perceive the objects in a scene from information that arrives fragmented not only in space but in time.

In recent years, my colleagues and I have sought to understand visual processes that assemble objects from information fragmentary in time and space. Early work showed that illusory figures may arise from inducing elements that are partially occluded in sequence (Kellman & Cohen, 1984; see also Bruno & Bertamini, 1990; Kojo, Liinasuo, & Rovamo, 1993). Perception under these circumstances requires that the visual system not only integrate information over time but also interpolate because some parts of the object never project to the eyes.

Existing models of visual interpolation are not set up to handle inputs that arrive fragmented over time (but see Shipley & Kellman, 1994). One issue in broadening both our understanding and our models is the difficulty of characterizing the stimulus relationships in both space and time that lead to the perception of complete, unified objects. The extra degrees of freedom given by motion make the problem formidable.

My colleagues and I approached this problem by assuming that spatiotemporal interpolation in object perception may build on the same basic geometry that underlies static, spatial interpolation. Palmer, Kellman, and Shipley (1997, 2000) proposed two hypotheses that connect the geometry of spatial relatability to the problem of spatiotemporal interpolation. Fig. 5.15 illustrates these ideas. The *persistence hypothesis* (Fig. 5.15A) suggests that the position and edge orientations of a briefly viewed fragment are encoded in a buffer, such that they can be integrated with later-appearing fragments. In Fig. 5.15A, an opaque panel containing two apertures moves in front of an object, revealing one part of an occluded object at time t_1 and another part at time t_2. If information concerning the part seen at t_1 persists in the buffer until the part at t_2 appears, then the standard spatial relatability computation can be performed to integrate the currently visible part with the part encoded earlier.

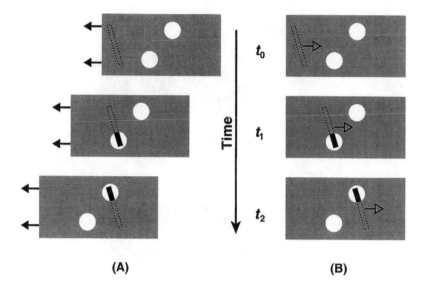

(A)   **(B)**

FIG. 5.15. Illustrations of (A) the persistence hypothesis and (B) the spatial updating hypothesis in spatiotemporal interpolation. (See text.) (A) The moving occluder reveals relatable parts of the rod sequentially in time (t_1 and t_2). Perceptual connection of parts requires that the initially visible part persists over time in some way. (B) Parts of the moving rod become visible through apertures sequentially in time. Perceptual connection of the parts requires not only persistence of the initially visible part but also positional updating based on velocity information. From Kellman, Guttman & Wickens "Geometric and Neural Models of Object Perception." In *From Fragments to Objects: Segmentation and Grouping in Vision* (p. 238), by T. F. Shipley and P. J. Kellman (Eds.), 2001, Amsterdam: Elsevier. Copyright 2001 by Elsevier Science. Reprinted with permission.

In Fig. 5.15B, the object moves behind a stationary occluder, again revealing one part through the bottom aperture at t_1 and a second part through the top aperture at t_2. This figure illustrates the *spatial updating hypothesis*. According to this idea, the visual system encodes a velocity signal of any moving objects or surfaces, in addition to their positions and edge orientations; once these surfaces become occluded, the visual system uses the velocity signal to update their spatial position over time. Thus, when a later-appearing object part (upper aperture at t_2) becomes visible, it can be combined with the updated position of the earlier-appearing part (lower aperture at t_1) using the standard spatial relatability computation. Together with the spatial notion of relatability, the persistence and spatial updating hypotheses comprise the notion of *spatiotemporal relatability*.

Palmer, Shipley and I (1997) developed an experimental paradigm to test spatiotemporal relatability. On each trial, an object passed once back and forth behind

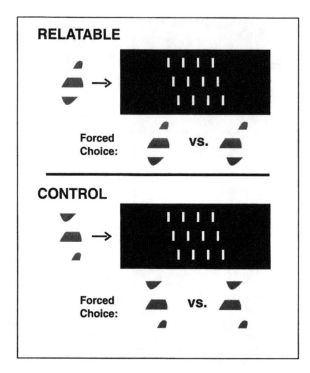

FIG. 5.16.   Design of a spatiotemporal interpolation experiment. (See text.) From Kellman, P. J. "An Update on Gestalt Psychology." *Essays in Honor of Henry and Lila Gleitman* by B. Landau, J. Jonides, E. Newport, and J. Sabini (Eds.), 2000, Cambridge, MA: MIT Press. Copyright 2000 by MIT Press. Reprinted with permission.

an occluder with several narrow slits, vertically separated so that some parts of the object never projected to the eyes. This feature makes the task a completion or interpolation task as opposed to only an integration task (where visible parts are integrated over time). Subjects made a forced choice between two test displays, choosing which matched the moving target display. The design is illustrated in Fig. 5.16.

Three display conditions were used. Relatable displays (apart from the shift manipulation; see later text) met the criterion of spatiotemporal relatability. The upper test display in Fig. 5.16 is an example. The other test display differed from the first by having one of the three fragments shifted by some amount. Five different amounts of shift (ranging from 1.67 arcmin to 8.33 arcmin of visual angle) were used. The target matched unshifted and shifted test displays each equal numbers trials.

We predicted that relatability would facilitate encoding of the visible parts in the target display. If three parts moving behind slits were grouped into a single, coherent object, this might lead to more economical encoding and memory than for control displays, in which three detached pieces were encoded. For simplicity, I will consider here only the cases in which either a test display or both the target and a test display were relatable. In these cases, it was predicted that the greater ease of encoding a relatable display would lead to better performance.

Displays in two control conditions were compared with the first. Nonrelatable displays consisted of the identical three pieces as in the relatable condition, but the top and bottom pieces were permuted. (See Fig. 5.16.) It was hypothesized that visual completion would not occur with these nonrelatable displays. Because each nonrelatable target might have to be encoded as three distinct pieces, it would lead to greater encoding demands and lower sensitivity to the relative spatial positions of the three parts. The third condition left the overall geometry of the relatable displays but sought to disrupt interpolation by rounding the tangent discontinuities of the visible parts. To make the rounded corners visible, the occluder was moved away slightly from visible parts.

A series of experiments has confirmed the usefulness of spatiotemporal relatability in describing relations over space and time that produce representations of connected objects. Fig. 5.17 shows accuracy data (discrimination d') from two experiments. In Fig. 5.17, part A, the data show means for 16 subjects for relatable and nonrelatable displays as a function of shift. Relatable displays were far more accurately discriminated than displays made of the identical physical parts but placed in nonrelatable (permuted) positions. The control group in which the corners or visible parts were rounded to eliminate tangent discontinuities provided additional confirmation that the initial results were due to interpolation effects. As predicted, rounding of tangent discontinuities weakened performance, despite the figure fragments appearing in the same positions and relations as in the relatable displays. Performance was not reduced as much as in the nonrelatable condition, however; this result may indicate that junction detectors at low spatial frequencies still signal junctions in these rounded displays.

Results of later experiments showed that illusory contour versions of these displays produced nearly identical speed and accuracy data as in the occluded case (Fig. 5.17B). This suggests that the identity hypothesis in contour interpolation applies to spatiotemporal interpolation.

The results support the notion of spatiotemporal relatability as a description of the geometry of object formation over time. There are numerous issues yet to be addressed. These and other studies in the spatiotemporal domain, however, are beginning to reveal the details of the persistence and spatial updating aspects of spatiotemporal object formation. The results suggest that connecting dynamic object perception to previous work with static displays is plausible in terms of the

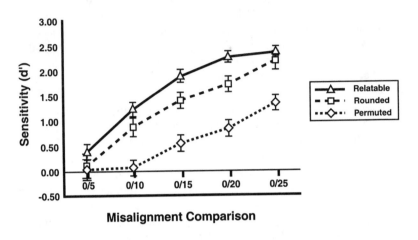

(A) Dynamic Occlusion Displays

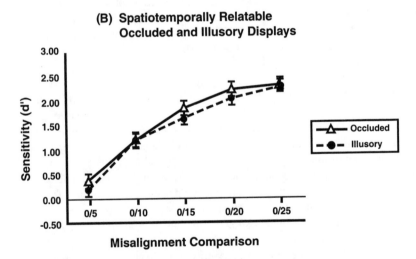

(B) Spatiotemporally Relatable Occluded and Illusory Displays

FIG. 5.17. Results of spatiotemporal interpolation experiments. Sensitivity (d′) is plotted as a function of the amount of shift distinguishing the aligned and misaligned choices presented to the subject. (A) Results from dynamic occlusion displays with spatiotemporally relatable and nonrelatable (permuted) displays, as well as relatable displays in which interpolation was disrupted by rounding off tangent discontinuities. (B) Results from dynamic occlusion and illusory contour versions of the experiment. (Displays had identical physically specified edges and gaps.) From Palmer, Kellman & Shiplay (2003).

underlying geometry, over space and time, that allows fragments to be connected perceptually.

GLOBAL AND LOCAL PROCESSING
IN INTERPOLATION

Most of our discussion to this point has focused on relatively local determinants of object perception. It has often been argued that in addition to these, there are more global influences. Perhaps the original idea of this type is the Gestalt principle of *good form,* which suggests that perceptual processes tend toward simple or regular (symmetric) outcomes (e.g., Koffka, 1935). Subsequent research attempted to formalize this notion (e.g., Buffart, Leeuwenberg, & Restle, 1981), and some provided empirical support for a role of symmetry in object completion (Sekuler, Palmer, & Flynn, 1994).

Both the role of global factors and the relationship between global and local factors in object formation remain unsettled. In object completion, Kanizsa (1979) argued that that global symmetry is a questionable or weak determinant, based on demonstrations that pitted global factors against local edge continuity. Evidence from priming studies, however, tends to show global effects (Sekuler, Palmer, & Flynn, 1994), along with local ones (Sekuler et al., 1994; van Lier, van der Helm, & Leeuwenberg, 1995). Van Lier et al. interpreted their results in terms of dual or multiple representations activated by partly occluded displays.

An example of a display for which global completion has been claimed is shown in Fig. 5.18, part A. Global completion entails seeing a fourth articulated part behind the occluder, making the display radially symmetric. The argument is that the process of contour interpolation somehow takes into account the potential for a symmetric shape in cases like this and represents boundaries consistent with that shape. In this example, the local completion (via relatability) would consist of a smooth, monotonic, constant curvature connection. (See Kellman, Guttman, & Wickens, 2001, for a discussion of several variants of claims about global completion.)

Does the visual system really interpolate edges to construct symmetric object representations? Here is a case in which the identity hypothesis can shed light on interpolation processes (or at least raise an interesting question). Recall the argument that a common contour interpolation process underlies occluded and illusory contours. If so, we might learn something by examining the idea of global completion not just under occlusion but in the illusory contour domain. Fig. 5.18B shows an illusory contour display that has physically given edges equivalent to the occlusion display in Fig. 18A. If completion operates to produce symmetric perceived objects, the four-lobed figure should be obvious, complete with clear illusory contours, in Fig. 5.18B. In fact, however, no global completion is evident in Fig. 5.18B. To my knowledge, there is not a single report of completion based on global symmetry of this sort in illusory object displays among all the hundreds of published reports on this topic. What might account for subjective reports and priming data indicating at least some tendency toward global completion under occlusion, but none in illusory object cases?

I have suggested the hypothesis that the discrepancy indicates the operation of two distinct categories of processing (e.g., Kellman, 2001). One is a bottom-up, relatively local process that produces representations of boundaries according to the relatability criterion. This process is *perceptual* in that it involves a modular process that takes stimulus relationships as inputs and produces boundaries and forms as outputs. The other process is more top-down, global, and cognitive, coming into play when familiar or symmetric forms can be recognized. For lack of a more concise label, we call it *recognition from partial information (RPI)*.

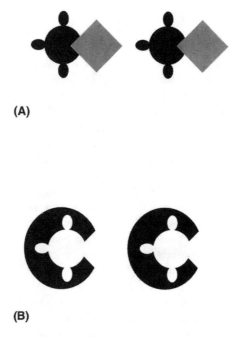

(A)

(B)

FIG. 5.18. (A) Example of an occlusion display used to study global completion. (B) Illusory contour version of the occlusion display in (A). Displays are stereo pairs, which may be free-fused by crossing the eyes. (The stereoscopic effect enhances the effect but is not necessary, as can be seen by viewing any single image.) According to the recognition-from-partial information hypothesis (see text), contour interpolation processes do not produce global (symmetric) completion (appearance of a fourth lobe of the central figure) in either display. In the occlusion display, observers perceive that part of the figure is out of sight, allowing the possibility of reports of symmetric completion.

If the identity hypothesis is true, why should global completion occur in occluded but not illusory object displays? The answer may be that the displays are the same in terms of the perceptual process of contour interpolation but different in terms of RPI. An occluded surface is an interpolated surface that is not nearest to the observer in some visual direction (i.e., there is something in front of it). An illusory surface is nearest to the observer among all surfaces in a certain visual direction. The crucial consequence of the difference is this: An observer viewing an occluded display is aware that part of the object is hidden from view. This allows certain kinds of reasoning and responses that are not sensible when no part of an object is occluded. In particular, despite any local completion process, *the observer can notice what parts are visible (unoccluded) and whether they are consistent with some familiar or symmetric object.*

Consider a concrete example. If you see the tail of your calico cat protruding from under the sofa, you may easily recognize and report that the cat is present, even though the particular contours and surfaces of the hidden parts of the cat are not given perceptually. A stored representation of the cat may be activated and a belief about its presence may be formed. But RPI differs from perceptual processes that actually specify the positions of boundaries and surfaces behind an occluder.

This separation of processes might explain the continuing disagreements about global and local processing. First, objective data supporting global outcomes have come solely from priming studies. It is well-known that priming occurs at many levels, from the most basic representation of the stimulus to higher conceptual classifications involving the stimulus (e.g., Kawaguchi, 1988). To my knowledge, no attempts have been made to specify the locus of priming influences in occlusion studies. Studies reporting global completion have typically used large numbers of trials with a small set of familiar and symmetric figures, such as circles and squares. Even if the subjects start out with little familiarity or do not notice the possibility of symmetry under occlusion, repeated exposure may produce familiarity or symmetry responses.

The observation that different levels have not been teased apart in priming studies on occlusion is not meant as a criticism. Priming may not be suitable for separating perceptual processes from more cognitive influences in this realm. Testing the possibility of different processes may require a different experimental paradigm. My colleagues and I developed such a paradigm, focusing on the idea that perceptual boundary completion processes lead to relatively specific representations of boundary locations; RPI will not do so, as in our occluded cat example. We measured the precision of boundary location by showing an occluded display and briefly flashing a probe dot in front of the occluder. Subjects were instructed to respond on each trial whether the probe dot fell inside or outside the occluded object's boundaries (i.e., whether the projection of the occluded object to the eye would or would not encompass the dot).

Adaptive staircase procedures were used. The stimulus value for each trial changed depended on the subject's responses. Systematic changes allowed estimation of particular points on a psychometric function. For each display, we used both a two-up, one-down and a one-up, two-down staircase to estimate two points: the .707 probability of seeing the dot as outside the boundary and .707 probability of seeing the dot inside the boundary (= .293 probability of outside). We took the *difference* between these estimates as a measure of the *precision* of boundary perception, and the *mean* of these estimates as an estimate of the perceived *location* of the boundary. Staircases for several stimulus patterns were interleaved, (i.e., patterns appeared in a random order, and screen position was varied randomly).

We realized that competing perceptual and recognition processes might lead to different strategies across subjects. Therefore, we gave subjects explicit strategy instructions. In the *global instruction condition,* we told subjects that they should see the display as symmetric; for the display in Fig. 5.18A, for example, they were told that there was a fourth protrusion behind the occluder identical to the three visible protrusions around the circle. In the *local instruction condition,* we told them that we wanted them to see the display as containing a simple curve connecting the two visible edges. In this manner, we sought to find the subjects' *best* ability to localize boundaries under a global or local set.

A number of interesting findings emerged (Kellman, Temesvary, Palmer, & Shipley, 2000). Localization of boundaries in displays where completion is predicted by relatability is extremely precise. This is true for both straight (collinear) and curved completions. The outcomes in cases where completion is predicted to follow global symmetry are quite different. Here, the range (difference between out and in thresholds) is far greater (approaching an order of magnitude greater). Not only is localization imprecise in the global cases, but it is also inaccurate. The estimate of subjects' perceived position of the boundary is consistently and substantially different from its theoretically predicted location. This result has shown up consistently in a variety of displays testing symmetry and related global notions of object completion. Many questions are still being investigated in this paradigm. What is already clear is that global influences do not lead to specification of precise boundary position in the way local perceptual completion does. These outcomes are consistent with the idea of separate perceptual completion and more cognitive RPI processes. For a more extensive discussion of these ideas, see Kellman (2001).

CONCLUSIONS

We have examined a wide range of phenomena, theories, and issues in object perception. Perhaps the most conspicuous conclusion of our tour is that this fundamental and active area of research poses a vast array of challenges to scientists interested in vision and cognition. It will take a great deal of work just to fill in the details of the framework given in Fig. 5.1. Moreover, it is a certainty that some of its processes, representations, and relations will be altered or reconfigured as progress occurs.

The other conclusion that pulls together most threads of our discussion is the idea that object perception is a four-dimensional process, in the sense that it depends on all three spatial dimensions as well as time. Researchers have come a long way in terms of understanding the phenomena of two-dimensional segmentation, grouping, and object formation. Our models of these processes have progressed in specifying their geometry, computations, and, to some degree, their neural implementation.

Yet the frontiers beckon. Truly realistic and comprehensive explanations will incorporate the ideas of the perceiver and the objects to be perceived existing in a three-dimensional world and moving relative to each other. The data are already clear in showing that we have capacities to detect relationships and produce representations that involve three-dimensional space and time. Achieving a detailed understanding of the information, processes, and neural circuitry involved will require considerably more work.

In exploring these frontiers, however, there is reason for early optimism. Investigations suggest that a simple piece of geometry, the notion of contour relatability, may account for many of the cases in which the visual system connects fragments into objects, not only in static, two-dimensional arrays but also, with simple extensions, in the three- and four-dimensional space-time in which we must perceive and act.

ACKNOWLEDGMENTS

Preparation of this chapter was supported in part by research grants from the National Science Foundation (SBR 9496112) and the National Eye Institute (R01 EY13518) to P. Kellman. I thank Patrick Garrigan, Sharon Guttman, and Evan Palmer for helpful discussions, Marlene Behrmann and Rutie Kimchi for useful comments on an earlier draft, and Jennifer Vanyo for general assistance. Correspondence should be addressed to Philip J. Kellman, UCLA Department of Psychology, 405 Hilgard Avenue, Los Angeles, CA 90095-1563 or via email (Kellman@cognet.ucla.edu).

REFERENCES

Anderson, B. L., Singh, M., & Fleming, R. W. (2002). The interpolation of object and surface structure. *Cognitive Psychology, 44,* 148–190.

Banton, T., & Levi, D. M. (1992). The perceived strength of illusory contours. *Perception and Psychophysics, 52,* 676–684.

Barrow, H. G., & Tenenbaum, J. M. (1986). Computational approaches to vision. In K. R. Boff, L. Kaufman, & J. P. Thomas (Eds.), *Handbook of perception and human performance: Vol. 2. Cognitive processes and performance* (pp. 38.1–38.70). New York: Wiley.

Biederman, I. (1995). Visual object recognition. In S. M. Kosslyn & D. N. Osherson (Eds), *Visual cognition: An invitation to cognitive science* Vol. 2, 2nd ed., (pp. 121–165). Cambridge, MA: MIT Press.

Bruno, N., & Bertamini, M. (1990). Identifying contours from occlusion events. *Perception & Psychophysics, 48,* 331–342.

Buffart, H., Leeuwenberg E., & Restle, F. (1981). Coding theory of visual pattern completion. *Journal of Experimental Psychology: Human Perception & Performance. 7*(2), 241–274.

Campbell, F. W., Cooper, G. F., & Enroth-Cugell, C. (1969). The spatial selectivity of the visual cells of the cat. *Journal of Physiology, 203,* 223–235.

Field, D., Hayes, A., & Hess, R. F. (1993). Contour integration by the human visual system: Evidence for a local "association field." *Vision Research, 33,* 173–193.

Fischer, B., & Poggio, G. F. (1979). Depth sensitivity of binocular cortical neurons of behaving monkeys. *Proceedings of the Royal Society of London B, 1157,* 409–414.

Geisler, W. S., Perry, J. S., Super, B. J., & Gallogly, D. P. (2001). Edge co-occurrence in natural images predicts contour grouping performance. *Vision Research, 41,* 711–724.

Gibson, J. J. (1966). *The senses considered as perceptual systems.* Boston: Houghton-Mifflin.

Gibson, J. J. (1979). *The ecological approach to visual perception.* Boston: Houghton-Mifflin.

Gibson, J. J., Kaplan, G. A., Reynolds, H. N., & Wheeler, K. (1969). The change from visible to invisible: A study of optical transitions. *Perception and Psychophysics, 5,* 113–116.

Gillam, B., Chambers, D., & Russo, T. (1988). Postfusional latency in stereoscopic slant perception and the primitives of stereopsis. *Journal of Experimental Psychology: Human Perception and Performance, 14*(2), 163–175.

Gold, J. M., Murray, R. F., Bennett, P. J., & Sekuler, A. B. (2000). Deriving behavioural receptive fields for visually completed contours. *Current Biology, 10* (11), 663–666.

Gregory, R. L., & Harris, J. P. (1974). Illusory contours and stereo depth. *Perception and Psychophysics, 15*(3), 1974, pp. 411–416.

Grossberg, S. (1994). 3-D vision and figure-ground separation by visual cortex. *Perception and Psychophysics, 55,* 48–120.

Grossberg, S., & Mingolla, E. (1985). Neural dynamics of form perception: Boundary completion, illusory figures, and neon color spreading. *Psychological Review, 92,* 173–211.

Guttman, S. E., & Kellman, P. J. (2000). Seeing between the lines: Contour interpolation without perception of interpolated contours. *Investigative Ophthalmology and Visual Science, 41*(4), S439.

Guttman, S. E., & Kellman, P. J. (2003). *Contour interpolation: Necessary but not sufficient for the perception of interpolated contours.* Manuscript in preparation.

Heitger, F., Rosenthaler, L., von der Heydt, R., Peterhans, E., & Kübler, O. (1992). Simulation of neural contour mechanisms: From simple to end-stopped cells. *Vision Research, 32,* 963–981.

Heitger, F., von der Heydt, R., Peterhans, E., Rosenthaler, L., & Kübler, O. (1998). Simulation of neural contour mechanisms: Representing anomalous contours. *Image and Vision Computing, 16,* 407–421.

Hoffman, D. D. (1998). *Visual intelligence: How we create what we see.* New York: W. W. Norton.

Hubel, D. H., & Wiesel, T. N. (1968). Receptive fields and functional architecture of monkey striate cortex. *Journal of Physiology, 195,* 215–243.

Humphreys, G. W., Cinel, C., Wolfe, J., Olson, A. & Klempen, A. (2000). Fractionating the binding process. Neuropsychological evidence distinguishing binding of form from binding of surface features. *Vision Research, 40,* 1569–1596.

Johansson, G. (1970). On theories for visual space perception: A letter to Gibson. *Scandinavian Journal of Psychology, 11*(2), 67–74.

Julesz, B. (1971). *Foundations of cyclopean perception*. Chicago: University of Chicago Press.

Kanizsa, G. (1979). *Organization in vision*. New York: Praeger.

Kawaguchi, J. (1988). Priming effect as expectation. *Japanese Psychological Review, 31*, 290–304.

Kellman, P. J. (2000). An update on Gestalt psychology. In B. Landau, J. Jonides, E. Newport, & J. Sabini (Eds.), *Essays in honor of Henry and Lila Gleitman* (pp. 157–190). Cambridge, MA: MIT Press.

Kellman, P. J. (2001). Separating processes in object perception. *Journal of Experimental Child Psychology, 78*(1), 84–97.

Kellman, P. J. (2003). *Relatability and good continuation*. Manuscript in preparation.

Kellman, P. J. & Arterberry, M. (1998). *The Cradle of Knowledge: Perceptual Development in Infancy*. Cambridge, MA: MIT Press.

Kellman, P. J., & Cohen, M. H. (1984). Kinetic subjective contours. *Perception and Psychophysics, 35*, 237–244.

Kellman, P. J., Guttman, S., & Wickens, T. (2001). Geometric and neural models of contour and surface interpolation in visual object perception. In Shipley, T. F. & Kellman, P. J. (Eds.) *From fragments to objects: Segmentation and grouping in vision.* (pp. 183–245). Elsevier Press.

Kellman, P. J., & Loukides, M. G. (1987). An object perception approach to static and kinetic subjective contours. In S. Petry & G. E. Meyer (Eds.), *The perception of illusory contours* (pp. 151–164). New York: Springer-Verlag.

Kellman, P. J., Machado, L. J., Shipley, T. F., & Li, C. C. (1996). 3-D determinants of object completion. *Investigative Ophthalmology and Visual Science, 37*, S685.

Kellman, P. J., & Shipley, T. F. (1991). A theory of visual interpolation in object perception. *Cognitive Psychology, 23*, 141–221.

Kellman, P. J., & Shipley, T. F. (1992). Visual interpolation in object perception. *Current Directions in Psychological Science, 1*(6), 193–199.

Kellman, P. J., Shipley, T. F., & Kim, J. (1996, November). *Global and local effects in object completion: Evidence from a boundary localization paradigm.* Paper presented at the 37th Annual Meeting of the Psychonomic Society, Chicago, IL.

Kellman, P. J., Temesvary, A., Palmer, E. M., & Shipley, T. F. (2000). Separating local and global processes in object perception: Evidence from an edge localization paradigm. *Investigative Ophthalmology and Visual Science, 41*(4), S741.

Kellman, P. J., Yin, C., Garrigan, P., Shipley, T. F., & Machado, L. J. (2003). *Visual interpolation in three dimensions*. Manuscript in preparation.

Kellman, P. J., Yin, C., & Shipley, T. F. (1998). A common mechanism for illusory and occluded object completion. *Journal of Experimental Psychology: Human Perception and Performance, 24*, 859–869.

Koffka, K. (1935). *Principles of Gestalt Psychology*. NY: Harcourt.

Kojo, I., Liinasuo, M., & Rovamo, J. (1993). Spatial and temporal properties of illusory figures. *Vision Research, 33*, 897–901.

Marr, D. (1982). *Vision*. San Francisco: W. H. Freeman.

Marr, D., & Hildreth, E. (1980). Theory of edge detection. *Proceedings of the Royal Society of London B, 207*, 187–217.

Michotte, A., Thines, G., & Crabbe, G. (1964). *Les complements amodaux des structures perceptives*. Louvain, Belgium: Publications Universitaires de Louvain.

Morrone, M. C., & Burr, D. C. (1988). Feature detection in human vision: A phase-dependent energy model. *Proceedings of the Royal Society of London B, 235*, 221–245.

Nakayama, K., Shimojo, S., & Silverman, G. (1989). Stereoscopic depth: Its relation to image segmentation, grouping, and the recognition of occluded objects. *Perception, 18*, 55–68.

Palmer, E. M., Kellman, P. J., & Shipley, T. F. (1997). Spatiotemporal relatability in dynamic object completion. *Investigative Ophthalmology and Visual Science, 38*(4), S256.

Palmer, E. M., Kellman, P. J., & Shipley, T. F. (2000). Modal and amodal perception of dynamically occluded objects. *Investigative Ophthalmology and Visual Science, 41*(4), S439.

Palmer, E. M., Kellman, P. J., & Shipley, T. F. (2003). Contour relatability in spatiotemporal object perception. Manuscript in preparation.

Palmer, S., & Rock, I. (1994). Rethinking perceptual organization: The role of uniform connectedness. *Psychonomic Bulletin & Review, 1,* 29–55.

Peterhans, E., & von der Heydt, R. (1989). Mechanisms of contour perception in monkey visual cortex. II. Contours bridging gaps. *Journal of Neuroscience, 9,* 1749–1763.

Peterhans, E., & von der Heydt, R. (1991). Subjective contours: Bridging the gap between psychophysics and physiology. *Trends in Neurosciences, 14,* 112–119.

Peterhans, E., & von der Heydt, R. (1993). Functional organization of area V2 in alert macaque. *European Journal of Neuroscience, 5,* 509–524.

Peterson, M. A. (1994). Object recognition processes can and do operate before figure-ground organization. *Current Directions in Psychological Science, 3*(4), 105–111.

Peterson, M. A., & Gibson, B. S. (1991). The initial identification of figure-ground relationships: Contributions from shape recognition processes. *Bulletin of the Psychonomic Society, 29,* 199–202.

Peterson, M. A., & Gibson, B. S. (1994). Must figure-ground organization precede object recognition? An assumption in peril. *Psychological Science, 5,* 253–259.

Petter, G. (1956). Nuove ricerche sperimentali sulla totalizzazione percettiva. *Rivista di Psicologia, 50,* 213–227.

Ringach, D. L., & Shapley, R. (1996). Spatial and temporal properties of illusory contours and amodal boundary completion. *Vision Research, 36,* 3037–3050.

Rock, I. (1977). In defense of unconscious inference. In W. Epstein (Ed.), Stability and constancy in visual perception. (pp. 321–373), NY: Wiley.

Rubin, E. (1915). *Synsoplevede figurer.* Copenhagen: Gyldendal.

Sekuler, A. B., Palmer, S. E., & Flynn, C. (1994). Local and global processes in visual completion. *Psychological Science, 5,* 260–267.

Shimojo, S., Silverman, G. H., & Nakayama, K. (1989). Occlusion and the solution to the aperture problem for motion. *Vision Research, 29,* 619–626.

Shipley, T. F., & Kellman, P. J. (1990). The role of discontinuities in the perception of subjective figures. *Perception and Psychophysics, 48,* 259–270.

Shipley, T. F., & Kellman, P. J. (1992a). Perception of partly occluded objects and illusory figures: Evidence for an identity hypothesis. *Journal of Experimental Psychology: Human Perception and Performance, 18,* 106–120.

Shipley, T. F., & Kellman, P. J. (1992b). Strength of visual interpolation depends on the ratio of physically-specified to total edge length. *Perception and Psychophysics, 52,* 97–106.

Shipley, T. F., & Kellman, P. J. (1994). Spatiotemporal boundary formation. *Journal of Experimental Psychology: General, 123,* 3–20.

Singh, M., & Hoffman, D. D. (1999). Completing visual contours: The relationship between relatability and minimizing inflections. *Perception and Psychophysics, 61,* 943–951.

van Lier, R. (1999). Investigating global effects in visual occlusion: From a partly occluded square to the back of a tree-trunk. *Acta Psychologica, 102,* 203–220.

van Lier, R. J., van der Helm, P. A., & Leeuwenberg, E. L. J. (1995). Competing global and local completions in visual occlusion. *Journal of Experimental Psychology: Human Perception and Performance, 21,* 571–583.

Wertheimer, M. (1958). Principles of perceptual organization. In D. C. Beardslee & M. Wertheimer (Eds.), *Readings in perception.* Princeton, NJ: Van Nostrand. (Original work published 1923)

Wurtz, R. P., & Lourens, T. (2000). Corner detection in color images through a multiscale combination of end-stopped cortical cells. *Image and Vision Computing, 18,* 531–541.

Yarbus, A. L. (1967). *Eye movements and vision.* New York: Plenum Press.
Yen, S. C., & Finkel, L. H. (1998). Extraction of perceptually salient contours by striate cortical networks. *Vision Research, 38,* 719–741.
Yin, C., Kellman, P. J., & Shipley, T. F. (1997). Surface completion complements boundary interpolation in the visual integration of partly occluded objects. *Perception, 26,* 1459–1479.
Yin, C., Kellman, P. J., & Shipley, T. F. (2000). Surface integration influences depth discrimination. *Vision Research, 40,* 1969–1978.

II

Development and Learning
in Perceptual Organization

6 The Development of Object Segregation During the First Year of Life

Amy Needham
Susan M. Ormsbee
Duke University

The processes of perceptual organization involve the observer imposing order on stimuli that have many possible interpretations, only one of which is veridical. This order is presumably based to some extent on the stimulus itself but also on the observer's knowledge about the world. As many perceptual theorists have acknowledged, visual perception is a process of interpreting the available visual information, with both correct and incorrect interpretations possible. One question that has intrigued scientists and philosophers for hundreds of years is whether (and if so, to what extent) human infants share adults' ability to organize the visual world. Do infants impose order on visual stimuli in much the same way as adults do? Or do they experience visual arrays as confused collections of shapes, colors, and patterns? These questions, especially as they concern infants' perception of objects, are what motivate this research.

SEGREGATING OBJECTS

How do we tell where one object ends and another begins? The study of object segregation seeks answers to this question. When considering adult perceptions, researchers disagree about the extent to which what we know about objects affects how we perceive objects (see Palmer, 1999; this volume, for interesting discussions of this issue). Some researchers believe that perception is not influenced by knowledge, either because everything necessary for veridical perception of the objects in the world is contained in the light reflected from those objects (e.g., Gibson, 1979) or because information processing is assumed to take place in individual, cognitively impenetrable modules (e.g., Fodor, 1983). Other researchers argue that the information contained in the visual image is not sufficient to ensure accurate perception and must be augmented with stored knowledge about objects and events (e.g., Biederman, 1987; Kimchi & Haddad, 2002; Peterson, 1994, this volume; Rock, 1983; Shepard, 1983). According to this view, there are many top-down influences from higher to lower levels of visual processing so that knowledge influences even early stages of visual processing. Through our research, we hope to learn more about cognitive and perceptual development by studying the cognitive factors that affect object perception in infancy.

OBJECT SEGREGATION IN INFANCY

Although adults' perception of objects has been studied for some time and has led to many important discoveries about the processes underlying this ability, infants' object perception has been studied for only the past 20 years or so. Kellman and Spelke (1983) were the first to systematically study how infants segregate objects. These investigators asked what sources of information would lead 4-month-old infants to visually unite the visible portions of a partly occluded object. Would infants use the common motion of the object surfaces or the features of the objects' surfaces (i.e., their shapes, colors, alignment)? They concluded that infants used the common motion, but not the common features, of the visible object surfaces to perceive these surfaces as connected behind the occluder. These findings, along with those of other studies of object segregation (e.g., Kestenbaum, Termine, & Spelke, 1987), led researchers to believe that for most of the 1st year of life, infants could use only object motion and spatial gaps between objects as cues for object boundaries.

However, more recent research (see Johnson, 1997, and Needham, 1997, for reviews) suggested that this characterization of infants' visual world is too bleak. Specifically, this research showed that infants use a variety of sources of information to segregate displays, including object features. In this paper, we describe studies that investigate infants' use of different sources of information and discuss the factors that affect infants' use of these sources of information when segregating objects.

METHOD USED IN THE PRESENT RESEARCH

In the experiments reported in this chapter, infants participated in a procedure consisting of a familiarization phase and a test phase. During the familiarization phase, the infants were given the opportunity to observe a stationary display composed of real, three-dimensional objects and to form an interpretation of its composition. During the test phase (except where noted), the infants saw test events in which a gloved hand took hold of one part of the display and moved it a short distance. For half of the infants, a portion of the display remained stationary (move-apart event); for the other infants, the two parts moved as a whole (move-together event). If the infants perceived the stationary display as a single unit (an object), their expectation would be violated if the object broke into pieces when pulled. In contrast, if the infants viewed the stationary display as composed of more than one unit, their expectation would be violated if the pieces moved together when one was pulled.

We thus assume that infants form an interpretation of the (stationary) display and that their reaction to the test event, as reflected by the length of their looking, depends on their interpretation of the display. It has been well established that infants tend to direct more attention toward novel or surprising events than toward familiar or expected events (see Bornstein, 1985, and Spelke, 1985, for a discussion of experimental methodologies based on this phenomenon). We use this aspect of infants' looking behavior to help us determine whether infants expect a display to be composed of a single object or of two separate objects.

One important facet of the work reported in this paper is that we reveal to each infant only one possible composition of the display (i.e., we use a between-subjects design) so that no cross-trial contamination of infants' surprise reactions would occur. For example, if infants perceived a particular display as composed of a single unit, they would presumably respond with relatively lengthy looking on the first test trial if the display were shown to consist of two separate units. However, if the second test trial revealed that the display was composed of a single unit, this event could be seen as surprising not because it contradicted their initial expectations about the display but because it contradicted the composition just revealed in the first test trial. Because these surprise reactions over trials could mask infants' true responses to the displays, we reveal to each infant only one of the two possible compositions of the display.

Control studies are not described here (and were not always necessary, depending on the design of the study and the nature of the test events), but they typically involve showing a separate group of infants the test events without a preceding familiarization trial. Because infants tend to watch the test events about equally in these experiments, their results suggest that infants do not have superficial preferences for one event over the other, and they need some familiarization time to examine the display and formulate an interpretation of the display as composed of one or two units.

INFANTS' USE OF PHYSICAL AND FEATURAL INFORMATION

Prior research on physical reasoning in infants (see Baillargeon, 1994, and Spelke, Breinlinger, Macomber, & Jacobson, 1992, for reviews) showed that infants as young as 4.5 months of age share many of adults' most basic beliefs about the behavior of objects. Thus, infants expect objects to continue to exist when hidden; collide with, rather than pass through, other objects; and fall when their supports are removed. With this in mind, Needham and Baillargeon (1997) explored the possibility that infants would use this physical knowledge when determining the locations of object boundaries. For example, because the handle of a drawer seems to rely on the drawer for its support, would infants consider the drawer and handle to be a single unit? Needham and Baillargeon also asked whether infants would use the featural information present in the display (i.e., the shapes, colors, and patterns of the object surfaces) if the physical information of support were not informative regarding the composition of the display. So, to continue our example, if the handle was no longer supported by the drawer, because both drawer and handle lay on the floor, would infants segregate these objects in the same way as before? Finally, the researchers were curious about how infants would integrate information from these two sources when they led to different interpretations of the display (i.e., when physical information contradicted featural information, or vice versa).

In one study, 8-month-old infants' use of information about the solidity of objects was examined (Needham & Baillargeon, 1997). In this study, infants were shown a display with highly similar parts: two adjacent octagons (see Fig. 6.1). At the beginning of each test event, half of the infants were given information about the connection between the octagons: a thin metallic blade encased in a bright red wooden frame was placed beside the octagons for one group of infants (Fig. 6.1A) and between the octagons for another group (Fig. 6.1B). Next, a gloved hand took hold of the right octagon and pulled it a short distance to the side. Half of the infants saw both octagons move as a single unit (move-together event) and half saw the left octagon remain stationary as the right one was pulled (move-apart event). If the infants used the featural information to segregate the display, the infants who saw the blade pass beside the octagons would have seen the octagons as connected and looked longer at the move-apart than at the move-together event. If the infants used the physical information to segregate the display (and if they selected this interpretation in the face of conflicting featural information) the infants who saw the blade pass between the octagons would have seen the octagons as separate objects and looked longer at the move-together than at the move-apart event.

The results showed that the infants who saw the blade pass beside the octagons looked reliably longer at the move-apart than at the move-together event, suggesting that they perceived the octagons as comprising a single object. In contrast, the infants who saw the blade pass between the octagons looked

Blade-Beside Condition

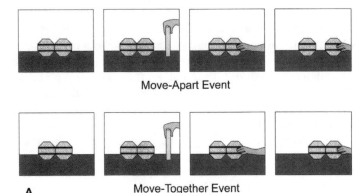

Move-Apart Event

A Move-Together Event

Blade-Between Condition

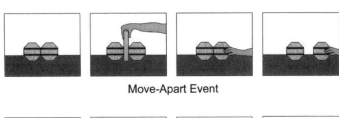

Move-Apart Event

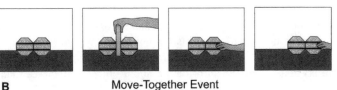

B Move-Together Event

FIG. 6.1. Test events involving octagons whose features indicate they compose a single unit. This information was all the infants in the blade-beside condition (Fig. 6.1A) presumably had to interpret the display. The infants in the blade-between condition (Fig. 6.1B) were also given information about the lack of a solid connection between the octagons as the blade passed through the two octagons. Reprinted from *Cognition, 62*, Needham, A. & Baillargeon, R. Object Segregation in 8-month-old infants, pp. 121–149. Copyright 1997, with permission from Elsevier Science.

reliably longer at the move-together than at the move-apart event, suggesting that they perceived the octagons as two separate units. These results suggest that the infants used both the featural and the physical information in the display to segregate the adjacent objects; when there was a conflict between the interpretations suggested by the two sources of information, infants chose the interpretation based on physical information over that based on featural information.

In a related study, Needham & Baillargeon (1997) examined 8-month-old infants' use of information about the support relations between two adjacent objects to segregate the display. The infants were shown two adjacent objects, a box and a cylinder, with markedly different featural properties (see Fig. 6.2). Half of the infants saw the cylinder resting on the apparatus floor (cylinder down), and half saw the cylinder suspended above the floor, with the box as its only visible means of support (cylinder up). If the infants used the features of the objects to segregate the display, they would see the cylinder-down display as composed of two separate units. However, if the infants used the physical information to segregate the display, they would see the cylinder-up display as composed of a single unit because the cylinder must have support and it must receive its support from the box. Once again, half of the infants saw the move-together event and half saw the move-apart event.

The results showed that the infants who saw the cylinder-down display looked reliably longer at the move-together than at the move-apart event, suggesting that they perceived the cylinder and box as separate objects. In contrast, the infants who saw the cylinder-up display looked reliably longer at the move-apart than at the move-together event, suggesting that they perceived the display as composed of a single unit. These results suggest that, by 8 months of age, infants can use the featural and physical information present in displays of adjacent objects to group their surfaces into separate units. Furthermore, when a conflict exists between the interpretations suggested by featural and physical information, infants choose the interpretation consistent with the physical information. These results also suggest that, like adults, infants may consider physical information to be a more accurate source of information about object boundaries than featural information.

Considered together, the results from these two experiments provide strong evidence that, by 8 months of age, infants can use both featural and physical information to form an interpretation of a display as consisting of one or two objects. When featural information is the only information available to form a clear interpretation of the display's composition, infants use this information to interpret the display. When both types of information are available, infants use physical information preferentially to interpret the displays, even if the featural information suggests a different interpretation. Like adults, infants may consider physical cues a more accurate source of information about object boundaries than featural cues, allowing the former to override the latter when determining the display's composition.

Cylinder-Down Condition

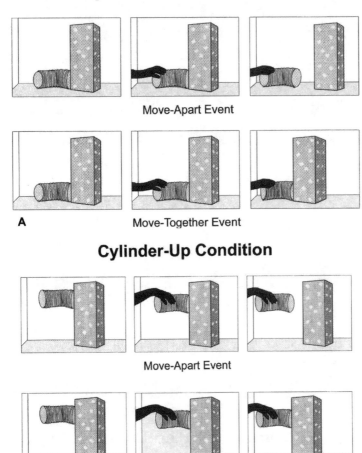

Move-Apart Event

A   Move-Together Event

Cylinder-Up Condition

Move-Apart Event

B   Move-Together Event

FIG. 6.2. Test events involving objects whose features indicate they compose separate units. This information was all the infants in the cylinder-down condition (Fig. 6.2A) presumably had to interpret the display. The infants in the cylinder-up condition (Fig. 6.2B) were also given information about the presence of a connection between the cylinder and box as the box seemed to provide the cylinder's only means of support. Reprinted from *Cognition, 62,* Needham, A. & Baillargeon, R. Object Segregation in 8-month-old infants, pp. 121–149. Copyright 1997, with permission from Elsevier Science.

Similar – Parallel Condition

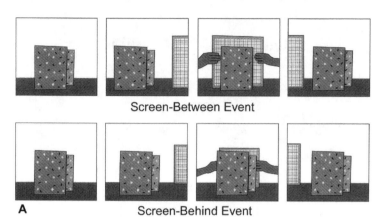

Screen-Between Event

A Screen-Behind Event

Similar – Angled Condition

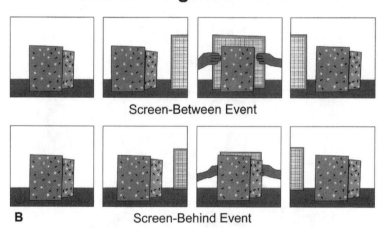

Screen-Between Event

B Screen-Behind Event

Dissimilar – Angled Condition

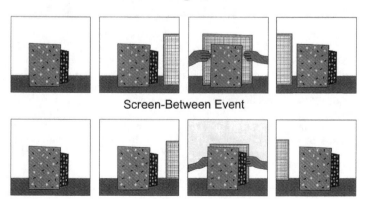

Screen-Between Event

212 **C** Screen-Behind Event

INFANTS' USE OF SPATIAL AND FEATURAL INFORMATION

Additional evidence to support this claim comes from a study on infants' use of spatial information (derived from the spatial layout of the objects in the display) and featural information to segregate a display. We investigated the interaction of infants' use of spatial and featural information in a set of experiments in which 9.5-month-old infants were shown one of three displays (see Fig. 6.3). In the similar-parallel display, two identical boxes, one partially in front of the other, were positioned with their front surfaces parallel to each other (and perpendicular to the infants' line of sight). There were two angled displays, in which the back box was angled toward the front box in such a way that it was not clear whether the boxes intersected. One of the angled displays consisted of two identical boxes (similar-angled display) and the other consisted of two boxes with highly discrepant colors and patterns (dissimilar-angled display).

In the test events, the objects were stationary, while a large screen moved either between or behind the objects. If the infants posited a connection between the boxes, they would look longer when the screen passed between the boxes than when it passed behind the boxes. The results showed that the infants who saw the similar-angled display looked reliably longer when the screen passed between the boxes than when it passed behind them, indicating that the infants saw the boxes as connected and were surprised to see the screen pass through the connection. In contrast, the infants who saw the similar-parallel display and those who saw the dissimilar-angled display looked about equally whether the screen passed between or behind the boxes, indicating that the infants who saw these displays expected no connection between the boxes.

These results suggest two conclusions about infants' use of different sources of information in object segregation. First, because the infants saw the similar-parallel display as composed of two separate units, despite the similarity in the featural properties of the boxes, it seems that infants use spatial information instead of featural information to segregate the display. Second, when spatial information

---

FIG. 6.3. (facing page) Test events involving objects whose spatial arrangements indicate no connection between them (the parallel display shown in Fig. 6.3A) or are ambiguous as to whether there is a connection (the angled displays shown in Fig. 6.3, parts B and C). The objects in the similar-angled display (shown in Fig. 6.3B) had features indicating they were connected; the objects in the dissimilar-angled display (shown in Fig. 6.3C) had features indicating they were separate. Reprinted from *Early Development and Parenting*, 6, Needham, A. & Kaufman, J., Infants' integration of information from different sources in object segregation, pp. 137–147. Copyright 1997, with permission from John Wiley and Sons.

did not lead to a clear interpretation of the display, as in the similar-angled and dissimilar-angled displays, the infants did use the featural information to accomplish this task. Specifically, different featural information (similar or dissimilar boxes) led infants to different interpretations of the displays (as composed of one or two units, respectively). As with physical information, when clear spatial information was available, the infants used this information preferentially to segregate the display. When the spatial information was ambiguous, the infants resorted to using the featural information to accomplish this task.

Together, the results of these three experiments support the claim that, by 8 to 9.5 months of age, infants have a hierarchy of kinds of information used to segregate displays. When multiple sources of information are available, infants tend to use the information that will provide the most accurate interpretation of the display (i.e., either physical or spatial information). However, when a source of information with high ecological validity is not available, infants will form interpretations based only on the available information (in these experiments, featural information).

DEVELOPMENT OF THE USE OF FEATURAL INFORMATION

The experiments described in the previous sections indicate that, by 8 months of age, infants use featural information to group object surfaces into units. But at what point in development does this ability arise? A recently proposed model suggests that the use of featural information to segregate displays depends on a few accomplishments (Needham et al., 1997). First, the infants must be able to detect the features in the display, so basic visual capacities such as acuity and color perception must be sufficiently developed. Second, the infants must have the knowledge that would allow them to interpret the featural information. That is, the infants must have featural knowledge, or the knowledge that abrupt changes in surfaces' featural properties are indications of an object boundary, and that similarity in surfaces' featural properties is an indicator that the surfaces belong to the same unit. And last, infants must be able to process (encode, compare, represent) the featural information present in a display. Lacking any of these three abilities (i.e., a failure in the detection or the processing of the featural information or a lack of featural knowledge) would lead to an indeterminate perception of a display. Conversely, a failure to use featural information to segregate a display could be the result of a failure in any of these three processes.

Because prior research led to conflicting estimates of the age at which infants begin to use object features to segregate displays (e.g., Craton, 1996; Spelke, Breinlinger, Jacobson, & Phillips, 1993), one possibility was that success in segregation tasks could depend on the specific features of the objects in the displays used in these studies. To investigate this possibility, Needham (1998) explored the development of infants' segregation of more and less complex displays.

In this series of studies, Needham (1998) used the cylinder-and-box display that had been used in a prior study of 8-month-old infants' object segregation (see Fig. 6.2A). This set of studies examined 4.5-, 6.5-, and 7.5-month-old infants' segregation of the display by presenting them with the same events as the 8-month-olds saw in the previous study (Needham, 1998; Needham & Baillargeon, 1998). The results showed that the 4.5- and the 6.5-month-old infants looked about equally at the move-apart and move-together events, suggesting that the prominent differences in the objects' shapes, colors, and patterns did not clearly indicate to the infants that the cylinder and box were separate objects. In contrast, the 7.5-month-old infants, like the 8-month-old infants in the previous study, looked reliably longer at the move-together than at the move-apart event, indicating that they saw the display as composed of two separate units.

These results could lead one to conclude that infants develop the ability to use featural information to segregate objects between 6.5 and 7.5 months of age, a finding that is in agreement with some prior research using partly occluded objects (Craton, 1996). However, when the features of the cylinder and box were simplified somewhat (the cylinder was straightened and the box was turned so that a side, rather than a corner, faced the infants; see Fig. 6.4), both the 4.5- and 6.5-month-old infants looked reliably longer at the move-together than at the move-apart event,

Simplified Cylinder-and-Box Condition

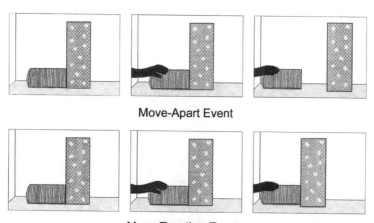

Move-Apart Event

Move-Together Event

FIG. 6.4. Test events featuring the simplified version of the cylinder-and-box display, in which a straightened cylinder was paired with the test box, which was oriented such that one of its sides faced the infant. Reprinted from *Infant Behavior and Development, 21*, Needham, A., Infants' use of featural information in the segregation of stationary objects, pp. 47–76. Copyright 1998, with permission from Elsevier Science.

indicating that they perceived the simplified display as consisting of two separate units. These and control results indicated that infants as young as 4.5 months of age have the knowledge that different-looking surfaces typically belong to different objects, but they are only able to use this knowledge to form clear interpretations of displays when the features of the objects in the display are simple to process.

We believe that the best interpretation of these findings is that when the features in a display are too difficult for infants to process, infants are unable to go further in the segregation process and instead produce an ambiguous interpretation for the display. The finding that young infants can use object features to segregate displays has been extended to partly occluded displays as well. In this work, Needham (1998) determined that infants perceive partly occluded versions of the cylinder and box display (see Fig. 6.5) just as they perceive the fully visible cylinder and box. If infants' perception of fully visible and boundary occluded versions of these displays is identical, then infants' interpretations of these displays cannot depend critically on the appearance of the boundary itself. Also, another set of studies indicates that infants perceive partly occluded displays with visible portions that are either highly similar or highly dissimilar in accordance with their featural properties (see Fig. 6.6; see Needham, Baillargeon, & Kaufman, 1997).

Occluded Cylinder-and-Box Displays

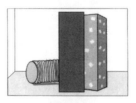

Curved

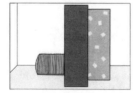

Simplified

FIG. 6.5. Boundary-occluded versions of the displays involving the curved and straight cylinders. Infants interpreted these displays in the same way they interpreted fully visible versions of the displays, indicating that the boundary information was not critical to their interpretation of the displays.

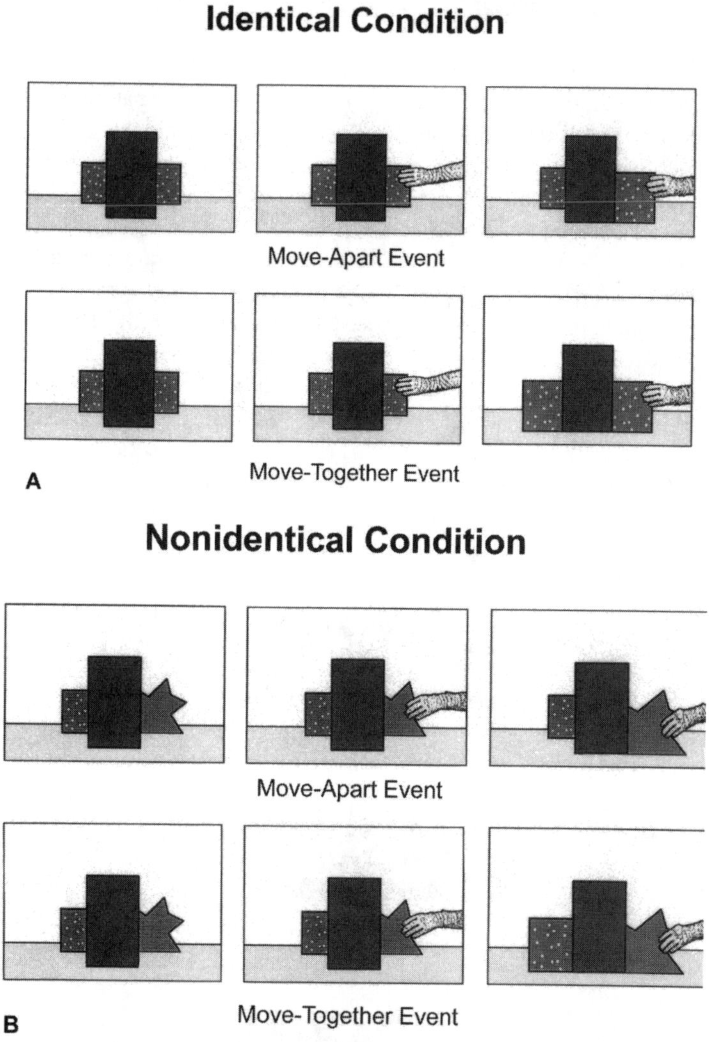

Identical Condition

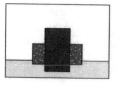 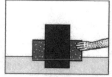 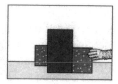

Move-Apart Event

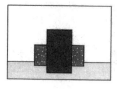 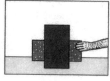 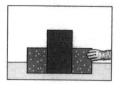

A   Move-Together Event

Nonidentical Condition

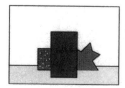 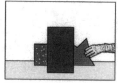 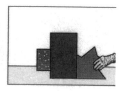

Move-Apart Event

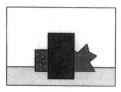 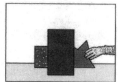 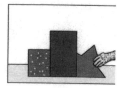

B   Move-Together Event

FIG. 6.6. Test events involving partly occluded objects whose visible portions were either identical to each other (identical condition shown in Fig. 6.6A) or were different in shape, color, and pattern (nonidentical condition shown in Fig. 6.6B). Four-month-old infants perceived the identical display as a single object behind the screen; they perceived the nonidentical display as two objects behind the screen. Reprinted from *Advances in Infancy Research*, Vol. 11, Needham, A., Baillargeon, R., & Kaufman, L., Object segregation in infancy, pp. 1–44. Copyright 1997, with permission from Greenwood Publishing Group.

USE OF INDIVIDUAL FEATURES

So far, we have referred to featural information as though it were a single unitary source of information. It is possible that infants use the information in a global or aggregate way as this term suggests, but it also seems possible that certain features of the objects are used and others are ignored. This question of which features are most useful to infants, and whether that changes with development, is the focus of this section of the chapter.

Our approach to this question was informed by the literature on adult object segmentation, which focused considerable attention on the use of object shape to parse displays (e.g., the minima rule, Hoffman & Richards, 1984). Thus, in the first study, Needham (1999) chose to ask whether 4-month-old infants would use shape or color and pattern to segregate two adjacent objects. In one display (similar display), all of the features that could reasonably be manipulated on a real object were designed to lead to the interpretation of the display as a single unit (see Fig. 6.7). Two conflict displays were also created (dissimilar-shape display and dissimilar-color-and-pattern display), in which shape led to one interpretation of the display and color and pattern led to a different interpretation. The research

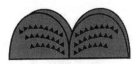

Similar Display

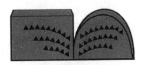

Dissimilar-Shape Display

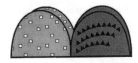

Dissimilar-Color-
and-Pattern Display

FIG. 6.7. Displays used to investigate infants' use of individual features when segregating objects. The top display involves no conflict between features: Shape, color, and pattern lead to the interpretation of a single unit. In the middle and bottom displays, shape leads to an interpretation different from color and pattern.

goal was that using these conflict displays would help determine whether one of these sources of featural information was relied on more than the other. Such a strategy has proved successful in previous research (Needham & Baillargeon, 1997; Needham & Kaufman, 1997).

As in previous studies, half of the infants seeing each display saw the move-apart event, and half saw the move-together event. Again, the reasoning was that infants' interpretation of the displays would reveal itself by producing longer looking at the unexpected event: Longer looking at the move-apart event would indicate an interpretation of a single unit, whereas longer looking at the move-together event would indicate an interpretation of two separate units. The results showed that the infants who saw the similar display and the dissimilar-color-and-pattern display looked reliably longer at the move-apart than at the move-together test event, indicating that they perceived the display as composed of a single unit. In contrast, the infants who saw the dissimilar-shape display looked reliably longer at the move-together than at the move-apart event, indicating that they perceived the display as composed of two separate units. These results (and those from a control condition) suggest that at 4 months of age, when infants may be just beginning to use features to define object boundaries, object shape may be the feature they attend to most.

To further explore this conclusion, another study was conducted using analogous displays with a more salient color and pattern (Kaufman & Needham, 2003). In this study, 4-month-old infants were shown move-apart or move-together test events featuring one of the displays shown in Fig. 6.8. The top display shows the dissimilar-shape version of the display, and the bottom display shows the similar-shape version. Another goal of this study was to explore infants' use of the boundary seam dividing the two portions of the display as a source of information to segregate the display. Accordingly, versions of both displays were created that did not have a boundary seam. Thus, for each display, the infants' looking times at three events were compared: (1) the move-apart event, (2) the move-together event featuring a display with a boundary seam, and (3) the move-together event featuring a display without a boundary seam. Infants' use of boundary seam, shape, and color and pattern was assessed by comparing the boundary seam and no-boundary seam conditions, as well as the dissimilar-shape and similar-shape displays.

The results were somewhat similar to those described in the previous study, in that it was clear that the infants used shape, rather than color and pattern, to segregate the objects in these displays. So it seems unlikely that the results from the initial study were related to the specific manipulation of color and pattern that was undertaken in that study. Second, the results indicated that the infants did make use of the boundary seam when segregating the dissimilar-shape, but not the similar-shape, display. This result may reflect an interdependence of these two sources of information. Specifically, the boundary seam may be salient when following the outer edge of the objects brings one's eye right to the boundary

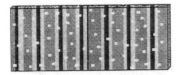

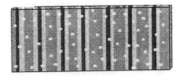

Box-Box Display
(With Boundary Seam)

Box-Box Display
(Without Boundary Seam)

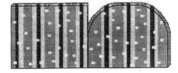

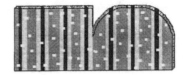

Box-Hump Display
(With Boundary Seam)

Box-Hump Display
(Without Boundary Seam)

FIG. 6.8.   Displays used to examine infants' use of shape, boundary seam, and color and pattern in determining the boundaries between objects. The displays contained parts of the same shape (the displays on the top) or different shape (the displays on the bottom) and either contained a boundary seam between the parts (the displays on the left side) or did not (the displays on the right side).

seam. In contrast, the boundary seam in the similar-shape display may be camouflaged by the series of vertical lines on the surface of the display, so it may not be seen as a seam that could carry information about the composition of the display. Finally, consistent with Needham's (1999) findings, object shape is the source of information infants rely on most when determining the boundaries in a display.

We are currently investigating the development of infants' use of shape and color and pattern later in infancy, and we are focusing on the question of when infants develop the ability to use color and pattern to define object boundaries (Ormsbee & Needham, 2003). Our initial findings regarding this question using the same displays as Needham (1999) are that they have begun to do so by 8 months of age. Infants may even overuse color and pattern at this age, relying on these features even more than shape. This phenomenon is reminiscent of overregularization in language development, in which children temporarily overuse rules for forming past tenses or plurals, extending them to irregular forms (e.g., "goed" or "wented" instead of "went"). Further study involving infants older than 8 months of age will explore infants' use of these sources of featural information toward the end of the 1st year of life.

THE ROLE OF INFANTS' OBJECT
EXPLORATION SKILLS

One contributor to the development of infants' object segregation abilities could be improvements in their object exploration abilities. Research by Rochat (1989) indicates that infants go through major advances in their oral, visual, and manual object exploration between 2 and 5 months of age. Specifically, infants at 5 months of age direct significantly more oral and visual exploration toward objects they are holding than they did at 2 months of age, and this exploration becomes more coordinated, with more switching back and forth between the oral and visual modalities. Further, there is evidence for a transition in the modality infants choose for initial exploration of an object between 3 and 4 months of age: At 2 and 3 months, infants choose to explore an object orally first; at 4 and 5 months, infants choose to explore an object visually first. Finally, at around 4 months of age, infants begin to coordinate visual and manual exploration through a more complex behavior Rochat calls fingering, in which infants run their fingers over the edges of an object. All of these findings point to important transitions in infants' object exploration skills occurring around 3 to 4 months of age.

To explore possible connections between infants' object exploration and object segregation abilities, the segregation abilities of infants younger than 4 months of age needed to be examined to determine whether this was in fact a period of transition in this domain as well. Prior research from other labs (Kestenbaum, Termine, & Spelke, 1987) suggested that 3-month-old infants tend not to use object features to define object boundaries, but Needham (2000) wanted to assess these abilities using a display that had been shown to be accurately segregated by 4-month-old infants.

In this study (Needham, 2000), older and younger 3-month-old infants were shown the simplified cylinder and box display and either the move-apart or the move-together test events used in previous research (see Fig. 6.4; Needham, 1998). The results showed that the younger 3-month-olds tended to see the display as a single unit, whereas the older 3-month-olds tended to see the display as composed of two separate units. In a second study, the display was changed to one in which the two parts of the display had very similar features (see Fig. 6.9). The infants' responses to the move-apart and move-together test events involving this display suggested that both older and younger infants perceived the display as consisting of a single unit. Together, the results of these two experiments suggest that in the weeks prior to turning 4 months of age, infants begin to use object features to define object boundaries. With this new ability, infants are able to segregate the cylinder-box display into two separate units, while their perception of the box-box display remains unchanged. This pattern of results is consistent with the notion that prior to using features to define object boundaries, infants

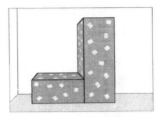

Box-Box Display

FIG. 6.9.   Display with two similar parts used to investigate the early
development of infants' object segregation.

perceive adjacent surfaces as connected in a single unit. Once object features
begin to be used, more accurate feature-based interpretations replace the primitive interpretations that are based only on whether the objects are adjacent or
not. This developmental framework is consistent with that formulated by Alan
Slater and his colleagues to characterize the development of infants' perception
of partly occluded objects (Slater, Morison, Somers, Mattock, Brown, & Taylor,
1990).

The findings from this study suggest that infants' ability to use features to segregate at least some objects from each other develops at or just before 4 months
of age. The correspondence in ages between the transition in infants' object exploration and the transition in infants' object segregation led us to further explore
the possible connection between these two abilities. Needham (2000) chose to
examine this connection by giving the same group of infants an exploration task
and a segregation task to see whether there would be a correspondence between
their performance in the two tasks.

In this study, infants were first given a series of objects to explore orally, visually, and manually (see Fig. 6.10). Each object was placed in the infant's hands
and his or her exploration behavior was videotaped. Next, the infant was given
an object segregation task using the simplified cylinder-box display used in previous research (Needham, 1998). As in prior work, each infant was shown either the move-apart or the move-together test event, and their looking time was
measured. Because completely different objects were used in the exploration and
segregation phases of the study, the goal was to determine whether a given infant was a more or less active explorer of objects in general and then determine
whether this corresponded to a particular kind of performance in the segregation
task.

Infants' object exploration strategies were characterized as more or less active
by measuring the percentage of the time they chose to visually or orally explore
an object that was placed in their hands. Infants who spent more than two thirds
of their time exploring the objects were classified as more-active explorers, and
those who spent less than two thirds of their time exploring were classified as

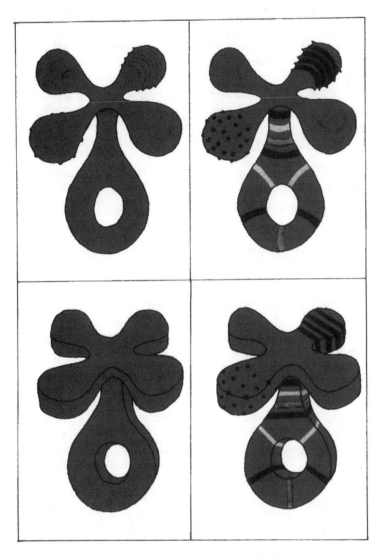

FIG. 6.10. Red teether objects used to assess infants' exploration skills. Infants were classified as high or low explorers, depending on the proportion of time they spent visually or orally exploring the objects. Reprinted from *Journal of Cognition and Development, 1,* Needham, A., Improvements in object exploration skills facilitate the development of object segregation in early infancy, pp. 131–156. Copyright 2000, with permission from Lawrence Erlbaum Associates.

less-active explorers. Looking at the more- and less-active exploring infants' performance in the object segregation task revealed that the more-active explorers looked reliably longer at the move-together than at the move-apart event, indicating that they had successfully segregated the cylinder and box into separate units. In contrast, the less-active exploring infants looked about equally at the two test events, indicating that they were unsure of the composition of the display. These findings indicate a connection between infants' exploration and segregation abilities. The hypothesis we are currently pursuing is that more-actively exploring infants learn more about the objects in their environment and as a result begin to use object features to define object boundaries earlier than less-actively exploring infants.

These findings offer preliminary, but intriguing, evidence that infants' own exploration of objects facilitates their learning about how object features can be used to define object boundaries.

USE OF PRIOR EXPERIENCE IN OBJECT SEGREGATION

One might be concerned that young infants would perceive all displays for which shape did not clearly specify object connections as ambiguous, but our work has shown that this is unlikely to be true. Specifically, infants' prior encounters with objects help them interpret displays that would otherwise be ambiguous. In one series of studies, infants who were not be able to segregate the objects in a display during their first encounter with it could segregate the objects if the infants had even a brief prior exposure to one of the objects in the display alone (Needham & Baillargeon, 1998). Further studies have indicated that changes in the features of the objects between infants' first and second encounters with them seem to prevent this facilitative effect, although changes in the spatial orientation of an object do not prevent the effect (Needham, 2001).

We are currently exploring how object knowledge is generalized over collections of objects. Specifically, as infants acquire knowledge about the categories of objects that make up the world, they may use this knowledge to help them interpret displays that would otherwise be ambiguous or that would be incorrectly parsed using object features (Needham, Dueker, & Lockhead, 2003). As in the hierarchy of information use described previously, infants may rely on the general rules about featural information to interpret displays if no additional knowledge can be brought to bear. However, when parsing a display consisting of categories of previously seen objects, infants may bypass these general rules and use category knowledge instead. This process is probably similar to that studied by Goldstone (this volume) in adults.

LIMITATIONS IN INFANTS' OBJECT SEGREGATION: KNOWLEDGE SPECIFICITY

Knowledge specificity has been found in a number of other domains, both within infant cognitive development (e.g., Baillargeon, 1994) and in other areas of infant development (e.g., motor development; see Adolph, 1997). The main idea here is that infants develop knowledge or ability in one narrow area and then fail to generalize to other areas that seem to rely on the same knowledge. For example, Baillargeon proposed that infants acquire separate tracks of knowledge about a variety of different event categories—superficially different kinds of events that may actually rely on the same underlying physical principle. For example, she found that infants are much better at forming expectations about when an object should be visible or not when it is in an occlusion context rather than a containment context (Hespos & Baillargeon, 2001). In seemingly unrelated work, Karen Adolph (1997) found that knowledge infants acquire about traversing potentially dangerous slopes as crawlers does not help them in these same situations once they begin to walk. Rather, infants seem to need to learn all over again which slopes are safe and which are dangerous once they begin walking.

This notion of knowledge specificity discussed by both Baillargeon and Adolph could be relevant for the development of object segregation as well. Specifically, the results of a set of recent studies from our lab suggest that infants develop skills that allow them to segregate objects setting side by side (as all of the studies we have described from our lab have involved), but that these skills may not allow them to segregate objects setting on top of other objects (Needham, 2003).

As described previously, when infants around 4 months of age are shown a simple, straight cylinder next to a tall, rectangular box (Fig. 6.11 top), they expect the two objects to be separate. However, when the display is turned on its side so that the cylinder is on top of, rather than next to the box, infants do not parse the display until they are somewhat older—about 12.5 months of age.

In these studies, infants were shown a display composed of the same two objects as in previous research (e.g., Needham 1998, 2000), but, instead of both objects being supported by the floor of the apparatus, the cylinder was supported by the box (see Fig. 6.11 bottom). The infants were shown test events in which a gloved hand grasped the cylinder and raised it into the air: Half of the infants saw the cylinder move apart from the box, which remained stationary throughout the event, and half saw the box move with the cylinder when it was pulled. Infants at four different ages were used in this study: 4.5-month-old infants, 6.5-month-old infants, 8-month-old infants, and 12.5-month-old infants.

The results showed an interesting developmental progression. The 4.5-month-old infants looked reliably longer at the move-apart event than at the move-together event, indicating that they perceived the display as clearly composed of a single

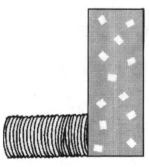

Side-by-Side Display

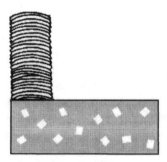

Stacked Display

FIG. 6.11.   Displays used to examine knowledge specificity in object segregation. Both displays were composed of the same cylinder and box. The top display shows them setting side by side; the bottom display shows the cylinder stacked on top of the box.

object. Both the 6.5- and 8-month-old infants looked about equally at the two test events, suggesting that the display was ambiguous for them. Finally, the infants at 12.5 months of age looked reliably longer at the move-together than at the move-apart event, indicating that they interpreted the display to consist of two separate objects, one setting on top of the other.

Thus, when the objects are stacked rather then placed side by side, the age at which infants can clearly interpret the display as two separate objects is 12.5 months rather than 4 months. This set of results suggests that infants may learn how to segregate specific kinds of object scenarios rather than developing and using very general rules for parsing objects regardless of orientation.

One reason for this discrepancy could be that infants probably often see stacked objects moving together, such as when food is carried on a plate, a doll rides in a toy car, or a stack of towels is carried in a laundry basket. Examples of separate side-by-side objects moving together in this way are much harder to imagine.

Infants' own actions on objects may not clarify the situation, either: Depending on whether they grasp the top or the bottom object, stacked objects that are separate may or may not move together. Because common motion is likely to be a very strong cue for object connectedness, infants may initially learn different rules for parsing side-by-side and stacked objects.

MECHANISMS OF DEVELOPMENT IN OBJECT SEGREGATION

What processes contribute to the development of object segregation in infancy? Three kinds of factors may influence the developmental changes described in this chapter: observational factors, basic visual development, and neural factors. First, we think it is likely that infants learn about the presence and absence of connections between adjacent object surfaces from their observations of other people interacting with objects. These observations could occur at some distance (i.e., not performed for or even near the infant), limited only by infants' attention and visual acuity. In addition, we presented evidence to suggest that infants' object exploration skills contribute to their segregation abilities, presumably by giving them more opportunities to learn about the relation between feature changes and object boundaries firsthand. As other researchers have recently noted, self-produced observations may be especially useful in learning (Campos, Anderson, Barbu-Roth, Hubbard, Hertenstein, & Witherington, 2000). In this context, infants' own object explorations may provide them with salient and well-timed information from which to learn about the relation between object features and object boundaries.

Second, the developing visual system also constrains and shapes infants' behaviors. The obvious limitations of the infant's visual system, as exemplified by relatively poor visual acuity and oculomotor control, have been well documented and will not be repeated here. It is worth noting, however, that particular visual development trajectories may underlie the hierarchy of useful object information detailed previously. For example, infants' early tendency to use object shape rather than color may be explained by the lag in infants' color perception abilities compared with overall visual acuity. Infants' ability to see color is not fully mature until 4 months of age (Teller & Bornstein, 1987). Moreover, infants' ability to use color information in cognitive tasks such as object individuation seems to lag even further behind, with infants not succeeding until almost 12 months of age (Tremoulet, Leslie, & Hall, 2000; Wilcox, 1999). These findings are also consistent with the idea that infants prefer to use more ecologically valid cues when given the choice: Shape is a fairly reliable indicator of object boundaries, whereas color, with its massive variability, is not. This may also reflect that shape is multimodal information, available visually, orally, and manually; color, on the other hand, is a purely visual phenomenon.

Third, and most speculatively at this point, is the role of the developing neural system. The brain continues to develop and organize well into childhood, and the role of the brain in behavior continues to tantalize researchers. Some speculation, we believe, is warranted and will doubtless be supplanted as more research examines this exciting topic.

In visual perception, two processing pathways have been identified in primate brains: a dorsal or where/action pathway and a ventral or what/sensation pathway (Livingstone & Hubel, 1988; Milner & Goodale, 1995; Ungerleider & Mishkin, 1982). Each pathway is thought to receive different types of information about the visual world, but the integration and rate of development of each remains largely unknown. (For a detailed discussion of what is known, see Johnson et al., 2001.)

It is attractive to suppose that the progression of infants' object segregation abilities, as well as the hierarchy of information used in this task, is reflected by the relative development of these two different pathways. For example, the ventral pathway subserves featural information such as shape and color, whereas the dorsal pathways subserves spatial and motion information. Could infants' prioritizing of spatial/physical information be due to the earlier development of the dorsal pathway, as compared with the ventral pathway? Further, the relation among types of featural information (shape, color, pattern) suggests that components of the ventral pathway develop individually and in progression, rather than as a unit.

This formulation remains somewhat simplistic, but at this early stage in the new field of developmental cognitive neuroscience, simple ideas must be tested to discover more complex truths. It seems clear that the study of these pathways is relevant for object segregation—after all, our tasks require infants to use these very components of visual perception. However, the relationships here are still tentative and await further study.

CONCLUSIONS

There are a number of conclusions we would like to focus on from the research presented previously, which will be discussed in turn.

Combining of Physical and Featural Information in Object Segregation

By 8 months of age, and possibly earlier, infants use both featural (e.g., shape, color, pattern) and physical (e.g., support, solidity, spatial arrangement) information to segregate objects. Even though features are available and interpretable by infants at this age, they tend not to use that information if (more reliable) physical information about the relations between objects is also available. Thus, we found that 8- to 9.5-month-old infants systematically use physical information instead of featural information to interpret displays, when both sources of information are available.

Development of Use of Object Features to Define Object Boundaries

Infants regard object features as indicators for object boundaries as early as 4 months of age for simple displays. We have some evidence that this early ability may develop at least in part because of improvements in infants' object exploration skills. Thus, improvements in infants' exploration of object features may lead to learning about the relations between object features and object boundaries.

Further experiments show that early in development, object shape seems to be the most useful feature for infants as they determine the boundaries between objects. Preliminary data from older infants suggests that color and pattern become more important (and shape less important) later in the 1st year of life as infants learn more about the multiple ways in which object boundaries can be predicted.

Learning and Object Segregation

Our research shows that infants use prior experiences with specific objects and groups of objects to facilitate their segregation of the objects in a display. The results of these studies suggest that (a) infants attend to object features, rather than irrelevant cues such as their spatial orientation, when determining whether they have seen an object before as an individual entity; (b) when infants believe they have seen an object before as an individual entity, they expect it will be an individual entity in its current display as well; and (c) infants acquire knowledge pertaining to categories of objects (e.g., the shape of an individual entity in this category) that they then apply to new members considered to belong to that category.

The role of learning in object segregation is also demonstrated by noting the differences in infants' segregation of objects that set side by side and those that are stacked on top of each other. Our findings suggest that infants know quite a bit about how features can be used to segregate objects that are side by side by 4.5 months of age but that this knowledge is not extended to objects that are stacked on top of each other until the end of the 1st year of life.

Final Thoughts

The findings presented in this paper highlight the many strengths and weaknesses in infants' early object segregation abilities and point to some interesting developmental processes that may underlie these changes. Future research on these and related topics will add much to our understanding of the development of perceptual organization during the 1st year of life and how developments in brain and behavior influence these changes.

ACKNOWLEDGMENTS

The research described in this chapter was supported by NICHD grants (FIRST grant HD-32129 and grant HD-37049) to the first author. We would like to thank the following individuals for their contributions to the research presented in this chapter: Tracy Barrett, Gwenden Dueker, Jordy Kaufman, Avani Modi, Ruth Ormsbee, Lubna Zaeem, the undergraduate students working in the Infant Perception Lab at Duke University, and the parents and babies who participated in the studies summarized here. Contact the first author at the Department of Psychological and Brain Sciences, Duke University, Durham, NC 27708-0086. E-mail: amy.needham@duke.edu.

REFERENCES

Adolph, K. E. (1997). Learning in the development of infant locomotion. *Monographs of the Society for Research in Child Development, 62* (Serial No. 251).

Baillargeon, R. (1994). How do infants learn about the physical world? *Current Directions in Psychological Science, 3,* 133–140.

Biederman, I. (1987). Recognition-by-components: A theory of human image understanding. *Psychological Review, 94,* 115–147.

Bornstein, M. H. (1985). Habituation of attention as a measure of visual information processing in human infants. In G. Gottlieb & N. Krasnegor (Eds.), *Measurement of audition and vision in the first year of postnatal life* (pp. 253–300). Norwood, NJ: Ablex.

Campos, J. J. Anderson, D. I., Barbu-Roth, M. A., Hubbard, E. M., Hertenstein, M. J., & Witherington, D. (2000). Travel broadens the mind. *Infancy, 1,* 149–219.

Craton, L. G. (1996). The development of perceptual completion abilities: infants' perception of stationary, partly occluded objects. *Child Development, 67,* 890–904.

Fodor, J. (1983). *The modularity of mind.* Cambridge, MA: MIT Press.

Gibson, J. J. (1979). *The ecological approach to visual perception.* Boston: Houghton Mifflin.

Hespos, S. J., & Baillargeon, R. (2001). Infants' knowledge about occlusion and containment events: A surprising discrepancy. *Psychological Science, 121,* 141–147.

Hoffman, D. D., & Richards, W. A. (1984). Parts of recognition. *Cognition, 18,* 65–96.

Johnson, S. P. (1997). Young infants' perception of object unity: Implications for development of attentional and cognitive skills. *Current Directions in Psychological Science, 6,* 5–11.

Johnson, M. H., Mareschal, D., & Csibra, G. (2001). The functional development and integration of the dorsal and visual pathways: a neurocomputational approach. In C. A. Nelson and M. Luciana (Eds.), *Handbook of Developmental cognitive neuroscience.* Cambridge. Mass: MIT Press.

Kaufman, J., & Needham, A. (2003). *The role of shape and boundary seam in 4-month-old infants' object segregation.* Manuscript submitted for publication.

Kellman, P. J., & Spelke, E. S. (1983). Perception of partly occluded objects in infancy. *Cognitive Psychology, 15,* 483–524.

Kestenbaum, R., Termine, N., & Spelke, E. S. (1987). Perception of objects and object boundaries by three-month-old infants. *British Journal of Developmental Psychology, 5,* 367–383.

Kimchi, R., & Hadad, B.-S. (2002). Influence of past experience on perceptual grouping. *Psychological Science, 13,* 41–47.

Livingstone, M., & Hubel, D. (1988). Segregation of form, color, movement, and depth: Anatomy, physiology, and perception. *Science, 240,* 740–749.

Milner, A. D., & Goodale, M. A. (1995). *The visual brain in action.* Oxford, UK: Oxford University Press.

Needham, A. (1997). Factors affecting infants' use of featural information in object segregation. *Current Directions in Psychological Science, 6,* 26–33.

Needham, A. (1998). Infants' use of featural information in the segregation of stationary objects. *Infant Behavior and Development, 21,* 47–76.

Needham, A. (1999). The role of shape in 4-month-old infants' segregation of adjacent objects. *Infant Behavior and Development, 22,* 161–178.

Needham, A. (2000). Improvements in object exploration skills may facilitate the development of object segregation in early infancy. *Journal of Cognition and Development, 1,* 131–156.

Needham, A. (2001). Object recognition and object segregation in 4.5-month-old infants'. *Journal of Experimental Child Psychology, 78,* 3–24.

Needham, A. (2003). *Knowledge specificity in object segregation: Infants' perception of side-by-side versus stacked objects.* Manuscript submitted for publication.

Needham, A., & Baillargeon, R. (1997). Object segregation in 8-month-old infants. *Cognition, 62,* 121–149.

Needham, A., & Baillargeon, R. (1998). Effects of prior experience in 4.5-month-old infants' object segregation. *Infant Behavior and Development, 21,* 1–24.

Needham, A., Baillargeon, R., & Kaufman, L. (1997). Object segregation in infancy. In C. Rovee-Collier & L. Lipsitt (Eds.), *Advances in infancy research* (Vol. 11, pp. 1–44). Greenwich, CT: Ablex.

Needham, A., Dueker, G. & Lockhead, G. (2003). I've seen that kind of thing before: Infants' formation and use of categories to segregate objects. Manuscript submitted for publication.

Needham, A., & Kaufman, J. (1997). Infants' integration of information from different sources in object segregation. *Early Development and Parenting, 6,* 137–147.

Ormsbee, S. M., & Needham, A. (2003). *The development of infants' use of shape, color, and pattern in object segregation.* Manuscript submitted for publication.

Palmer, S. E. (1999). *Vision science: Photons to phenomenology.* Cambridge, MA: MIT Press.

Peterson, M. A. (1994). Object recognition processes can and do operate before figure-ground organization. *Current Directions in Psychological Science, 3,* 105–111.

Rochat, P. (1989). Object manipulation and exploration in 2- to 5-month-old infants. *Developmental Psychology, 25,* 871–884.

Rock, I. (1983). *The logic of perception.* Cambridge, MA: MIT Press.

Shepard, R. (1983). Ecological constraints on internal representation: Resonant kinematics of perceiving, imagining, thinking, and dreaming. *Psychological Review, 91,* 417–447.

Slater, A., Morison, V., Somers, M., Mattock, A., Brown, E., & Taylor, D. (1990). Newborn and older infants' perception of partly occluded objects. *Infant Behavior and Development, 13,* 33–49.

Spelke, E. S. (1985). Preferential looking methods as tools for the study of cognition in infancy. In G. Gottlieb & N. Krasnegor (Eds.), *Measurement of audition and vision in the first year of postnatal life* (pp. 323–363). Norwood, NJ: Ablex.

Spelke, E. S., Breinlinger, K., Jacobson, K., & Phillips, A. (1993). Gestalt relations and object perception: A developmental study. *Perception, 22,* 1483–1501.

Spelke, E. S., Breinlinger, K., Macomber, J., & Jacobson, K. (1992). Origins of knowledge. *Psychological Review, 99,* 605–632.

Teller, D. Y., & Bornstein, M. H. (1987). Infant color vision and color perception. In P. Salapatek & L. Cohen (Eds.), *Handbook of infant perception: From sensation to perception* (Vol. 1, pp. 185–236). New York: Academic Press.

Tremoulet, P. D., Leslie, A. M., & Hall, D. G. (2000). Infant individuation and identification of objects. *Cognitive Development, 15,* 499–522.

Ungerleider, L. G., & Mishkin, M. (1982). Two cortical systems. In D. J. Ingle, M. A. Goodale, & R. J. W. Mansfield (Eds.), *Analysis of visual behavior* (pp. 549–585). Cambridge, MA: MIT Press.

Wilcox, T. (1999). Object individuation: Infants' use of shape, size, pattern, and color. *Cognition, 72,* 125–166.

7 Learning to Perceive While Perceiving to Learn

Robert L. Goldstone
Indiana University

The world we experience is formed by our perceptual processing. However, it is not viciously circular to argue that our perceptual systems are reciprocally formed by our experiences. In fact, it is because our experiences are necessarily based on our perceptual systems that these perceptual systems must be shaped so that our experiences are appropriate and useful for dealing with our world.

The notion that our perceptions are experience driven has been construed as everything from mundane to magical. At the mundane (at least, well-understood) pole, much is known of the mechanisms underlying simple sensitization and habituation. Through sensitization, repetitive presentation of a stimulus leads to increased sensory response to the stimulus. Through habituation, repetitive presentation of a stimulus leads to decreased responsiveness. The neurochemical circuitry underlying the sensitization of the aplysia's gill withdrawal response is well understood (Frank & Greenberg, 1994). Closer to the magical end of the continuum, scholars have argued for profound perceptual consequences of experience. Kuhn (1962) described how scientists, when exposed to a particular theoretical paradigm, see physical phenomena in new ways: "Though the world does not change with a change of paradigm, the scientist afterward works in a different world" (p. 121), and "during [scientific] revolutions, scientists see new and different things when looking with familiar instruments in places they have looked before" (p. 111).

233

Similarly, the new look movement in psychology (Bruner, Postman, & Rodriguez, 1951) and cultural anthropologists (Whorf, 1941/1956) have claimed that learned culture and experiences constrain our perceptions, partially blinding us to alternative perceptual descriptions that are inconsistent with our expectations.

TUNED PERCEPTUAL SYSTEMS

Before describing my laboratory's experiments on and models of experience-induced perceptual learning, it is useful to remember why an adaptive perceptual system is beneficial. Flexibility is beneficial when the world is variable. If everyone were confronted with the same environment, and this environment remained unchanged millennium after millennium, then perceptual systems could become hardwired for this particular environment. These perceptual systems would be efficient because they are specifically tuned to the unchanging environment. At a first pass, this does describe human perceptual systems. Humans from different cultures possess highly similar apparati for vision (Kay & McDaniel, 1978, but see Schafer, 1983 for some apparent exceptions). Many general environmental factors, such as color characteristics of sunlight, the position of the horizon, and the change in appearance that an approaching object makes, have all been mostly stable over the time that the human visual system has developed.

However, if we look more closely, there is an important sense in which different people face different environments. Namely, to a large extent, a person's environment consists of animals, people, and things made by people. Animals and people have been designed by evolution to show variability, and artifacts vary widely across cultures. Evolutionary pressures may have been able to build a perceptual system that is generally adept at processing faces (Bruce, 1998; Farah, 1992), but they could not have hardwired a neural system that was adept at processing a particular face, such as John Kennedy's, for the simple reason that there is too much generational variability among faces. Individual faces show variability from generation to generation, and variability is apparent over only slightly longer intervals for artifacts, words, ecological environments, and animal appearances. Thus, we can be virtually positive that tools show too much variability over time for there to be a hardwired detector for hammers. Words and languages vary too much for there to be a hardwired detector for the written letter *A*. Biological organisms are too geographically diverse for people to have formed a hardwired cow detector, for example. When environmental variability is high, the best strategy for an organism is to develop a general perceptual system that can adapt to its local conditions.

There is an even deeper sense in which people face different environments. People find themselves in different worlds because they choose to specialize. English-speaking people become specialized at hearing and seeing English words. People familiar with a particular race become specialized at recognizing faces from that race (Shapiro & Penrod, 1986). Experts at wine tasting, chick sexing, X-ray diagnosing, identical twin identifying, and baseball pitch judging all have unique perceptual capabilities because of the tasks they perform. Experts typically have highly specialized skills, many of which are perceptual (Sowden, Davies, & Roling, 2000). Moreover, the examples of word and face recognition suggest that every person has domains in which they show expertise. Even if all people confronted the same world initially, they would create distinctive communities with unique languages, artifacts, and objects of importance. In large part, individuals decide for themselves what objects they will be exposed to, and one's identity is defined by the particular specialized niche one assumes. One's niche will depend on many factors, including proclivity, community needs, local support, random accidents, and positive feedback loops. Thus, it is again advisable to build a perceptual system with the flexibility needed to support any one of a large number of niches.

This argument is that evolutionary forces drive a perceptual system to not only adapt but also to have mechanisms that allow for adaptation within an organism's lifetime when the environmental stability required for hardwiring is not present. An information theoretic perspective suggests additional computational advantages for perceptual systems that become tuned to organisms' environments within their lifetime. In particular, perceptual systems can create highly efficient, compressed encodings of stimuli if the encodings are tuned to statistical structures across a set of stimuli. One particularly powerful method of doing this is to devise a set of elements that, if combined together, would generate the set of objects in one's world. Part of the power from this approach stems from compositionality—creating representations by composing building blocks. An exceedingly large number of objects can be created from a surprisingly small set of building blocks if the building blocks can be combined in different arrangements. A set of 10 building blocks can be combined to form 10^5 objects that each contains 5 building blocks simply superimposed on top of each other. If there are eight different relations (i.e., left-of, right-of, above, below, inside, attached-to, behind, and in-front-of relations) that specify how these five building blocks within an object interrelate, then there would be 107,374,182,400,000 possible configurations of these five building blocks. The number of configurations that P parts, sampled from a set of S parts, create when potentially related to every other part in one of R ways is

$$R^{\frac{P(P-1)}{2}} S^P . \tag{1}$$

A moral that should be drawn from this combinatorial explosion of potential configurations is that complex stimuli should often be represented in terms of parts and their relations (Biederman, 1987; Hummel, 2000; Markman, 1999), rather than in terms of nondecomposed configurations. This is particularly true when there are a large number of possible stimuli and the stimuli share often-repeated parts or relations. However, the moral that is typically drawn from these considerations is slightly different—that stimuli ought to be represented in terms of fixed and a priori parts. A frequent strategy in cognitive science has been to represent entities in terms of hardwired primitive features. In linguistics, phonemes have been represented by the presence or absence of fewer than 12 features such as voiced, nasal, and strident (Jakobson, Fant, & Halle, 1963). Scenarios, such as ordering food in a restaurant, have been represented by Schank (1972) in terms of a set of 23 primitive concepts such as Physical-transfer, Propel, Grasp, and Ingest. In the field of object recognition, Biederman (1987) proposed a set of 36 geometric shapes such as wedge and cylinder to be used for representing objects such as telephones and flashlights. Wierzbicka (1992) proposed a set of 30 semantic primitives, including good, want, big, and time, to be composed together in structured phrases to generate all other words. To summarize, in this widespread and successful approach toward representation, the ability to represent new entities derives from combining a fixed set of a priori primitives, features, or parts in novel arrangements.

In what follows, I will argue that the building blocks an observer uses for construing their world depends on the observer's history, training, and acculturation. These factors, together with psychophysical constraints, mold one's set of building blocks. The researchers who proposed fixed sets of hardwired primitives are exactly right in one sense—the combinatorics of objects, words, scenes, and scenarios strongly favor componential representations. However, this does not necessitate that the components be hardwired. By developing new components to subserve particular tasks and environments, a newly important discrimination can generate building blocks that are tailored for the discrimination. Adaptive building blocks are likely to be efficient because they can be optimized for idiosyncratic needs and environments.

A neural network that provides an excellent initial conception of how a system can acquire useful building blocks is the expectation maximization (EM) algorithm for factorial learning (Dempster, Laird, & Rubin, 1977; Ghahramani, 1995; Hinton, Dayan, Frey, & Neal, 1995; Tenenbaum, 1996). This approach considers the statistics of component parts across a set of inputs. When presented with a set of inputs, this approach finds an underlying set of independent components that, when combined in different arrangements, reproduces the set of inputs. For example, Ghahramani (1995) created a set of 160 patterns by combining a horizontal line in any one of four positions with a vertical line in any one of four positions, together with added noise. The complete set of patterns is shown in Fig. 7.1. From these patterns, an EM algorithm could generate the set of eight horizontal and vertical lines that suffice for generating the 160 patterns. It does so by finding the weightings of different hidden dimensions (such as a bar) that would be most likely to have produced the 160 patterns. The algorithm is able to discover both the hidden dimensions and their weightings by iterating between two steps: (1) computing the expected hidden dimensions given the current weights and (2) maximizing the likelihood of the weights given these expected dimensions. Finding decompositions into parts is a useful enterprise in terms of information demands. Imagine wanting to represent each of the 16 basic configurations of four

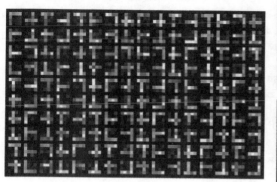 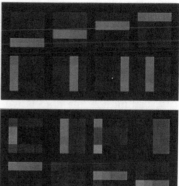

FIG. 7.1. EM simulations by Ghahramani (1995). On the left is a set of 160 patterns created by combining a horizontal line in any one of four positions, a vertical line in any one of four positions, and randomly distributed noise. The panels on the right show two separate runs of his EM algorithm trained on the 160 patterns. Feature detectors are created that, when combined together, can approximately reconstruct all of the input patterns. From "Factorial Learning and the EM algorithm," by Z. Ghahramani, 1995, *Advances in Neural Information Processing Systems*, p. 622, Cambridge, MA: MIT Press. Copyright 1995 by MIT Press. Reprinted with permission.

horizontal and four vertical lines. Rather than creating 16 different complex configurations, the componential representation requires only eight simpler parts to be stored. Although the storage requirements are only halved in this case, the savings becomes far greater as the number of composed dimensions and the number of values per dimension increases. The neural network modeling that I later report will differ from the EM algorithm in several ways. The network will develop building blocks that are modulated online by categorization feedback and perceptual constraints. Still, my later modeling borrows the basic insight from this application of the EM algorithm. It is efficient to represent objects in terms of building blocks, particularly if exactly those building blocks can be discovered that would provide compressed encodings of the objects.

Considering perceptual learning from an information theoretic perspective, this claim about the advantages of learned componential representations should be qualified. Whether or not the objects comprising an observer's world are efficiently represented by composing together parts or by nondecomposed, configural units will depend on the amount and kinds of similarity shared by objects. A well-spaced set of objects that uniformly covers an abstract stimulus space will typically be efficiently represented by a compositional set of parts. It is the factorial combination of horizontal and vertical parts in Fig. 7.1 that makes it useful to extract them out as parts. If each horizontal line occurred with only one particular vertical line, then it would be more efficient to represent only the four pairings of two lines rather than eight individual lines (Edelman, 1999; Kohonen, 1995). As such, the distribution of objects can inform whether the objects ought to be represented in terms of parts or holistically.

The choice between compositional and holistic representations is also influenced by how the objects will be used. Parts may need to be extracted if they predict an important categorization or use of the object (Gibson, 1969). Conversely, if a single complex configuration dictates the use of an object, then there should be a bias to represent the configuration holistically rather than by its parts. By analogy, if the efficacy of a medicine in treating a skin disease depends only on the skin's dryness, then dryness should be extracted as an isolated component for representing patients. However, if the medicine is only effective for a particular combination of dryness, body location, radius, and patient age, then there should be a bias to connect together these diverse attributes into a single functional feature. The general principle for creating efficient codes for stimuli is to find the level of representation that captures the systematicities present between and within objects.

VARIETIES OF PERCEPTUAL LEARNING

In arguing for flexible tuning of perceptual systems, one natural question to ask is, "Is the adaptation truly perceptual, or does it perhaps occur at postperceptual stages?" I have argued elsewhere for a deliberate blurring of the boundary between perception and cognition (Goldstone & Barsalou, 1998). There are deep similarities between perceptual unitization and chunking in memory and between perceptual differentiation and association building (Hall, 1991). Although downplaying a definite boundary where perception leaves off and true cognition begins, it is still useful to highlight learned changes in processing that involve adjusting initial representations of stimuli. Perceptual learning exerts a profound influence on behavior precisely because it occurs early during information processing and thus shifts the foundation for all subsequent processes.

The neurological evidence fails to support the notion that cortical areas involved with early perceptual processes are fairly fixed, context insensitive, and stable, whereas more central cortical processes show most of the lability. Consistent with an early stage of adaptation, Weinberger (1993) describes evidence that cells in the primary auditory cortex become tuned to the frequency of often-repeated tones. Practice in discriminating among small visual motions in different directions significantly alters electrical brain potentials that occur within 100 ms of the stimulus onset (Fahle & Morgan, 1996). These electrical changes are centered over the primary visual cortex, suggesting plasticity in early visual processing. Karni and Sagi (1991) find evidence, based on the specificity of training to eye (interocular transfer does not occur) and retinal location, that is consistent with early, primary visual cortex adaptation in simple discrimination tasks (see also Fahle & Morgan, 1996; Shiu & Pashler, 1992). Changes in the primary somatosensory areas in the cortex are observed when environmental or cortical changes occur (Garraghty & Kaas, 1992). When cortical areas are lesioned, neighboring areas newly respond to sensory information formerly controlled by the lesioned area; when external sensory organs are disabled, cortical areas formerly activated by the organ become sensitive to sensory stimulation formerly controlled by its neighboring areas (Kaas, 1991). When two fingers are surgically fused, creating highly correlated inputs, a large number of cortical areas develop that respond to both fingers (Allard, Clark, Jenkins, & Merzenich, 1991). In sum, there is an impressive amount of converging evidence that training leads to changes to very early stages of information processing.

This neurophysiological evidence makes a good case for relatively early changes to perception with laboratory training or general experience. This case having been briefly made, the evidence that follows focuses not on the locus of changes within the brain or the stage of information processing but on the mechanisms that underlie some of these changes. I describe these mechanisms at a functional rather than concrete level. Even though neurological details are known in some cases, a functional level of description is appropriate for interpreting the results from cognitive experiments and for unifying the accounts of human and computational learning. The following mechanisms of perceptual change are not exhaustive (a more complete organization is provided by Goldstone, 1998). Instead, mechanisms of perceptual change are described that will have particular relevance to a subsequently presented model of the interaction between perceptual and conceptual change.

Imprinting

By imprinting, perceptual detectors or receptors are developed that are specialized for stimuli or parts of a stimuli. Internalized detectors develop for repeated stimuli, and these detectors increase the speed, accuracy, and general fluency with which the stimuli are processed. In computational learning terms, imprinting is an unsupervised learning mechanism in that there is no need for a parent, teacher, or programmer to tell the learner what a stimulus is called. Learning proceeds by adapting internal detectors to become better specialized for the imprinting stimulus. The advantages of developing a detector that increasingly resembles an input stimulus are that small deviations from the input stimulus can be easily detected, particularly, strong responses can be quickly produced when the stimulus is presented again, and shorter codes can represent often-presented stimuli. Detectors may imprint on either a whole stimulus or a subset of the whole stimulus.

Imprinting on an entire stimulus is tantamount to developing a functional detector that is specialized for a specific stimulus. One of the most common paradigms for studying this has been to show subjects a briefly presented stimulus and ask them to identify it. Such stimuli are more accurately identified when the subject has been previously exposed to them (Schacter, 1987). The identification advantage for previously familiarized instances lasts at least 3 weeks, is found for both words and pictures, requires as few as one previous presentation of an item, and is often tied to the specific physical properties of the item during its initial exposure. Several models in psychology and computer science have exploited the power of storing individual exposures to stimuli in a relatively raw, unabstracted form. Exemplar, instance-based, view-based, case-based, nearest neighbor, configural cue, and vector quantization models all share the fundamental insight that novel patterns can be identified, recognized, or categorized by giving the novel patterns the same response that was learned for similar, previously presented patterns. By creating detectors for presented patterns not only is it possible to respond to repetitions of these patterns, but it is also possible to give novel patterns responses that are likely to be correct by sampling responses to old patterns, weighted by their similarity to the novel pattern. Consistent with these models, psychological evidence suggests that people show good transfer to a new stimulus in perceptual tasks just to the extent that the new stimulus superficially resembles previously learned stimuli (Kolers & Roediger, 1984; Palmeri, 1997).

In addition to imprinting on entire stimuli, unsupervised information from the environment can also lead to imprinting on selected parts or features from a stimulus. Whereas imprinting to whole stimuli supports configural, holistic processing, imprinting to parts supports componential processing of a stimulus by piecing it together out of a perceptual vocabulary. If a stimulus part varies independently of other parts, or occurs frequently, people may develop a specialized detector for that part. Schyns and Rodet (1997) found unfamiliar parts (arbitrary curved shapes within an object) that are important in one task are more likely to be used to represent subsequent categories. Their subjects were more likely to represent a conjunction of two parts, X and Y, in terms of these two components (rather than as a whole unit or a unit broken down into different parts) when they received previous experience with X as a defining part for a different category. Neural networks have proved to be highly effective at creating building blocks for describing sets of stimuli. In addition to the previously described work by Ghahramani (1995), researchers have discovered that simple exposure to photographs of natural scenes suffices to allow neural networks to create a repertoire of oriented line segments to be used to describe the scenes (Miikkulainen, Bednar, Choe, & Sirosh, 1997; Obermayer, Sejnowski, & Blasdel, 1995; Schmidhuber, Eldracher, & Foltin, 1996). These feature detectors bear a strong resemblance to neural detectors found in the primary visual cortex and are created by learning algorithms that develop units that respond to independent sources of regularity across photographs.

Human and computer systems that develop perceptual vocabulary elements based on the objects in their environment have an advantage over systems that employ only fixed features. One difficulty with fixed sets of features is that it is hard to choose exactly the right features that will suffice to accommodate all possible future entities. On the one hand, if a small set of primitive elements is chosen, then it is likely that two entities will eventually arise that must be distinguished but cannot with any combination of available primitives. On the other hand, if a set of primitives is sufficiently large to accommodate all entities that might occur, then it will likely include many elements that lie unused, waiting for their moment of need to possibly arise (Schyns, Goldstone, & Thibaut, 1998). If entities are represented by a smaller set of fixed features that are composed as building blocks in different arrangements to accommodate a wide range of entities, then very small building blocks will be required, resulting in large and inefficient representations of whole entities. However, by developing new components as needed, newly important discriminations can cause the construction of detectors that are tailored for the discrimination.

Task-Dependent Perceptual Learning

In imprinting, the stimuli themselves shape the perceptual change and can do so irrespective of what must be done with the stimuli. Not only is the perceptual change unsupervised in the sense of not requiring a label or response to be associated with the stimuli, but it is task independent in the more general sense of proceeding without any regard for context or the observer's goals. However, in many situations, what is to be done with a stimulus influences what information is extracted from the stimulus (Gibson, 1969; Goldstone, Lippa, & Shiffrin, 2001; Pick, 1992).

People can dynamically shift their attention to different stimulus features depending on their perceived importance. One way that perception becomes adapted to tasks and environments is by increasing the attention paid to perceptual features that are important, or by decreasing attention to irrelevant dimensions and features, or both. Whether accomplished by moving one's eyes or more covertly, shifts of visual attention play an important role in allowing us to learn needed categories. As such, it comes as no surprise that most successful theories of categorization and learning incorporate selective attention. In Sutherland and Mackintosh's (1971) analyzer theory, learning a discrimination involves strengthening the tendency to attend to relevant analyzers. In Nosofsky's (1986) exemplar model of categorization, the categorization of an object depends on its similarity to previously stored category members in a multidimensional space (see also Medin & Shaeffer, 1978). Critically, distances between objects are compressed and expanded along dimensions in this space depending on the categorization required. Distances between objects on relevant dimensions are expanded, and irrelevant dimensions are compressed. For example, Nosofsky (1986) found that if participants are given a categorization where the angle of a line embedded in a circular form is relevant while the size of the circular form is irrelevant, then distances between objects on the angle dimension are increased and distances on the size dimension are decreased.

The next two mechanisms of perceptual learning I describe produce dynamic changes to the sizes of perceptual units used in representing an object. One of the mechanisms creates larger units out of smaller units, and the other mechanism divides a larger unit into smaller units. However, before describing these mechanisms, it is important to be clear about what it means for a system to have a perceptual unit. What could it mean for a system to learn a new feature? When writing of features, I am concerned with psychologically internalized rather than external features of an object. This is the only possible strategy because the only awareness of an object that we have is necessarily filtered through our perceptual system. The only way an objective property of an object can influence us is if it influences a psychologically represented feature. Even if a physicist can measure the illuminance of an object or a chemist can measure the tannin content of a Bordeaux, these stimulus properties are not psychological features unless the perceiving organism can isolate them as well. A psychological feature, then, is a set of stimulus elements that are responded to together, as an integrated unit. That is, a feature is a package of stimulus elements that is separated from other sets of elements and reflects the subjective organization of the whole stimulus into components.

In my usage of the term feature, I purposefully encompass several terms typically treated as distinct: features, dimensions, and parts. Features are typically understood as qualitative stimulus values that are either present or absent. Dimensions are stimulus values that have quantitative levels. Parts are spatially localized regions of a stimulus. One reason to define features as psychologically isolated packages of stimulus elements with the intention of referring to all three types of stimulus organization is that a clear distinction between these organizations is often hard to justify. For example, "has wings" is typically described as a feature of birds, but wings are also spatially localized parts. Does a red patch on an object count as a part but suddenly become a feature if it covers the entire object? Does the difference between a circle and a square suddenly shift from being featural to dimensional as soon as shapes with intermediate levels of curvature are introduced? A unified account of all three structures is desirable.

This definition corresponds closely to standard operationalizations of features. Garner (1976) measures the extent to which two stimulus elements are psychologically fused by determining how much categorizations made on the basis of one of the elements are slowed by irrelevant variation on the other. Treisman and Gelade (1980) argue for a vocabulary of features that includes color, orientation, and closure elements. Their empirical task involves visually searching for a target defined by a simple feature or conjunction of features, among a set of distractor objects. Features are empirically identified by response times to targets that are not influenced by the number of distracters if the targets are distinguished by a feature. Tests for featurehood typically involve showing that some information is dependent on other information (in the same feature) but is independent of still other information (in different features). For feature learning to occur simply means that the organization of elements into sets has changed. For example, although the saturation and brightness of a color are not strong psychological features for most people, they may be for color experts (Burns & Shepp, 1988), if the color expert can demonstrate that they can attend to saturation without being very influenced by brightness. In the modeling presented later, features are implemented as acquired detectors in a hidden layer of a neural network model, and two stimulus elements belong to the same feature to the extent that a single unit responds selectively to those elements. Thus, there need not be anything more magical about the development of novel features than reorganizing functional detectors so that they are influenced by only some sources of information.

Unitization. One result of category learning is to create perceptual units that combine stimulus components that are useful for the categorization. Such a process is one variety of the more general phenomenon of unitization, by which single functional units are constructed and triggered when a complex configuration arises. Cattell (1886) invoked the notion of perceptual unitization to account for the advantage that he found for tachistoscopically presented words relative to nonwords. Gestalt psychologists proposed the perceptual principle that objects tend to be perceived in terms of components that have acquired familiarity (Koffka, 1935). Weisstein and Harris (1974) found that briefly flashed line segments are more accurately identified when they are part of a set of lines forming a unitary object rather than an incoherent pattern. They interpreted this effect as showing that arrangements of lines can form configural patterns that are perceived before the individual lines are perceived. More recently, Gauthier and Tarr (1997; see also Gauthier, Williams, Tarr, & Tanaka, 1998) found that prolonged experience with a novel object leads to a configural representation of it that combines all of its parts into a single, viewpoint-specific, functional unit. Their evidence for such a representation is that recognition of these familiarized objects improved considerably with practice and was much more efficient when the object was in its customary upright form rather than inverted.

Unitization has also been explored in the field of attention. Using a task where participants decided whether or not two visual objects were identical, LaBerge (1973) found that when stimuli were unexpected, participants were faster at responding to actual letters than to letterlike controls. Furthermore, this difference diminished as the unfamiliar letterlike stimuli became more familiar over practice. He argued that the shape components of often-presented stimuli become processed as a single functional unit with practice. More recently, Czerwinski, Lightfoot, and Shiffrin (1992) referred to a process of perceptual unitization in which conjunctions of stimulus features are chunked together so that they become perceived as a single unit. Shiffrin and Lightfoot (1997) argued that separated line segments can become unitized following prolonged practice with the materials. Their evidence comes from the slopes relating the number of distracter elements to response time in a feature search task. When participants learned a conjunctive search task in which three line segments were needed to distinguish the target from distracters, impressive and prolonged decreases in search slopes were observed over 20 hourlong sessions. These prolonged decreases were not observed for a simple search task requiring attention to only one component.

Unitization is also important during the development of object perception. Newborn infants fail to integrate the separate regions of an object that is occluded (Slater et al., 1990). However, by 4.5 months of age, babies form the same interpretation of displays whether they are fully visible or occluded (Johnson, 1997; Needham, 1997, this volume). This developed ability to integrate different parts into a single object representation depends on the featural similarity of these parts (Needham, 1999).

I recently completed experiments designed to test whether category learning can lead to stimulus unitization and to explore the boundary conditions on unitization related to stimulus characteristics and amount of training (Goldstone, 2000). Whenever the claim for the construction of new units is made, two objections must be addressed. First, perhaps people already possessed the unit before categorization training. My stimuli were designed to make this explanation unlikely. Each unit to be sensitized was constructed by connecting five randomly chosen curves. There were 10 curves that could be sampled without replacement, yielding 30,240 ($10 \times 9 \times 8 \times 7 \times 6$) possible different units, an implausibly large number under the constraint that all units preexisted. The second objection is that no units need be formed; instead, people analytically integrate evidence from the five separate curves to make their categorizations. However, this objection was shown to be untenable because subjects, at the end of 20 hours of training, were faster at categorizing the five-element units than would be expected by an analytic approach. In this analytic account, the response time required to respond to a unit was predicted by the response times required to respond to individual components within the unit. The response-time modeling involved Fourier deconvolutions for isolating component processes within response-time distributions and is too involved to describe here (for discussions, see Goldstone, 2000, or Goldstone, Steyvers, Spencer-Smith, & Kersten, 2000). For present purposes, I simply treat pronounced response time improvements to respond to a multicomponent unit as suggestive evidence for unitization, setting aside the more elaborate analyses.

In the experiments, subjects saw objects appear on the screen and were required to categorize them as quickly as possible. The categorization was designed so that evidence for five components had to be received before certain categorization responses were made. The stimuli and their category memberships are shown in Fig. 7.2. Each of the letters refers to a particular segment of a doodle. Each doodle was composed of five segments, with a semicircle below the segments added to create a closed figure. To reliably place the doodle labeled "ABCDE" into Category 1, all five components, "A," "B," "C," "D," and "E," must be processed. For example, if the right-most component were not attended, then ABCDE could not be distinguished from ABCDZ, which belongs in Category 2. Not only does

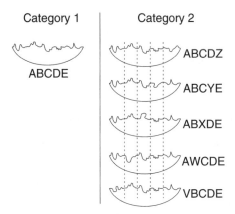

FIG. 7.2. Stimuli used by Goldstone (2000). Each letter represents a particular stimulus segment, and each stimulus is composed of five segments. To categorize the item represented by ABCDE as belonging to Category 1, it is necessary to process information associated with each of its segments because every single-segment distortion from ABCDE belongs in Category 2. The dashed lines in the right column were not part of the stimuli but show the decomposition of the stimuli into their five components.

no single component suffice for accurate categorization of ABCDE, but two-way, three-way, and four-way conjunctions of components also do not suffice.

If unitization occurs during categorization, then the stimulus ABCDE should become efficiently processed with practice. It is the only object that belongs to Category 1, and to reliably classify this item the entire object must be processed. Results from a speeded categorization task, shown in Fig. 7.3, show exactly this pattern. When all five components must be attended to reliably categorize "ABCDE" as belonging in Category 1, then there is a large improvement in speed over the course of four blocks and 1.5 hours (see the ordered-five condition in Fig. 7.3). This large improvement was not found when only one of the components was required to make a Category 1 response. In the ordered-one task, only one object, such as ABCDZ, belongs to Category 2, so detecting component "E" is sufficient for making a Category 1 response. The large improvement in speed was also not found when each of the five components of ABCDE needed to be identified but were randomly ordered. That is, ABCDE, DEBAC, and any other permutation of the five components A–E, were treated as equivalent. In this condition, a single photograph-like image cannot serve to represent ABCDE because many different images produce this pattern. The lack of impressive improvement in this random-five condition suggests that components that are not combined in a consistent manner to create a coherent image are not effectively unitized. Thus, the first constraint on the unitization process, illustrated in the top panel of Fig. 7.4, is that unitization only proceeds when a photograph-like template can be constructed for

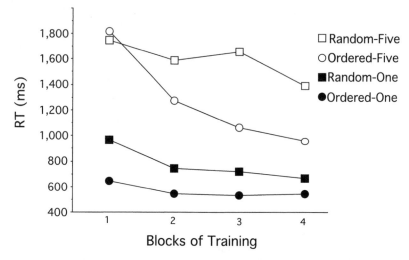

Blocks of Training

FIG. 7.3. Results from Goldstone (2000), Experiment 1. The most pronounced practice effects were observed for the "ordered-five" task, where a subject can only make a Category 1 response when they have detected five doodle segments, but the segments occur in the same order on each trial. In the one tasks, subjects only need to attend to one of the five segments. In the random tasks, the segments were spatially randomized on each trial, preventing a single image from being useful for categorization.

the unit. Unitization apparently consists in establishing templates for patterns that are diagnostic for categorization.

The nature of these templates was tested in a second experiment that compared speed improvements for detecting conjunctions of five components that were either separated or spatially contiguous. The same components were used for the contiguous and separated displays, and the distance between the endpoints was equated, but in the separated condition the components were stacked on top of each other so that they no longer touched (as shown in the second panel of Fig. 7.4). As shown in Fig. 7.5, there was a small advantage found for contiguous over separated displays, found when either all five or only one component(s) needed to be identified for a Category 1 response. However, both the separated-five and contiguous-five conditions improved dramatically over blocks of practice, with almost equal rates of improvement for each. As such, the unitization process is not constrained to form images for contiguous images. Separating the components of an image does not interfere with unitization in the manner that randomly permuting the components did.

However, the third panel in Fig. 7.4 shows a constraint on people's ability to unitize across discontiguous components. In a third experiment, a conjunction

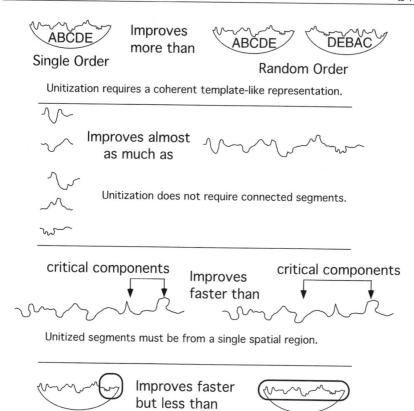

FIG. 7.4. Four constraints on category-dependent unitization studied by Goldstone (2000). See text for details.

of two (rather than five) components was critical for categorization. These two components were either contiguous to each other or were separated by a third irrelevant component. More precisely, in the Together condition, ABCDE belonged to Category 1, and ABCDZ and ABCYE belonged to Category 2. In the Apart condition, ABCDE belonged to Category 1, and ABCDZ and ABYDE belonged to Category 2, and, hence, Components C and E were critical for making a Category 1 response. Category 1 response times improved much more quickly in the Together than in the Apart condition. In fact, the pattern of improvement in the Apart condition closely resembled the improvement shown when a conjunction of three components was required. Apparently, in the Apart condition, subjects form a unit by combining the two disconnected components and the irrelevant component between them. This result can be reconciled with the previous paragraph by hypothesizing that units are formed for components within a single spatially

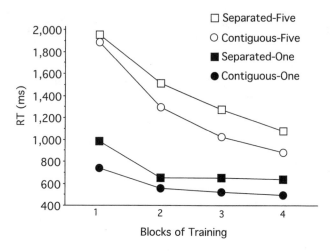

FIG. 7.5. Results from Goldstone (2000), Experiment 2. Large practice effects were found for conjunctive tasks that involved either contiguous or separated segments, although the influence of practice
was slightly greater for the conjunctive task involving contiguous segments. Subjects appear to be able to form units even if the parts are
not touching, as long as the parts fall in one spatial region.

delineated region. The unitized components need not be physically connected,
but, if they are not, then the region between the components will be incorporated
into the unit as well. Eriksen and Murphy (1987) report a similar constraint of
contiguity for spatial attention, although there is also evidence that this constraint
can be violated in some situations (Egly & Homa, 1984).

The bottom panel of Fig. 7.4 illustrates a final constraint on unitization. As
the size of the unit that needs to be created increases, so does the period of time
required to construct it. In a fourth experiment, I varied the number of components
that needed to be conjoined to make a reliable Category 1 response from 1 to 5.
Response times for all five tasks were well fit by a power function that takes the form
$RT = a + bN^c$, where N is the trial number, a is the asymptotic response time, b is the
difference between the initial and asymptotic response times, and c is the learning
rate (which controls the steepness of the learning curve[1]). Finding best-fitting
parameters for a, b, and c revealed that as the number of components to be unitized
increased, parameter b increased, but c decreased. That is, the total amount of
improvement became greater, but the course of improvement was more prolonged.

---

[1] In everyday language people often speak of tasks that show very slow improvement as showing a
steep learning curve, but this usage is exactly wrong. A steep learning curve (high absolute value of c)
is a learning curve where there is a fast rate of improvement. Presumably, when people informally refer
to a steep learning curve, they are intending to claim that the total amount of improvement required to
go from novice to expert performance is large, which is a claim that the parameter b, not c, is large.

Impressively complex units can be formed, but as unit complexity increases, so does the time required for unitization. The important implicit message from this result is that unitization is not like taking photographic film to be developed. Although the end result of each may be similar, an imagelike template recording an environmental input, the process by which these results are obtained is dissimilar. A photograph of a crowd takes no longer to develop than a photograph of a single face, but for human unitization development time is proportional to stimulus complexity. Once constructed, units of different complexity may be identified almost equally quickly, but this belies the large differences in time required for constructing the units.

Dimension Differentiation. Selective attention, described earlier, is a critical component of adaptive learning, but it may not be the only process that dynamically alters the description of an object in a categorization task. A second candidate process is dimension differentiation, by which dimensions that are originally psychologically fused together become separated and isolated. Selective attention presumes that the different dimensions that make up a stimulus can be selectively attended. To increase attention to size but not color, one must be able to isolate size differences from color differences. In his classic research on stimulus integrality and separability, Garner argued that stimulus dimensions differ in how easily they can be isolated or extracted from each other (Garner, 1976, 1978). Dimensions are said to be separable if it is possible to attend to one of the dimensions without attending to the other. Size and brightness are classic examples of separable dimensions; making a categorization on the basis of size is not significantly slowed if there is irrelevant variation on brightness. Dimensions are integral if variation along an irrelevant dimension cannot be ignored when trying to attend a relevant dimension. The classic examples of integral dimensions are saturation and brightness, where saturation is related to the amount of white mixed into a color, and brightness is related to the amount of light coming off of a color. For saturation and brightness, it is difficult to attend to only one of the dimensions (Burns & Shepp, 1988; Melara, Marks, & Potts, 1993).

From this work distinguishing integral from separate dimensions, one might conclude that selective attention can proceed with separable but not integral dimensions. However, one interesting possibility is that category learning can, to some extent, change the status of dimensions, transforming dimensions that were originally integral into more separable dimensions. Experience may change the underlying representation of a pair of dimensions such that they come to be treated as relatively independent and noninterfering sources of variation that compose an object. Seeing that stimuli in a set vary along two orthogonal dimensions may allow the dimensions to be teased apart and isolated, particularly if the two dimensions are differentially diagnostic for categorization. There is developmental evidence that dimensions that are easily isolated by adults, such as the brightness and size of a square, are treated as fused together for 4-year old children (Kemler & Smith,

1978). It is relatively difficult for children to decide whether two objects are identical on a particular dimension but relatively easy for them to decide whether they are similar across many dimensions (Smith, 1989). Children show considerable difficulty in tasks that require selective attention to one dimension while ignoring another, even if the dimensions are separable for adults (Smith & Kemler, 1978). For example, children seem to be distracted by shape differences when they are instructed to make comparisons based on color. Adjectives that refer to single dimensions are learned by children relatively slowly compared with nouns (Smith, Gasser, & Sandhofer, 1997).

The developmental trend toward increasingly differentiated dimensions is echoed by adult training studies. Under certain circumstances, color experts (art students and vision scientists) are better able to selectively attend to dimensions (e.g., hue, chroma, and value) that comprise color than are nonexperts (Burns & Shepp, 1988). Goldstone (1994a) showed that people who learn a categorization in which saturation is relevant and brightness is irrelevant (or vice versa) can learn to perform the categorization accurately, and as a result of category learning, they develop selectively heightened sensitivity at making saturation, relative to brightness, discriminations. That is, categorization training that makes one dimension diagnostic and another dimension nondiagnostic can serve to split apart these dimensions, even if they are traditionally considered to be integral dimensions. These training studies show that to know how integral two dimensions are, one has to know something about the observer's history.

Goldstone and Steyvers (2001) recently explored whether genuinely arbitrary dimensions can become isolated from each other. They explored dimension differentiation by a category learning and transfer paradigm. Their subjects first learned to categorize a set of 16 faces into two groups by receiving feedback from a computer and then were transferred to a second categorization. The stimuli varied along arbitrary dimensions that were created by morphing between randomly paired faces. As shown in Fig. 7.6, Dimension A was formed by gradually blending from Face 1 to Face 2, and Dimension B was formed by gradually blending from Face 3 to Face 4. Using a technique described by Steyvers (1999), a set of faces can be created from these two dimensions such that each face is defined half by its value on Dimension A and half by its value on Dimension B. Dimensions are thus formed by creating negative contingencies between two faces—the more of Face A that is present in a particular morphed face, the less of Face B there will be. The 4×4 matrix of faces in Fig. 7.6 shows how a set of faces can be constructed that varies independently along the two arbitrary dimensions. However, using the same dimensions, one can create a set of stimuli with even less intrinsic dimensionality by assigning 16 faces to coordinates that fall on a circle, rather than a grid, in the abstract space defined by Dimensions A and B. A variable D was created and assigned 16 different values, from 0 to 360 in $22.5°$ steps. For each value assigned to D, the Dimension A value for a face was equal to cosine(D) and the

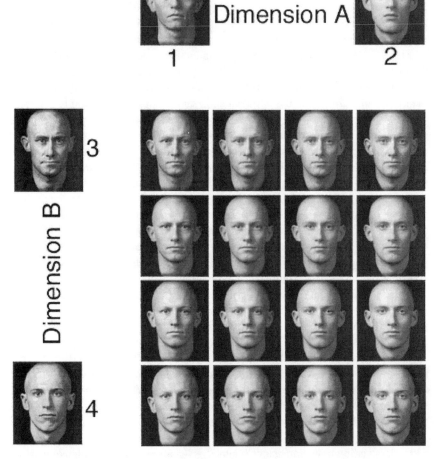

FIG. 7.6. Stimuli used by Goldstone and Steyvers (2001). Faces 1, 2, 3, and 4 are blended in different proportions to create a 4 × 4 matrix of faces. The proportions of Faces 1 and 2 are negatively correlated so that the more of Face 1 present in one of the 16 center faces, the less of Face 2 there will be. This negative correlation establishes Dimension A, and a similar negative correlation between Faces 3 and 4 establishes Dimension B. Each of the 16 center faces is defined half by its value on Dimension A and half by its value on Dimension B.

Dimension B value was sine(D). The end result, shown in Fig. 7.7, is a set of faces organized on a circle with no privileged dimensional axes suggested by the set of faces.

With these faces, Goldstone and Steyvers (2001) asked whether the organization of the faces into dimensions could be influenced by the required categorization. Subjects were shown faces, asked to categorize them, and then received feedback on the correctness of their categorization. The categorization rules all involved splitting the 16 faces into two equal piles with straight lines, such as those shown in Fig. 7.7. Each subject was given training with one categorization rule and then was transferred to a second rule. The critical experimental manipulation was whether the final categorization rule involved a rotation of 45° or 90° relative to the initial rule. Given that the initial categorization rules were randomly selected, the only difference between the 45° and 90° rotation conditions was whether the category boundary was shifted by two or four faces. The results from four similar experiments indicate that in the second phase of category learning, there was an advantage for the 90° over 45° rotation condition in all of the conditions that involved integral (psychologically fused) dimensions. This is somewhat surprising given that categorizations related by 90° are completely incompatible as far as their selective attention demands. The dimension that was originally completely irrelevant becomes completely relevant. In the 45° condition, the originally relevant dimension is at least partially relevant later. However, categorizations related by 90° do have an advantage as far as dimensional organization. The relevant dimensions for the two categorizations are compatible with each other in the sense of relying on independent sources of variation. For example, acquiring Dimension A in Fig. 7.6 is compatible with later acquiring Dimension B because both are independent dimensions that can coexist without interference. Learning that Dimension A is relevant and Dimension B is irrelevant should encourage isolating Dimension A from Dimension B to only attend to Dimension A. This is exactly the same isolation of dimensions that is useful for learning that Dimension B is relevant and Dimension A is irrelevant, albeit for opposite reasons. Thus, categorization rules separated by 90° are completely inconsistent with respect to their selective attention demands but are consistent with respect to their dimensional organization of stimuli.

Understanding how dimensions related by 90° are organizationally compatible may be difficult with the abstract dimensions of Fig. 7.7. However, consider representing the rectangles in Fig. 7.8. Categorizing rectangles on the basis of height is compatible with categorizing them on the basis of width because these two dimensions can each be separately registered and do not interfere with each other. Someone who thought about rectangles in terms of height would also be likely to think about them in terms of width. Organizing rectangles in terms of shape (ratio of width to height) and area is an alternative dimensional organization. A person who thinks in terms of rectangle shape might also be expected to think in terms of area because this is the remaining dimension along which rectangles vary

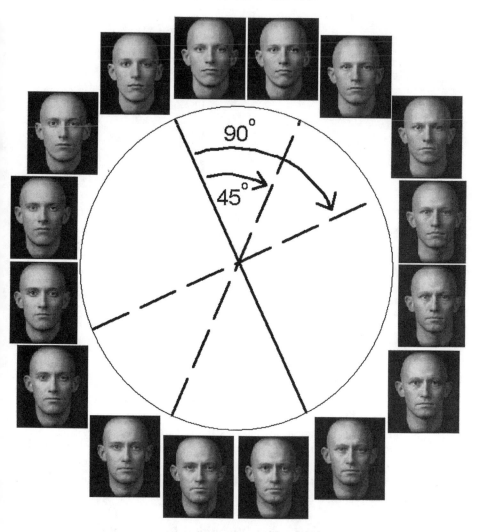

FIG. 7.7. Stimuli from Goldstone and Steyvers (2001), Experiment 3. Using the same dimensions as Fig. 7.6, a set of circularly arranged faces was created by varying degrees from 0° to 360°, assigning the face a value on Dimension A based on the cosine of the degrees, and assigning the face's Dimension B value based on the sine of the degrees. Subjects learned two successive categorizations involving the faces. Each categorization split the faces into two equal groups with a straight dividing line. The two category boundaries given to a subject were either related to each other by 45° or 90°.

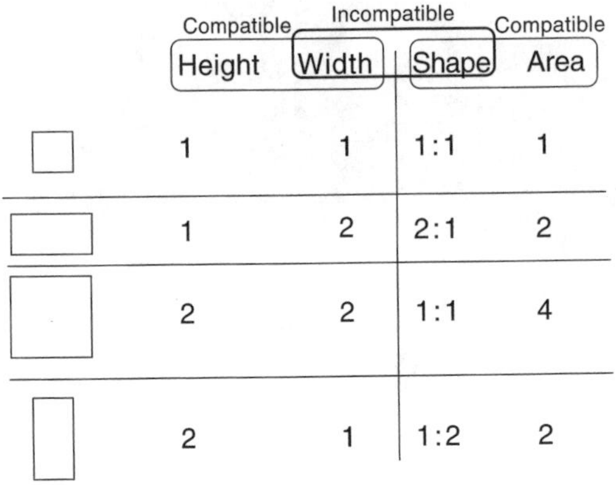

	Compatible	Incompatible		Compatible
	Height	Width	Shape	Area
	1	1	1 : 1	1
	1	2	2 : 1	2
	2	2	1 : 1	4
	2	1	1 : 2	2

FIG. 7.8. An illustration of how stimuli can be understood in terms of competing dimensional organizations. Rectangles can be understood in terms of height and width or in terms of their area and shape. An analysis in terms of width is compatible with an analysis in terms of height but is incompatible with an analysis in terms of shape because width and shape are cross-cutting, rather than nonoverlapping, dimensions of variation.

once shape has been extracted. However, organizing rectangles in terms of height is incompatible with organizing them in terms of area because area is partially dependent on height. In assessing the compatibility of dimensional organizations, two dimensions are compatible if they involve independent sources of variation and are incompatible if they do not. Dimensional axes related by 45° involve cross-cutting and, hence incompatible, dimensions. In summary, there appears to be more to learning than learning to selectively attend to existing dimensions. Perceptual learning also involves establishing which dimensions are available for selective attention. People learn not only appropriate weights for dimensions but also learn how to learn appropriate weights for dimensions.

Reconciling Unitization and Dimension Differentiation.   The two previous sections described apparently contrary ways in which category learning affects perceptual learning. Unitization involves the construction of a single functional unit out of component parts. Dimension differentiation divides wholes into relatively separable component dimensions. There is an apparent contradiction between experience creating larger chunks via unitization and dividing an object into more clearly delineated components via differentiation. This incongruity can be transformed into a commonalty at a more abstract level. Both mechanisms depend on the requirements established by tasks and stimuli. Objects will tend to be decomposed into their parts if the parts reflect independent sources of variation or if the parts differ in their relevancy. Parts will tend to be unitized if they co-occur frequently, with all parts indicating a similar response. Thus, unitization and differentiation are both processes that build appropriate sized representations for the tasks at hand.

Pevtzow and Goldstone (1994; also see Goldstone et al., 2000) reported a series of experiments illustrating the compatibility of unitization and differentiation by showing that both processes are probably involved when learning how to segment pictures into component parts. People often spontaneously segment objects into parts, thereby organizing their world. Palmer conducted several studies on the naturalness of parts within whole objects, exploring factors that make certain parts more natural than others (Palmer, 1977, 1978). Palmer also developed a quantitative model of part naturalness that included a number of objective factors about the parts and whole: how close the line segments within a part are to each other, whether they formed closed objects, whether they have similar orientations, and whether the line segments of a part are similar to line segments within other parts.

In addition to these objective properties that determine how psychologically natural a particular segmentation of an object into parts will be, researchers have found that segmentations also depend on subjective experience. Behrmann, Zemel, and Mozer (1998) found that judgments about whether two parts had the same number of humps were faster when the two parts belonged to the same object rather than different objects. Further work found an influence of experience on subsequent part comparisons. Two stimulus components are interpreted as belonging to the same object if they have cooccurred many times (Zemel, Behrmann, Mozer, & Bavelier, 1999). Pursuing a similar line of inquiry, Pevtzow and Goldstone (1994) explored the influence of category learning on segmentation using materials based on Palmer's stick figures and shown in Fig. 7.9. Naturalness was measured by how quickly subjects could confirm that a part was contained within a whole object (Palmer, 1978). To test the conjecture that how psychologically natural a part is depends on whether it has been useful for previous categorizations, we gave participants a categorization task, followed by part/whole judgments. During categorization, participants were shown distortions of the objects A, B, C, and D, shown in Fig. 7.9. The objects were distorted by adding a random line segment that connected to the five segments already present. Subjects were given extended training with either a vertical or horizontal categorization rule. For participants who learned that A and C were in one category and B and D were in another (a vertical categorization rule), the two component parts at the bottom of Fig. 7.9 were diagnostic. For participants who learned that A and B belonged in one category and C and D belonged to the other category (a horizontal rule), the components on the right were diagnostic.

During part/whole judgments, participants were shown a whole, and then a part, and were asked whether the part was contained in the whole. Participants were given both present and absent judgments, and examples of these judgments are shown in Fig. 7.10. Note that the two parts shown in Fig. 7.10 were both

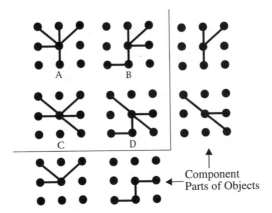

FIG. 7.9. Materials used by Pevtzow and Goldstone (1994). The four objects, A, B, C, and D, were categorized into two groups. When A and B were placed in one group, and C and D were placed in the other, the parts on the right were diagnostic. When A and C were placed in one group, and B and D were placed in the other, then the parts on the bottom were diagnostic.

potentially diagnostic during the earlier categorization training. Whether or not a part was diagnostic was independent of the appearance of the part itself, depending only on how the four objects of Fig. 7.9 were grouped into categories.

The major result, shown in Fig. 7.11, was that subjects were faster to correctly respond "present" when the part was diagnostic than when it was nondiagnostic (for a related result, see Lin & Murphy, 1997). To the extent that one can find response-time analogs of signal detection theory sensitivity and bias, this effect seems to be a sensitivity difference rather than a bias difference because absent judgments also tended to be faster for diagnostic than nondiagnostic parts. These results indicate that it is not simply the physical stimulus properties that determine how readily a person can segment an object into a particular set of components; segmentation is also influenced by the learned categorical diagnosticity of the components.

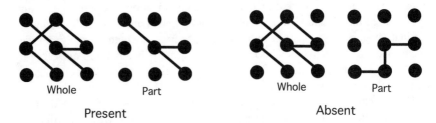

FIG. 7.10. Present and absent trials from Pevtzow and Goldstone (1994). In each case, the subject's task was to respond whether the part is present or absent in the whole stimulus.

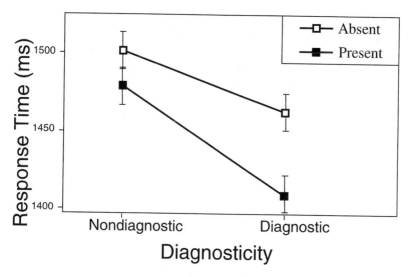

FIG. 7.11. Results from Pevtzow and Goldstone (1994). It is easier to detect the presence of a part within a whole object when the part was previously diagnostic for a categorization.

This experiment raises the strong possibility that the processes of composing parts into a single functional unit and differentiating a unit into several functional parts may be aspects of the same mechanism. Acquiring a diagnostic component involves both integrating its parts together into a single unit and separating this unit from other components. Both aspects are evident in the Pevtzow and Goldstone (1994) experiments because the units that are built up during category learning are not the entire five–line segment stimulus that is present on a trial. As such, the constructed units are complex configurations of multiple line segments yet are still only part of the entire stimulus. Both differentiation of a stimulus into parts and unitization could be incorporated in a model that begins with a specific featural description of objects, creates units for conjunctions of features if the features frequently occur together, and divides a feature into subfeatures if independent sources of variation in the original feature are detected. Describing such a model is the task now at hand.

MODELING INTERACTIONS BETWEEN CONCEPTUAL AND PERCEPTUAL LEARNING

In developing a computational model for perceptual learning, I have been drawn to neural networks that possess units that intervene between inputs and outputs and are capable of creating internal representations. For current purposes, these units can be interpreted as learned feature detectors and represent the organism's acquired perceptual vocabulary. The immediate goal of the modeling described is explaining the qualitative behavior that was observed in the experiments previously described. However, more general attributes of the model are also described and are relevant for information compression and adaptive coding. The specific goals of the modeling are to explain how (1) category learning alters the perceptual vocabulary that is derived for a set of objects, (2) perceptual descriptions are a joint function of category demands and perceptual constraints, (3) category learning can influence the subsequent segmentation of presented objects into parts, (4) detectors are built for complex configurations of parts (unitization), and (5) a perceptually constrained set of building blocks can be created in an online fashion to efficiently represent a set of objects (differentiation).

First, I describe a mutually interacting pair of neural networks that are designed to categorize and segment patterns, with an eye toward accounting for Pevtzow and Goldstone's (1994) results. As with the experiment, the network is first given categorization training and then is given a subsequent segmentation task, using the same network weights. The goal of the modeling is to show how categorization training can prime the segmentation network so that objects will tend to be segmented into parts that were previously diagnostic for categorization.

The Categorization Network

The categorization network has three layers of units: one representing the input patterns, one representing a bank of learned detectors, and one reflecting the category assignments of the inputs. Both of the weights from the input patterns to the detectors and the weights from the detectors to categories are learned. The categorization task uses a modified unsupervised competitive learning algorithm (O'Reilly & Munakata, 2000; Rumelhart & Zipser, 1985) but includes a top-down influence of category labels that incorporates supervised learning. The network begins with random weights from a two-dimensional input array to a set of detector units and from the detectors to the category units. When an input pattern is presented, the unit with the weight vector that is closest to the input pattern is the winner and will selectively adjust its weights to become even more specialized toward the input. By this mechanism, the originally homogenous detectors will become differentiated over time, splitting the input patterns into categories represented by the detectors. The competitive learning algorithm automatically learns to group input patterns into the clusters that the patterns naturally form. However, given that we want the detectors to reflect the experiment-supplied categories, we need to modify the standard unsupervised algorithm. This is done by including a mechanism that allows detectors that are useful for categorizing an input pattern to become more likely to win the competition to learn the pattern. The usefulness of a detector is assumed to be directly proportional to the weight from the detector to the presented category, which is provided as a label associated with an input pattern. The input-to-detector weights do not have to be set before the weights from detectors to categories are learned.

In addition to modifying the unsupervised development of hidden-layer detectors by considering their usefulness for categorization, a second modification of the standard competitive learning algorithm is required to fix one of its general problems in optimally making use of all detectors to cover a set of input patterns. This problem is that if multiple input patterns are presented that are fairly similar to each other, there will be a tendency for one detector to be the winner for all of the patterns. As a result, the winning detector's weight vector will eventually become similar to the average of the input patterns' activations, and the rest of the detectors will not learn at all. This situation is suboptimal because the input patterns are not covered as well as they would be if the unchanging detectors learned something. The standard solution to this problem is called leaky learning and involves adjusting both winning and losing detectors but adjusting losing detectors at a slower rate (Rumelhart & Zipser, 1985). To understand the more subtle problem with this solution, imagine, for example, that four input patterns naturally fall into two groups based on their similarities, and the network is given four detectors. Ideally, each of the detectors would become specialized for one of the input patterns. However, under leaky learning, one detector will tend to become specialized for one cluster, a second will become specialized for the other cluster, and the remaining two detectors will be pulled equally by both clusters, becoming specialized for neither. Note that it does not help to supplement leaky learning by the rule that the closer a detector is to an input pattern, the higher its learning rate should be. There is no guarantee that the two losing units will evenly split so that each is closer to a different cluster.

Other researchers noted related problems with competitive learning and suggested solutions (Grossberg, 1987). Our current solution is to conceptualize competitive learning as not simply a competition among detectors to accommodate a presented input pattern but also as a competition among input patterns to be accommodated by a given detector. Input patterns are presented sequentially to the network, and as they are presented the most similar input pattern to each detector is determined. The learning rate for a detector is set to a higher value for its most similar input pattern than for other inputs. In this manner, detectors that are not the winning detector for a pattern can still become specialized by becoming unequally influenced by different patterns. In addition, the learning rate for a detector when presented with an input pattern will depend on how well the input is currently covered by existing detectors. This dependency is required to allocate detectors to input regions where they are required. Putting these considerations together, the activation of detector i when presented with pattern p, is

$$A_{i,p} = \sum_{h=1}^{n} I_{h,p} W_{i,h} + \sum_{j=1}^{c} ST W_{j,i}, \qquad (2)$$

where $I_{h,p}$ is the activation of input unit h for pattern p, $W_{i,h}$ is the weight from input h to detector i, S is the strength of the top-down pressure on detector development, T is the teacher signal (if Pattern p belongs to Category j then $T = 1$, otherwise $T = -1$), and $W_{j,i}$ is the weight from Detector i to Category Unit j. The second term increases the activation of a detector to the extent that it is useful for predicting the input pattern's categorization. The detector activation will determine which detector is the winner for an input pattern. As such, detectors that are useful for categorization will tend to become winners, thus increasing their learning rate.

Input-to-detector weights are learned via top-down biased competitive learning using the following equation for changing weights from input pattern h to Detector i:

$$\Delta W_{i,h} = \left\{ \begin{array}{l} M(I_{h,p} - W_{i,h}) \text{ if } \forall x(A_{i,p} \geq A_{x,p}) \\ N(I_{h,p} - W_{i,h})K_p \text{ if } \forall y(A_{i,p} \geq A_{i,y}) \\ O(I_{h,p} - W_{i,h})K_p \text{ otherwise} \end{array} \right\} \text{otherwise,} \qquad (3)$$

where M, N, and O are learning rates $(M > N > O)$, and K_p is the distance between pattern p and its closest detector. This distance is inversely related to the cosine of the angle between the vector associated with the closest detector and p. This set of learning rules may appear to be nonlocal in that all detectors are influenced by the closest detector to a pattern and depend on previous presented inputs. However, the rules can be interpreted as local if the pattern itself transmits a signal to detectors revealing how well covered it is, and if detectors have memories for previously attained matches to patterns. When an input pattern is presented, it will first activate the hidden layer of detectors, and then these detectors will cause the category units to become activated. The activation of the category unit A_j will be

$$A_j = \sum_{i=1}^{d} A_i W_{j,i}, \qquad (4)$$

where d is the number of detectors. Detector-to-category weights are learned via the delta rule, $\Delta W_{j,i} = L(T - A_j)A_i$, where L is a learning rate and T is the teacher signal previously described.

We formed a network with two detectors units and two category units and presented it with four input patterns. We gave the network four patterns that were used in experiments with human subjects. These patterns are not identical to the patterns shown in Fig. 7.9 but are of the same abstract construction. When the patterns were categorized as shown in Fig. 7.12A, such that the first two patterns belonged to Category 1 and the second two patterns belonged to Category 2, then on virtually every run the detectors that emerged were those reflecting the diagnostic segments—those segments that were reliably present on Category 1 or Category 2 trials. The picture within a detector unit in Fig. 7.12 reflects the entire

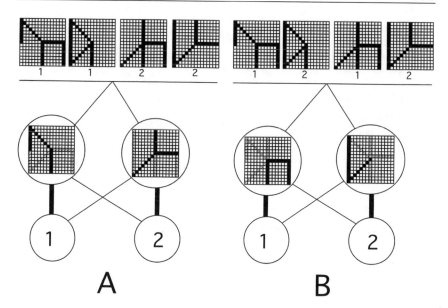

FIG. 7.12. A category learning network based on a supervised version of competitive learning was presented with patterns used by Pevtzow and Goldstone (1994). The same four patterns were categorized in two ways (panels A and B), and each pattern's categorization is shown by the number below it. Intervening between the inputs and the category-level units is a bank of acquired feature detectors. The acquired specialization of these detectors is shown by the matrix within each detector. These matrices show the strength of the connections from each of the 15 × 15 input units to each detector. Strong positive connections are shown in black. Detectors tend to emerge for segments from the inputs that are particularly diagnostic for the categorization. At the same time, strong connections (shown as thicker lines) between these detectors and the appropriate category are learned via a delta learning rule.

weight vector from the 15 × 15 input array to the detector. The darkness of a pixel is proportional to the strength of the input-to-detector connection. When the same patterns are presented, but are categorized in the orthogonal manner shown in Fig. 7.12B, then different detectors emerge that again reflect the category-diagnostic segments. In both cases, each detector will have a strong association to one and only one of the category units. This is expected given that one of the factors influencing the development of detectors was their categorical diagnosticity. For the results shown here, and the later simulations I report, the following parameter values were chosen: M = 0.1, N = 0.05, O = 0.02, and S = 0.1. Activation values were between −1 and +1. One hundred passes through the input materials were presented to the network.

The Segmentation Network

The basic insight connecting categorization and segmentation tasks is that segmentation can also be modeled using competitive learning, and thus the two tasks can share the same network weights and can consequently have an influence on each other. Competitive learning for categorization sorts complete, whole input patterns into separate groups. Competitive learning for segmentation takes a single input pattern and sorts the pieces of the pattern into separate groups. For segmentation, instead of providing a whole pattern at once, we feed in the pattern one pixel at a time, so instead of grouping patterns, the network groups pixels together. Thus, each detector will compete to cover pixels of an input pattern so that the detector with the pixel-to-detector weight that is closest to the pixel's actual value will adapt its weight toward the pixel's value and inhibit other detectors from so adapting. Panels A–D show the weights from the 15×15 input array to each of two detectors and reflect the specializations of the detectors. If the pattern in Fig. 7.13 is presented to the network, the network might segment it in the fashion shown in Panel A. The two segments are complements of each other—if one detector becomes specialized for a pixel, the other detector does not.

Unfortunately, this segmentation is psychologically implausible. No person would decompose the original figure into the parts in Fig. 7.13A. To create psychologically plausible segmentations, we modify the determination of winners. Topological constraints on detector creation are incorporated by two mechanisms: Input-to-detector weights leak to their neighbors in an amount proportional to their proximity in the 15×15 array, and input-to-detector weights also spread to each other as a function of their orientation similarity, defined by the inner product of four orientation filters. The first mechanism produces detectors that tend to respond to cohesive, contiguous regions of an input. The second mechanism produces detectors that follow the principle of good continuation, dividing the figure X into two crossing lines rather than two kissing sideways Vs because the two halves of a diagonal line will be linked by their common orientation. Thus, if a detector wins for pixel X (meaning that the detector receives more activation when pixel X is on than any other detector), then the detector will also tend to handle pixels that are close to, and have similar orientations to, pixel X. The segmentation network, augmented by spreading weights according to spatial and orientation similarity, produces segmentations such as the one shown in Panel B of Fig. 7.13. For an alternative approach to segmentation that uses synchronized oscillations rather than architecturally separated detectors to represent segmentations, see Mozer, Zemel, Behrmann, and Williams (1992).

Although the segmentation in Panel B is clearly superior to Panel A's segmentation, it is still problematic. The pixels are now coherently organized into line segments, but the line segments are not coherently organized into connected parts. Spreading weights according to spatial similarity should ideally create segmentations with connected lines, but such segmentations are often not found because

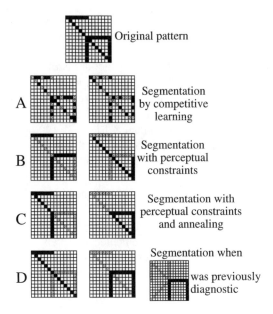

FIG. 7.13.   When a competitive learning segmentation network is supplied the original pattern at top, the detectors specialized for different pixels (panel A). When the network is supplemented with perceptual biases to develop spatially coherent, smooth features, segmentations such as the one shown in panel B are obtained. When this network is now supplemented with an annealing regime that gradually reduces the randomness in the input-to-detector weights as more coherent segments are formed, segmentations such as that shown in Panel C are obtained. When this latter network is run after it has already acquired a detector for a particular component during categorization training (see Fig. 7.12), then the segmentation shown in panel D is typically found.

of local minima in the harmony function (the value N defined later). Local minima occur when a detector develops specializations for distantly related pixels, and these specializations develop into local regions of mutually supporting pixels. Adjacent regions will frequently be controlled by different detectors. Each of the detectors may have sufficiently strong specializations for local regions that they will not be likely to lose their specialization due to the local relations of mutual support.

A common solution to local minima is to incorporate simulated annealing, by which randomness is injected into the system, and the amount of randomness decreases as an exponential function of time (Kirkpatrick, Gelatt, & Vecchi, 1983). Simulated annealing allows a system to settle into a good global minimum by ensuring a sufficient amount of randomness early on to explore the coarse solution landscape and sufficient regularity later on to ensure that the network will set-tle on a single solution. One dissatisfaction with simulated annealing is that the amount of randomness is time-locked. That is, it depends on the number of cy-cles executed by the network rather than the goodness of the network's solution per se. Other researchers have successfully developed annealing approaches that reduce the amount of randomness in the system over time but do so by basing the amount of randomness on the current structural goodness of a solution. For example, in the Copycat project (Hofstadter & Mitchell, 1994), the amount of ran-domness in the system is inversely proportional to the quality of the solution cur-rently found. The current network uses the same notion to create globally coherent segmentations.

The segmentation network works by fully connecting a 15×15 input array of pixel values to a set of N detectors. Although ideally the value of N would be dynamically determined by the input pattern itself, in the current modeling, we assume that each object is to be segmented into two parts (as did Palmer, 1978). When an input pattern is presented, the pixels within it are presented in a random sequence to the detectors, and the activation of detector i which results from presenting pixel p is

$$A_{i,p} = \sum_{h=1}^{n} I_h W_{i,h} S_{h,p}, \tag{5}$$

where I_h is the activation of pixel h, $W_{i,h}$ is the weight from pixel h to detector i, and S is the similarity between pixels h and p. As such, detectors are not only activated directly by presented pixels but are also activated indirectly by pixels that are similar to the presented pixels. Thus, a detector likely will be strongly activated by a certain pixel if it is already activated by other pixels similar to this pixel.

The similarity between two pixels h and p is determined by

$$S_{h,p} = T \frac{\sum\limits_{i=1}^{n} G_{ih} G_{ip} L_{i,h,p}}{n} + U e^{-D_{h,p} C}, \tag{6}$$

where T and U are weighting factors, G_{ih} is the response of orientation filter i to Pixel h, $L_{i,h,p}$ is the degree to which pixels h and p fall on a single line with an orientation specified by filter i, $D_{h,p}$ is the Euclidean distance between pixels h and p, and C is a constant that determines the steepness of the distance function. Four orientation filters were applied, at $0°$, $45°$, $90°$, and $135°$. The response of each filter was found by finding the inner product of the image centered around a pixel and a 5×5 window with the image of one of the four lines. Thus, the greater the overlap between the line and the image, the greater will be the output of the filter for the line. The alignment of two pixels along a certain direction was found by measuring the displacement, in pixels, between the infinite length lines established by the two pixel/orientation pairs.

Pixel-to-detector weights are learned via competitive learning:

$$\Delta W_{i,p} = \begin{cases} M(I_p - W_{i,p}) + Random(-N, +N) \text{ if } \forall x(A_{i,p} \geq A_{x,p}) \\ Random(-N, +N) \text{ otherwise} \end{cases}, \quad (7)$$

where M is a learning rate, and $Random(-N, +N)$ generates Gaussian random noise scaled by $+$ and $-N$. The amount of noise, N, in adjusting weights is a function of the harmony across all detectors relative to R, the maximal harmony in the system:

$$N = R - \sum_{i=1}^{n} \sum_{p=1}^{m} \sum_{h=1}^{m} I_h I_p W_{i,h} W_{i,p} S_{h,p} \quad (8)$$

As such, if similar pixels in similar states have similar weights to detectors, then the harmony in the system will be high, and the amount of noise will be low. Thus, the amount of randomness in the weight-learning process will be inversely proportional to the coherency of the current segmentation. These learning equations allow the network to regularly create segmentations like the one shown in Panel C of Fig. 7.13.

In the simulations of the segmentation network to be reported, no attempt was made to find optimal parameter values. T and U were set at 0.5, M was set at 0.1, and C was set to 1.

Combining the Networks

Considered separately, the categorization and segmentation networks each can be considered to be models of their respective tasks. However, they were also designed to interact, with the aim of accounting for the results from Pevtzow and Goldstone's (1994) experiments with human subjects. The segmentation network, because it shares the same input-to-detector weights that were used for the categorization network, can be influenced by previous category learning. Detectors that were diagnostic for categorization will be more likely used to segment a pattern because they have already been primed. Thus, if a particular shape is diagnostic and reasonably natural, the network will segment the whole into this shape most of the time, as shown in Panel D Fig. 7.13. In short, category learning can alter the perceived organization of an object. By establishing multisegment features along a bank of detectors, the segmentation network is biased to parse objects in terms of these features. Thus, two separate cognitive tasks can be viewed as mutually constraining self-organization processes. Categorization can be understood in terms of the specialization of perceptual detectors for particular input patterns, where the specialization is influenced by the diagnosticity of a segment for categorization. Object segmentation can be viewed as the specialization of detectors for particular parts within a single input pattern. Object segmentation can isolate single parts of an input pattern that are potentially useful for categorization, and categorization can suggest possible ways of parsing an object that would not otherwise have been considered.

To model the results from Pevtzow and Goldstone (1994), the network was first trained on distortions of the patterns A, B, C, and D shown in Fig. 7.9, with either a horizontal or vertical categorization rule. As with the human experiment, the distortions were obtained by adding one random line segment to each pattern in a manner that resulted in a fully contiguous form. Following 30 randomly ordered presentations of distortions of the four patterns, the segmentation network was then presented with the original pattern shown in Fig. 7.13. Segmentations were determined by examining the stable input-to-detector weight matrix for each of the two detector units. Simulation results showed that the segmentation of the ambiguous original object is influenced by category learning. In particular, the original object tended to be segmented into parts that were previously relevant during category learning. As such, the results from Pevtzow and Goldstone (1994) are predicted under the additional assumption that response times in a part/whole task are related to the likelihood of generating a segmentation that includes the probed part.

In a subsequent test of the networks, the actual wholes used by Pevtzow and Goldstone (1994) in their part/whole task were presented to the segmentation network. Each whole was presented 200 times, 100 times preceded by each of the two possible categorization rules. Out of the 24 whole objects tested, segmentations involving categorization-relevant parts were produced more often than segmentations involving irrelevant parts for 19 of the objects. This comparison controls for any intrinsic differences in naturalness between segmentations of a whole object because the parts that are categorization-relevant for half of the simulated subjects are irrelevant for the other half. As such, the reported simulation results generalize to the actual materials used in the experiment.

This modeling shows how learning to group objects into categories affects grouping parts from a single object into segments. Category learning causes detectors to develop, and once these detectors have developed there is a tendency to use these primed detectors when segmenting an object into parts. Future work will be necessary to compare the model to other existing models that allow for experience-dependent visual object segmentation (e.g., Behrmann et al., 1998; Mozer et al., 1992). Two extensions of the model would clearly be desirable: (1) allowing the model to determine for itself how many segments a pattern should be decomposed into and (2) allowing the computed segmentation of a single pattern to influence its categorization. The latter extension is required to fit human experimental evidence suggesting that not only does category learning influence segmentation, but also the perceived segmentation of an object influences its categorization (Schyns et al., 1998; Schyns & Rodet, 1997; Wisniewski & Medin, 1994).

Creating Building Blocks With the Segmentation Network

The categorization and segmentation networks both use principles derived from competitive learning for creating specialized detectors. Using these principles, detectors become specialized for either important classes of input patterns (with categorization) or for important segments within a single input pattern (with segmentation). In both cases, importance was both a function of the unsupervised statistical and psychophysical information in the stimuli and the task requirements involving the stimuli. The learning rules for the two networks were similar, although there were important differences to allow the categorization network to create optimally specialized detectors and the segmentation network to create psychologically plausible detectors. The main difference between the networks was that the categorization network was presented with multiple patterns, one pattern at a time, whereas the segmentation network was presented with only a single pattern, one pixel at a time. When the segmentation network is presented with multiple patterns, with each pattern still presented one pixel at a time, it shows some remarkable properties. The network is able to discover building blocks that can account for an entire set of patterns (as did Ghahramani, 1995), and it can do so while taking into account perceptual constraints to create coherent building blocks, and with an online (rather than batch) learning process.

To understand these properties of the segmentation network, it is helpful to return to the categorization network with a simple example. In Fig. 7.14A, I present four input patterns to a categorization network with two detectors. Like standard competitive learning algorithms (Rumelhart & Zipser, 1985), the network learns the unsupervised statistical structure of the inputs and will typically divide the inputs into two categories—objects with a vertical bar on the left and objects with a vertical bar on the right. In this figure, the pattern shown in each detector represents the 4×4 set of weights going to the detector (0 = white, 1 = black). Superficially, it may appear that this network is extracting out the vertical bars as components of the patterns, but these bars are only strongly present because these are the parts shared by the patterns for which a detector is specialized. The network does not isolate parts; it simply superimposes weight vectors from similar patterns. When this categorization network is given four rather than two detectors, as in Fig. 7.14B, then it will almost always develop a specialized detector for each of the patterns.

If the same patterns are presented to the segmentation network, then very different detectors emerge. Now, as shown in Fig. 7.14C, the segmentation network creates parts that, if combined, would generate each of the four patterns. Instead

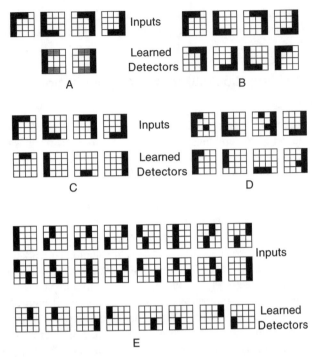

FIG. 7.14. Input patterns and the detectors that are created to accommodate them. When the categorization network is given two detectors and is presented the four shapes in panel A, it typically creates
detectors that are specialized for the two most obvious clusters of input patterns. When the categorization network is given four detectors
(panel B), then each detector becomes specialized for an entire input pattern. This contrasts with the segmentation network's solution
(panel C), which is to decompose the four input patterns into four
parts that can jointly reconstruct the patterns. This kind of componential solution is not found when the composing parts do not obey
Gestalt laws of good organization such as contiguity (panel D). An
advantage of the segmentation network in terms of information compression is shown in panel E, where a set of 16 patterns based on
two dimensions with four values per dimension can be represented
by composing only eight learned parts together.

of creating detectors specialized for entire patterns, it creates detectors for useful
parts—parts that consistently appear across the patterns. These useful parts are
created because a detector that is the winner for a pixel (is relatively specialized
for the pixel) will also tend to be the winner for pixels that cooccur with the pixel.
This is because the amount of activation of a detector when presented with a lit
pixel is not determined only by the connection strength of the link connecting the
pixel to the detector; it is also determined by other lit pixels, modulated by their

link to the detector and their similarity to the pixel in question. This simple leakage of activations between similar, cooccurring pixels suffices to create detectors that will win (have the highest activation) for all pixels of a coherent part that repeatedly recurs. The tendency for a single detector to respond to cooccurring pixels can be strengthened even more by making the similarity of two pixels be not only a function of their orientation and spatial similarity but also their cooccurrence similarity. This cooccurrence similarity is simply obtained by creating a side network that connects every pixel with every other pixel and uses Hebbian learning to alter the links connecting pixels. With this network, pixels that are simultaneously present will develop strong positive links connecting them, and these links represent high cooccurrence similarity.

The segmentation network is still influenced by the spatial and orientation similarity of pixels when creating detectors, with the consequence that statistically equivalent input sets are not treated equivalently. This is apparent in Fig. 7.14D. The input patterns have the same logical structure as those in Fig. 7.14C, but one of the pixels (on the top row, third from the left) has been shifted down by two pixels. However, the detectors no longer create four detectors that can combine in different arrangements to exactly recreate each of the input patterns. This would be possible if the network created a detector with two disconnected pixels, but such a detector is unlikely to be created even if the pixels perfectly predict each other's presence. The previously described EM algorithm does not have this constraint on creating perceptually coherent segments, but the empirical evidence suggests that people do indeed have such a constraint. In other work from my laboratory using exactly the grid materials shown in Fig. 7.14, we find that people rarely construct parts out of pixels that are separated by a chess knight's move. Instead, they either ignore one of the pixels, create a contiguous part by adding connecting pixels, or mentally distort the position of one of the pixels to make the part more coherent.

The detectors created in Fig. 7.14, parts B and C, are both reasonable solutions, and each has its place. Fig. 7.14B's detectors offer a more holistic solution, creating detectors that become imprinted on whole input patterns. The power of Fig. 7.14C's decompositional solution becomes apparent in Fig. 7.14E. Here, 16 input patterns can be represented in terms of conjunctions of eight acquired detectors. Again, the detectors that emerge combine pixels that are similar in their orientations and locations and reliably cooccur. Each of the 16 original patterns can be reconstructed exactly using only half as many detectors as would be required from a holistic solution. As a side benefit, the network also learns about negative contingencies between stimulus parts, for example, learning that a vertical bar on the top left predicts the absence of a vertical bar on the top right. This is a valuable first step in learning new dimension organizations, given that dimensions can be understood as sets of mutually exclusive alternative values. The feature values Red and Blue belong to the same Color dimension because an elementary object can only possess one of the values. The network implicitly extracts these relations, coming to represent the stimuli of Fig. 7.14E in terms two dimensions each of which has four mutually exclusive alternatives.

The segmentation network is capable of constructing part-based representations for a set of stimuli, but depending on the statistical structures present in a set of stimuli, it can also create the same kind of holistic representations as the categorization network. For example, in Fig. 7.15A, four patterns that have very little overlap are presented to the network. In this case, the detectors each become specialized for an entire input pattern because there are no useful, frequently recurring parts to extract. More interestingly, in Fig. 7.15B, the input patterns fall into two varieties. Four of the patterns are composed of recurring parts, and one of the patterns is isolated from the others in that it shares no pixels with any other pattern. The segmentation network accommodates these patterns by representing most of the patterns componentially (as the conjunction of two detectors) but one of the patterns holistically. Consistent with the complementary advantages of configural and analytic representations, the network will represent patterns that are composed of factorially combined parts in terms of their parts but will simultaneously represent sparsely distributed and isolated patterns in terms of entire patterns. As such, the network has a natural way of reconciling the empirical evidence for unitization and differentiation. Both representations can be created, depending on the categorical and statistical pressures.

The results from these last figures suggests that the segmentation network can provide an account of learned differentiation into parts, but a final example shows a more specific analog to the 90° and 45° rotation conditions. Recall that participants showed better transfer between categorization rules related by 90°, rather than 45°. I argued that this was because orthogonal dimensions (separated by 90°) are compatible in that their contributions to a stimulus can be independently determined and combined. An analog of this is shown in Fig. 7.15C, where three patterns are presented, and four detectors are assigned to the segmentation network. The learned detectors show that the box pattern on the left is broken down into four bars. The presence of the two horizontal bars should come as no surprise given that they were also presented as input patterns. However, the two vertical bars reveal the extraction of detectors that are complementary to, and hence compatible with, other extracted detectors. Just as a rectangle can be consistently organized in terms of height and width (see Fig. 7.8), the box on the left is consistently organized into horizontal and vertical bars—bars that have no overlapping pieces. Fig. 7.15D shows that this trend toward extracting consistent parts can overcome some preferences in terms of perceptual organization. In Fig. 7.15D, the same box pattern is presented with two diagonal segments, and the network extracts these diagonal segments and the other diagonal segments that can combine to form the box pattern. Similar to the strong transfer found between orthogonal (90° rotated) dimensions, priming the segmentation network with some parts of a pattern makes the network also extract the parts of the pattern that are consistent with these primed parts. The explanation for this behavior is the same competitive learning principle.

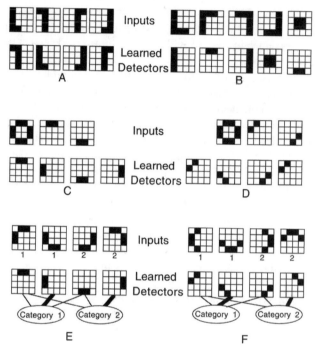

FIG. 7.15. Like the categorization network, the segmentation network can also develop detectors specialized for entire input patterns if the input patterns possess little overlap (panel A). In fact, it can also develop a hybrid representation, representing some objects in terms of their parts and other objects as configurations. Part-based representations will be used for objects that share several segments in common with other objects from the set, whereas whole-object representations will be used for isolated objects (panel B). In panels C and D, the boxlike input pattern on the left is decomposed into different parts by the segmentation network, depending on other patterns that are presented. Detectors are created for parts that are complements of presented patterns, even though the complements are never presented by themselves. When patterns are presented with category assignments (shown as numbers below input patterns), there is a tendency to extract parts that are diagnostic for the categorization and also to extract the compatible complements of those diagnostic parts. This is shown in panels E and F, as are the learned associations between detectors and category units. The connection strength between detectors and categories is shown by the thickness of the line connecting them.

When the patterns of Fig. 7.15D are presented, detectors will likely emerge for the two pairs of diagonally related pixels that always cooccur. Once these detectors are constructed, they will be likely to win the competition for the diagonal portions of the box pattern when it is presented, leaving the two other diagonal parts left to be claimed. These unclaimed parts will then be claimed by detectors that have not yet become specialized.

Fig. 7.15, Panels C and D, show that actions that promote attending a part (such as presenting it or making it diagnostic for a categorization) also promote attending to the complementary part that is consistent with it. Fig. 7.15, Panels E and F, shows that this occurs even with displays that are closer analogs to the stimuli shown in Fig. 7.9. In these figures, each input pattern is made up of two features, and each feature has two possible values. Unlike previous demonstrations of the segmentation network, the patterns are categorized into two groups so that the first two patterns belong to Category 1, and the second two patterns belong to Category 2. The network creates early detectors for the category-relevant parts and learns strong weights between these detectors and the appropriate category unit, as shown by the relatively thick lines connecting diagnostic detectors to category units. However, the network also learns the complements of these diagnostic parts exactly because the complements are the parts that remain in a stimulus once diagnostic parts have been accommodated.

Fig. 7.15, Panels C–F, are analogs to the dimension differentiation observed by Goldstone and Steyvers (2001) in that consistent rather than cross-cutting featural interpretations are generated. The simulations are only analogs because the experiments were concerned with the extraction of independent, complementary dimensions that influenced the whole stimulus rather than spatially isolated parts. There seems to be a close connection between organizing an object into dimensions and parts, but I leave it for future work to reveal whether the simulations reported here can be interpreted as more than mere analogies. At least the segmentation network provides a way of intuitively understanding the seemingly paradoxical positive transfer between orthogonal (90° rotated) categorization rules. When considering a physical part of an object, it is natural to notice the complement of the part—the parts that remain in the stimulus when the part is removed. It is easy to see that the complement requires the same parsing of the object into pieces as does the part itself. In the same way, a dimension is compatible with a second dimension that is removed from it by 90°.

CONCLUSIONS

On both empirical and theoretical grounds I have argued that the perceptual descriptions given to objects are influenced by the tasks for which the objects are used. Several types of perceptual change were empirically reported. Imprinting on whole objects happens if they occur frequently or on parts of objects if the parts are shared across several objects. These two types of imprinting can occur in the absence of any feedback. The stimuli themselves, and their statistical properties, can drive the perceptual learning. However, each of these two types of learning also has a parallel when the objects are learned in the context of categorization. Learning by imprinting on whole objects becomes particularly influential when a specific object belongs in an important category. In a process referred to as unitization, originally separated parts of an object are combined into a unified and coherent whole. Once constructed, the unit can be efficiently recognized and has properties similar to a photograph-like template. Category learning can also induce the opposite process to occur, separating originally integrated percepts into psychologically differentiated dimensions or parts. Rather than viewing unitization and differentiation as contradictory, they are best viewed as aspects of the same process that bundles stimulus components together if they diagnostically cooccur and separates these bundles from other statistically independent bundles. Under this conception, learning a featural or dimensional organization consists in learning how to carve a stimulus into useful components.

The empirical conclusion, generalized to unify differentiation and unitization, is that the perceptual building blocks used for representing objects adapt to unsupervised and supervised demands. This conclusion has a consequence for literature on the development of perception with age or expertise. Rather than trying to characterize development in terms of a single integral-to-separable or component-to-configural trend, this conclusion suggests that both of these trends should be expected and that which is found will depend on the nature of the stimuli and the feedback. Both trends potentially can be explained by a single process of creating useful building blocks. There are real and important differences between perceiving an object by breaking it down into parts and by matching it to a configural representation. However, in both cases units are formed so that the physical segments within the units interact and interfere with each other and are likely to be perceived together, whereas segments from different units are relatively independent. For example, regardless of whether a unit of perception exists at the line segment, letter, syllable, word, phrase, or sentence level (Wheeler, 1970), the same factors will probably determine the strength of the unit: How often do the unit's pieces cooccur, how important is that cooccurrence for a linguistic category, how often do the unit's pieces cooccur with pieces from other units, and what perceptual grouping principles support the unit?

The major theoretical contribution of the research has been to specify a model for how perceptual and conceptual learning might interact. In the neural network presented, feature detectors are developed that represent the network's set of acquired vocabulary elements. The network begins with homogenous, undifferentiated detectors that become specialized for different patterns or pattern parts over time. Furthermore, the model has a mechanism by which detector-to-category associations modify the nature of the detectors. It is not necessary to first develop detectors and then build associations between detectors and categories. These two types of learning can and should go on simultaneously (Goldstone, 1994b). The concepts to be learned can reach down and influence the very features that ground the concepts. This is done without requiring dynamic, online recurrent activation passing, as is found in McClelland and Rumelhart's (1981) interactive activation model. That is, when processing patterns, the network is purely feedforward, with input patterns triggering detectors, and detectors triggering categories. Categories influence the detectors that are created by making useful detectors more likely to be constructed. However, once constructed, categories do not need to send activation to detectors nor do detectors affect input representations (although these are interesting possibilities to explore). The feedforward nature of the network is advantageous with respect to speed and efficiency. The network's detectors can be quickly triggered before category-level information is available on a particular occasion, even though their nature has been adapted over longer time courses to categorization needs.

Like a good pair of Birkenstock shoes that provide support by flexibly conforming to the foot, perceptual object descriptions support our concepts by conforming to these concepts. Ironically, more stable shoes and perceptions would actually be less adequate as foundations. In these and other situations, flexible, not rigid, foundations make strong foundations. If flexibility in perceptual foundations is desirable, it is important to also remember that this flexibility is constrained by perceptual grouping principles (Kellman & Arterberry, 1998), informational requirements, patterns of repetition and cooccurrence, and task usefulness. Within these constraints, the building blocks of perception can show a surprising degree of adaptability. Human creativity requires a certain amount of conceptual block busting to be sure (Adams, 1974) but also benefits from a healthy dose of perceptual block building.

ACKNOWLEDGMENTS

The research reported in this chapter has benefited greatly from comments and suggestions by Marlene Behrmann, Rutie Kimchi, John Kruschke, Douglas Medin, Amy Needham, Robert Nosofsky, Mary Peterson, and Richard Shiffrin. This research was supported by National Institute of Health Grant R01 MH56871 and National Science Foundation Grant 0125287. The author can be reached by electronic mail at rgoldsto@indiana.edu and further information about the laboratory can be found at http://cognitrn.psych.indiana.edu/.

REFERENCES

Adams, J. L. (1974). *Conceptual blockbusting: A guide to better ideas*. New York: Freeman.
Allard, T., Clark, S. A., Jenkins, W. M., & Merzenich, M. M. (1991). Reorganization of somatosensory area 3b representation in adult Owl Monkeys after digital syndactyly. *Journal of Neurophysiology, 66*, 1048–1058.

Behrmann, M., Zemel, R. S., & Mozer, M. C. (1998). Object-based attention and occlusion: Evidence from normal participants and a computational model. *Journal of Experimental Psychology: Human Perception and Performance, 24,* 1011–1036.

Biederman, I. (1987). Recognition-by-components: A theory of human image understanding. *Psychological Review, 94,* 115–147.

Bruce, V. (1998). *In the eye of the beholder: The science of face perception.* New York: Oxford University Press.

Bruner, J. S., Postman, L., & Rodriguez, J. (1951). Expectations and the perception of color. *American Journal of Psychology, 64,* 216–227.

Burns, B., & Shepp, B. E. (1988). Dimensional interactions and the structure of psychological space: The representation of hue, saturation, and brightness. *Perception and Psychophysics, 43,* 494–507.

Cattell, J. M. (1886). The time it takes to see and name objects. *Mind, 11,* 63–65.

Czerwinski, M., Lightfoot, N., & Shiffrin, R. M. (1992). Automatization and training in visual search. *The American Journal of Psychology, 105,* 271–315.

Dempster, A., Laird, N., & Rubin, D. (1977). Maximum likelihood from incomplete data via the EM algorithm. *Journal of the Royal Statistical Society Series B, 39,* 1–38.

Edelman, S. (1999). *Representation and recognition in vision.* Cambridge, MA: MIT Press.

Egly, R., & Homa. D. (1984). Sensitization of the visual field. *Journal of Experimental Psychology: Human Perception and Performance, 10,* 778–793.

Eriksen, C. W., & Murphy, T. D. (1987). Movement of attentional focus across the visual field: A critical look at the evidence. *Perception & Psychophysics, 14,* 255–260.

Fahle, M., & Morgan, M. (1996). No transfer of perceptual learning between similar stimuli in the same retinal position. *Current Biology, 6,* 292–297.

Farah, M. J. (1992). Is an object an object an object? Cognitive and neuropsychological investigations of domain-specificity in visual object recognition. *Current Directions in Psychological Science, 1,* 164–169.

Frank, D. A., & Greenberg, M. E. (1994). CREB: A mediator of long-term memory from mollusks to mammals. *Cell, 79,* 5–8.

Garner, W. R. (1976). Interaction of stimulus dimensions in concept and choice processes. *Cognitive Psychology, 8,* 98–123.

Garner, W. R. (1978). Selective attention to attributes and to stimuli. *Journal of Experimental Psychology: General, 107,* 287–308.

Garraghty, P. E., & Kaas, J. H. (1992). Dynamic features of sensory and motor maps. *Current Opinion in Neurobiology, 2,* 522–527.

Gauthier, I., & Tarr, M. J. (1997). Becoming a "greeble" expert: Exploring mechanisms for face recognition. *Vision Research, 37,* 1673–1682.

Gauthier, I., Williams, P., Tarr, M. J., & Tanaka, J. (1998). Training "greeble" experts: A framework for studying expert object recognition processes, *Vision Research, 38,* 2401–2428.

Ghahramani, Z. (1995). Factorial learning and the EM algorithm. In G. Tesauro, D. S. Touretzky, & T. K. Leen (Eds.), *Advances in neural information processing systems 7* (pp. 617–624). Cambridge, MA: MIT Press.

Gibson, E. J. (1969). *Principles of perceptual learning and development.* New York: Appleton-Century-Crofts.

Goldstone, R. L. (1994a). Influences of categorization on perceptual discrimination. *Journal of Experimental Psychology: General, 123,* 178–200.

Goldstone, R. L. (1994b). The role of similarity in categorization: Providing a groundwork. *Cognition, 52,* 125–157.

Goldstone, R. L. (1998). Perceptual learning. *Annual Review of Psychology, 49,* 585–612.

Goldstone, R. L. (2000). Unitization during category learning. *Journal of Experimental Psychology: Human Perception and Performance, 26,* 86–112.

Goldstone, R. L., & Barsalou, L. (1998). Reuniting perception and conception. *Cognition, 65,* 231–262.

Goldstone, R. L., Lippa, Y., & Shiffrin, R. M. (2001). Altering object representations through category learning. *Cognition, 78,* 27–43.

Goldstone, R. L., & Stevyers, M. (2001). The sensitization and differentiation of dimensions during category learning. *Journal of Experimental Psychology: General, 130,* 116–139.

Goldstone, R. L., Steyvers, M., Spencer-Smith, J., & Kersten, A. (2000). Interactions between perceptual and conceptual learning. In E. Diettrich & A. B. Markman (Eds.), *Cognitive dynamics: Conceptual change in humans and machines* (pp. 191–228). Mahwah, NJ: Lawrence Erlbaum Associates.

Grossberg, S. (1987). Competitive learning: From interactive activation to adaptive resonance. *Cognitive Science, 11,* 23–63.

Hall, G. (1991). *Perceptual and associative learning.* Oxford, UK: Clarendon Press.

Hinton, G. E., Dayan, P., Frey, B. J., & Neal, R. M. (1995). The "wake-sleep" algorithm for unsupervised neural networks. *Science, 268,* 1158–1161.

Hofstadter, D. R., & Mitchell, M. (1994). The Copycat project: A model of mental fluidity and analogy-making. In K. J. Holyoak & J. A. Barnden (Eds.), *Advances in connectionist and neural computation theory, Volume 2* (pp. 31–112). Norwood, NJ: Ablex.

Hummel, J. E. (2000). Where view-based theories break down: The role of structure in human shape perception. In E. Diettrich & A. B. Markman (Eds.), *Cognitive dynamics: Conceptual change in humans and machines* (pp. 157–185). Mahwah, NJ: Lawrence Erlbaum Associates.

Jakobson, R., Fant, G., & Halle, M. (1963). *Preliminaries to speech analysis: The distinctive features and their correlates.* Cambridge, MA: MIT Press.

Johnson, S. P. (1997). Young infants' perception of object unity: Implications for development of attentional and cognitive skills. *Current Directions in Psychological Science, 6,* 5–11.

Karni, A., & Sagi, D. (1991). Where practice makes perfect in texture discrimination: Evidence for primary visual cortex plasticity. *Proceedings of the National Academy of Sciences of the United States of America, 88,* 4966–4970.

Kaas, J. H. (1991). Plasticity of sensory and motor maps in adult mammals. *Annual Review of Neuroscience, 14,* 137–167.

Kay, P., & McDaniel, C. (1978). The linguistic significance of the meaning of basic color terms. *Language, 54,* 610–646.

Kellman, P. J., & Arterberry, M. E. (1998). *The cradle of knowledge.* Cambrdige, MA: MIT Press.

Kemler, D. G., & Smith, L. B. (1978). Is there a developmental trend from integrality to separability in perception? *Journal of Experimental Child Psychology, 26,* 498–507.

Kirkpatrick, S., Gelatt, C. D., & Vecchi, M. P. (1983). Optimization by simulated annealing, *Science, 220,* 671–680.

Koffka, K. (1935). *Principles of Gestalt psychology.* New York: Harcourt Brace.

Kohonen, T. (1995). *Self-organizing maps.* Berlin: Springer-Verlag.

Kolers, P. A., & Roediger, H. L. (1984). Procedures of mind. *Journal of Verbal Learning and Verbal Behavior, 23,* 425–449.

Kuhn, T. S. (1962). *The structure of scientific revolutions.* Chicago: University of Chicago Press.

LaBerge, D. (1973). Attention and the measurement of perceptual learning. *Memory and Cognition, 1,* 268–276.

Lin, E. L., & Murphy, G. L. (1997). Effects of background knowledge on object categorization and part detection. *Journal of Experimental Psychology: Human Perception and Performance, 23,* 1153–1169.

Markman, A. B. (1999). *Knowledge representation.* Mahwah, NJ: Lawrence Erlbaum Associates.

McClelland, J. L., & Rumelhart, D. E. (1981). An interactive activation model of context effects in letter perception: Part 1. An account of basic findings. *Psychological Review, 88,* 375–407.

Medin, D. L., & Shaeffer, M. M. (1978). A context theory of classification learning. *Psychological Review, 85,* 207–238.

Melara, R. D., Marks, L. E., & Potts, B. C. (1993). Primacy of dimensions in color perception. *Journal of Experimental Psychology: Human Perception and Performance, 19,* 1082–1104.

Miikkulainen, R., Bednar, J. A., Choe, Y., & Sirosh, J. (1997). Self-organization, plasticity, and low-level visual phenomena in a laterally connected map model of primary visual cortex. In R. L. Goldstone, P. G. Schyns, & D. L. Medin (Eds.), *Perceptual learning: The psychology of learning and motivation* (pp. 257–308). San Diego: Academic Press.

Mozer, M. C., Zemel, R. S., Behrmann, M., & Williams, C. K. I. (1992). Learning to segment images using dynamic feature binding. *Neural Computation, 4,* 650–665.

Needham, A. (1997). Factors affecting infants' use of featural information in object segregation. *Current Directions in Psychological Science, 6,* 26–33.

Needham, A. (1999). The role of shape in 4-month-old infants' segregation of adjacent objects. *Infant Behavior and Development, 22,* 161–178.

Nosofsky, R. M. (1986). Attention, similarity, and the identification-categorization relationship. *Journal of Experimental Psychology: General, 115,* 39–57.

Obermayer, K., Sejnowski, T., & Blasdel, G. G. (1995). Neural pattern formation via a competitive Hebbian mechanism. *Behavioral Brain Research, 66,* 161–167.

O'Reilly, R. C., & Munakata, Y. (2000). *Computational explorations in cognitive neuroscience: Understanding the mind by simulating the brain.* Cambridge, MA: MIT Press.

Palmer, S. E. (1977). Hierarchical structure in perceptual representation. *Cognitive Psychology, 9,* 441–474.

Palmer, S. E. (1978). Structural aspects of visual similarity. *Memory & Cognition, 6,* 91–97.

Palmeri, T. J. (1997). Exemplar similarity and the development of automaticity. *Journal of Experimental Psychology: Learning, Memory, and Cognition, 23,* 324–354.

Pevtzow, R., & Goldstone, R. L. (1994). Categorization and the parsing of objects. *Proceedings of the Sixteenth Annual Conference of the Cognitive Science Society* (pp. 717–722). Hillsdale, NJ: Lawrence Erlbaum Associates.

Pick, H. L. (1992). Eleanor J. Gibson: Learning to perceive and perceiving to learn. *Developmental Psychology, 28,* 787–794.

Rumelhart, D. E., & Zipser, D. (1985). Feature discovery by competitive learning. *Cognitive Science, 9,* 75–112.

Schacter, D. L. (1987). Implicit memory: History and current status. *Journal of Experimental Psychology: Learning, Memory, and Cognition, 13,* 501–518.

Schafer, R. P. (1983). The synchronic behavior of basic color terms in Tswana and its diachronic implications. *Studies in African Linguistics, 14,* 112–123.

Schank, R. (1972). Conceptual dependency: A theory of natural language understanding. *Cognitive Psychology, 3,* 552–631.

Schmidhuber, J., Eldracher, M., & Foltin, B. (1996). Semilinear predictability minimization produces well-known feature detectors. *Neural Computation, 8,* 773–786.

Schyns, P. G., Goldstone, R. L., & Thibaut, J. (1998). Development of features in object concepts. *Behavioral and Brain Sciences, 21,* 1–54.

Schyns, P. G., & Rodet, L. (1997). Categorization creates functional features. *Journal of Experimental Psychology: Learning, Memory, and Cognition, 23,* 681–696.

Shapiro, P. N., & Penrod, S. D. (1986). Meta-analysis of face identification studies. *Psychological Bulletin, 100,* 139–156.

Shiffrin, R. M., & Lightfoot, N. (1997). Perceptual learning of alphanumeric-like characters. In R. L. Goldstone, P. G. Schyns, & D. L. Medin (Eds.), *The psychology of learning and motivation,* Volume 36 (pp. 45–82). San Diego: Academic Press.

Shiu, L., & Pashler, H. (1992). Improvement in line orientation discrimination is retinally local but dependent on cognitive set. *Perception and Psychophysics, 52,* 582–588.

Slater, A., Morison, V., Somers, M., Mattock, A., Brown, E., & Taylor, D. (1990). Newborn and older infants' perception of partly occluded objects. *Infant Behavior and Development, 13,* 33–49.

Smith, L. B. (1989). From global similarity to kinds of similarity: The construction of dimensions in development. In S. Vosniadou & A. Ortony (Eds.), *Similarity and analogical reasoning* (pp. 146–178). Cambridge, UK: Cambridge University Press.

Smith, L. B., Gasser, M., & Sandhofer, C. (1997). Learning to talk about the properties of objects: A network model of the development of dimensions. In R. L. Goldstone, P. G. Schyns, & D. L. Medin (Eds.), *The psychology of learning and motivation, Vol. 36* (pp. 219–255). San Diego, CA: Academic Press.

Smith, L. B., & Kemler, D. G. (1978). Levels of experienced dimensionality in children and adults. *Cognitive Psychology, 10,* 502–532.

Sowden, P. T., Davies, I. R. L., & Roling, P. (2000). Perceptual learning of the detection of features in X-ray images: A functional role for improvements in adults' visual sensitivity? *Journal of Experimental Psychology: Human Perception and Performance, 26,* 379–390.

Steyvers, M. (1999). Morphing techniques for generating and manipulating face images. *Behavior Research Methods, Instruments, & Computers, 31,* 359–369.

Sutherland, N. S., & Mackintosh, N. J. (1971). *Mechanisms of animal discrimination learning.* New York: Academic Press.

Tenenbaum, J. B. (1996). Learning the structure of similarity. In G. Tesauro, D. S. Touretzky, & T. K. Leen (Eds.), *Advances in neural information processing systems 8* (pp. 4–9). Cambridge, MA: MIT Press.

Treisman, A., & Gelade, G. (1980). A feature-integration theory of attention. *Cognitive Psychology, 12,* 97–136.

Weinberger, N. M. (1993). Learning-induced changes of auditory receptive fields. *Current Opinion in Neurobiology, 3,* 570–577.

Weisstein, N., & Harris, C. S. (1974). Visual detection of line segments: An object-superiority effect. *Science, 186,* 752–755.

Wheeler, D. D. (1970). Processes in word recognition. *Cognitive Psychology, 1,* 59–85.

Whorf, B. L. (1956). Languages and logic. In J. B. Carroll (Ed.), *Language, thought, and reality: Selected papers of Benjamin Lee Whorf* (pp. 233–245). Cambridge, MA: MIT Press. (Original work published 1941)

Wierzbicka, A. (1992). Semantic primitives and semantic fields. In A. Lehrer & E. F. Kittay (Eds.), *Frames, fields, and contrasts: New essays in semantic and lexical organization* (pp. 209–228). Hillsdale, NJ: Lawrence Erlbaum Associates.

Wisniewski, E. J., & Medin, D. L. (1994). On the interaction of theory and data in concept learning. *Cognitive Science, 18,* 221–281.

Zemel, R. S., Behrmann, M., Mozer, M. C., & Bavelier, D. (1999). *Experience-dependent perceptual grouping and object-based attention.* Unpublished manuscript.

III

Neural Approaches
to Perceptual Organization

8 Neural Coding of Border Ownership: Implications for the Theory of Figure-Ground Perception

Rüdiger von der Heydt
Hong Zhou
Howard S. Friedman
Johns Hopkins University

The interpretation of two-dimensional retinal images in terms of a three-dimensional world is a fundamental problem of vision, which, through evolution and experience, has shaped the neural processing mechanisms in our visual system. An example is the tendency to perceive contrast borders as part of one of the adjacent regions, as if they were contours of objects in three-dimensional space. Rubin's famous vase figure demonstrates this compulsion of the visual system (Fig. 8.1). The borders are perceived either as the contours of a vase or as the contours of two faces. Each border is perceived as belonging to one or the other side but rarely to both. In the case of a simple figure, such as the light square of Fig. 8.2A, the contrast borders are of course perceived as the contours of the square; they seem to belong to the enclosed light-textured region. The surrounding gray does not own the borders; therefore, it is perceived as extending behind the square, and hence is called the background. This tendency of perception was first described by the Gestalt psychologists (Koffka, 1935) and was termed the law of the interior (Metzger, 1953).

We can understand this compulsion of the visual system to assign borders unilaterally as a consequence of the main goal of its design: to infer a three-dimensional world from two-dimensional images. The images are usually projections of three-dimensional scenes in which objects in the foreground occlude others in the

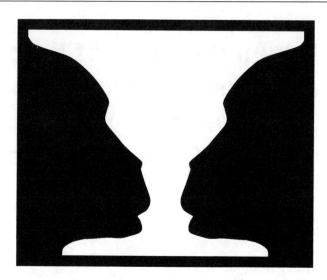

FIG. 8.1.   The visual system tends to interpret contrast borders as occluding contours. In this figure the black-white borders are perceived
either as contours of the vase or as contours of the faces.

background. In the image, foreground and background become adjacent regions.
The borders between foreground and background regions (the contours of the
silhouettes of objects) are called occluding contours. For the vision process the
detection of occluding contours is of fundamental importance because the features
of different objects have to be kept separate and because occluding contours carry
important shape information. This information has to be assigned unilaterally because the shape of an occluding contour gives information about the foreground
object but bears no relation to the background. Occluding contours usually appear as sharp contrast borders because foreground and background are generally
unrelated and will therefore likely differ in luminance or chromaticity. Although
contrast borders can also have other causes, such as surface texture and shading, they are most frequently produced by occlusion. Therefore, identifying sharp
contrast borders as occluding contours is an efficient strategy (Marr, 1982).

Because the assignment of borders to regions is a basic task of vision, we
wondered if and where signals in the visual cortex would indicate the ownership
of borders. In the experiments we review in this chapter, we recorded from cells
in the cortex of monkeys during behaviorally induced fixation and compared the
responses to contrast borders when these borders were displayed as part of different
visual objects (Zhou, Friedman, & von der Heydt, 2000). Fixation was induced
by having the animals respond quickly to an orientation change in a small target,
which occurred at a random time in each trial. Thus, the animal attended to the
fixation target rather than the test stimuli.

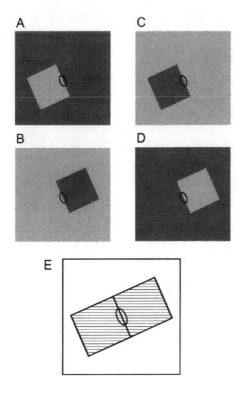

Predictions

(1) Local edge only: A = B and C = D

(2) Border ownership: A + C > B + D (left side), or B + D > A + C (right side)

FIG. 8.2. The standard test used in experiments by Zhou et al. (2000) to assess border ownership coding in neurons of the visual cortex. Ellipses represent the minimum response field of the cell under study. The same local edge was presented as the top right edge of a light square (A) and the bottom left edge of a dark square (B). (C–D), Analogous displays with contrast reversed. (E), Hatched area indicates region of identical stimulation in A–B and C–D. From "Coding of Border Ownership in Monkey Visual Cortex," by H. Zhou, H. S. Friedman, and R. von der Heydt, 2000, *Journal of Neuroscience, 20,* p. 6594–6611. Copyright 2000 by Society for Neuroscience. Adapted with permission.

The basic test is shown in Fig. 8.2. Once the action potentials of a cell were isolated and its minimum response field[1] determined (ellipse), an edge of a square at optimal orientation was centered in the field. For example, the edge could be the right side of a light square, as in Fig. 8.2A, or the left side of a dark square, as in Fig. 8.2B. Two colors or grays were used for square and background, namely, the previously determined preferred color of the cell (which could also be black or white) and a light gray. The colors of square and background, and the side of the square, were switched between trials, resulting in the four conditions shown in Fig. 8.2. Note that the contrast borders presented in the receptive field are identical in Fig. 8.2A and B and so are the contrast borders in Fig. 8.2C and D, which have reversed contrast compared to Fig. 8.2A and B.

The size of the square defined the neighborhood around the receptive field in which displays in Fig. 8.2A and B (or C and D) are identical, as illustrated by hatching in Fig. 8.2E. Thus, if the activity of a neuron were solely determined by local features, it would respond equally to Fig. 8.2, A and B, and equally to C and D. However, if the neural response carries border ownership information, there should be consistent differences depending on the side of the figure; the sum of the responses to Fig. 8.2, A and C, should be greater, for example, than the sum of the responses to Fig. 8.2, B and D. In principle, it would be sufficient to compare the responses between A and B (or C and D) to assess border ownership selectivity, but the effect of the local edge contrast polarity (A + B vs. C + D) is also of interest, as we will see.

RESULTS

Integration of Global Form Cues

Neurons in cortical areas V1, V2, and V4 were studied with this test. In V1 (the striate cortex) we focused on layers 2–3, which provide the main output to the extrastriate areas. An example of a cell recorded from V2 is shown in Fig. 8.3. The stimulus was a green square surrounded by gray in Fig. 8.3, parts A and D and a gray square surrounded by green in Fig. 8.3, parts B and C. The ellipses indicate the location and approximate size of the minimum response field, and the crosses mark the position of the fixation target. The raster plots at the bottom show the responses to repeated random presentations of the four stimuli. It can be seen that the cell responded more strongly to a display with the figure on the left side (Fig. 8.3A) than on the right side (Fig. 8.3B) although the local edge was identical. Furthermore, when the contrast was reversed, the cell again produced a stronger response to the figure on the left side (cf. Fig. 8.3, parts C and D). Thus, the cell

---

[1]The minimum response field is the minimum region of visual field outside which no response can be evoked with an optimized bar stimulus (Barlow et al., 1967). Fig. 8.13A of Zhou et al. (2000) illustrates the procedure for determining the minimum response field.

Cell 13id4 (V2)

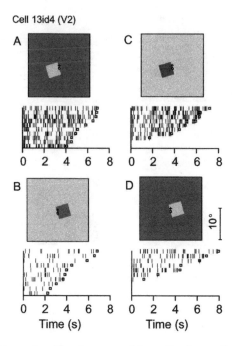

FIG. 8.3.   Example of border ownership coding in a cell recorded in area V2 in the behaving monkey. The stimuli are shown at the top, and event plots of the corresponding responses are at the bottom. Ellipses indicate location and orientation of minimum response field, and crosses show position of fixation target. In the event plots, each row represents a trial, and small vertical lines represent the times of action potentials relative to the moment of lever pulling (which generally indicated the beginning of fixation). Small squares indicate the time of target flip (end of fixation). For each condition, trials are sorted according to length of fixation period. (A–B), The cell responded better to the edge of a green square on the left side than to the edge of gray square on the right side of the receptive field, although both stimuli were locally identical (green depicted here as light gray). (C–D), When the colors were reversed, the cell again responded better to an edge that belonged to a square on the left than a square on the right. From "Coding of Border Ownership in Monkey Visual Cortex," by H. Zhou, H. S. Friedman, and R. von der Heydt, 2000, *Journal of Neuroscience, 20*, p. 6594–6611. Copyright 2000 by Society for Neuroscience. Reprinted with permission.

was selective for the side of the figure. Response strength and side preference were independent of the local contrast polarity.

Fig. 8.4 shows a second example of a V2 cell. This cell was color selective, preferring dark reddish colors, and brown and gray were used for the test (depicted here as dark and light gray). The cell responded to the top edge but not the bottom edge of the brown square, and it barely responded to the edges of the gray square.

Cell 12ij2 (V2)

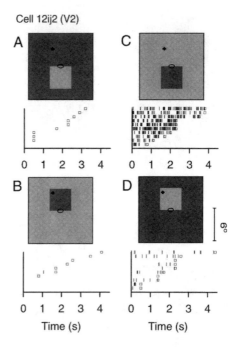

FIG. 8.4. Example of simultaneous coding of border-ownership and edge contrast polarity. This cell of area V2 was color selective with a preference for dark, reddish colors. Brown and gray were used for the test (here depicted as dark and light gray). Other conventions as for Fig. 8.3. The cell responded to the upper edge of a brown square (C) but hardly at all to the lower edge of a gray square (D), although in both cases the same gray/brown color boundary was presented in the receptive field. The cell did not respond at all to edges of the reversed contrast (A, B). From "Coding of Border Ownership in Monkey Visual Cortex," by H. Zhou, H. S. Friedman, and R. von der Heydt, 2000, *Journal of Neuroscience, 20*, p. 6594–6611. Copyright 2000 by Society for Neuroscience. Reprinted with permission.

The differences between Fig. 8.4, parts A and C and between B and D indicate that the cell was selective for edge contrast polarity. This is thought to be typical for simple cells (Schiller, Finlay, & Volman, 1976). However, the responses of this cell were much stronger in Fig. 8.4, part C than in D, in which the local edge contrast was the same, showing that the responses were not solely determined by the local edge but depended also on the side of figure location. The factors side of figure and local contrast polarity also interacted. As a result, the cell responded almost exclusively to displays in which a horizontal contrast border was present in the minimum response field, the border belonged to a figure below the field, and the figure was red.

In other cells the responses were determined solely by the local contrast border. These cells responded equally to displays in Fig. 8.4, parts A and B and to displays

C and D. Some of these were selective for the contrast polarity (differences between Fig. 8.4, parts A and C and between parts B and D).

An influence of figure side as demonstrated in Figs. 8.3–4 was found in about half of the cells tested (only orientation selective cells were studied). For any location and orientation of receptive field we found cells that responded better to figures on one or the other side, and this preference was invariant as long as we could record from a cell. Apparently, the responses of these cells carry information not only about the location and orientation of an edge but also about the side to which the edge belongs. We call this phenomenon border ownership coding.

Fig. 8.5 shows a summary of the results obtained in cortical areas V1, V2 and V4. For each cell the effects of border ownership and local contrast polarity were determined by ANOVA. (A three-factor ANOVA was performed on the spike

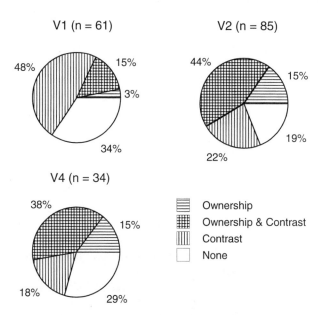

FIG. 8.5. The distribution of the types of contour responses found in cortical areas V1, V2, and V4. Classification based on significance of effects assessed by analysis of variance ($p < 0.01$). Ownership, responses modulated according to side of ownership, Contrast, responses modulated according to local contrast polarity, Ownership & contrast, modulation by either factor, None, no modulation. In V2 and V4, more than half of the cells showed border-ownership modulation. About one third of the cells also showed significant interaction between border ownership and local contrast. In most of these cases, cells responded nearly exclusively to one of the four conditions, as shown in Fig. 8.4. From "Coding of Border Ownership in Monkey Visual Cortex," by H. Zhou, H. S. Friedman, and R. von der Heydt, 2000, *Journal of Neuroscience, 20*, p. 6594–6611. Copyright 2000 by Society for Neuroscience. Reprinted with permission.

counts in 1-s bins, beginning at the time of stimulus onset, with the factors being border ownership, local contrast polarity, and time.) The figure represents the proportions of cells in each of the three areas in which the effects of border ownership and edge contrast polarity were significant ($p < 0.01$). (The effect of the time factor and its interactions with the other two factors were rarely significant). It can be seen that more than half of the cells of areas V2 and V4 showed selectivity for border ownership (V2, 59%; V4, 53%), compared with 18% of the cells of V1. A majority of these cells was also affected by the polarity of edge contrast, as in the example of Fig. 8.4. Cells that were influenced by border ownership irrespective of the contrast polarity, as in Fig. 8.3, were rare in V1 but made up 15% of the cells in V2 and V4. The p values for side of ownership differed significantly between the areas ($p < 0.0001$, Kruskal-Wallis); the differences V1–V2 and V1–V4 were significant ($p < 0.005$), but the difference V2–V4 was not ($p > 0.75$). On the other hand, there was no difference between areas regarding selectivity to local contrast polarity ($p > 0.17$).

The difference between upper layer V1 and V2 and the similarity between the V2 and V4 results indicate that significant processing of figure-ground cues occurs in V2. This was unexpected because the small size of receptive fields in this area seems to preclude the evaluation of figure-ground cues that require a larger view. That the coding of contrast polarity appears unchanged is also remarkable. If separation of the form and color aspects of the stimulus were a goal of processing at this level, then one would expect the orientation-selective cells to become more independent of contrast polarity at the higher levels, but this was not the case.

An important aspect of the results of Fig. 8.5 is the large proportion of cells in V2 and V4 that are selective for both local contrast polarity and border ownership. Besides the main effects, the ANOVA also indicated interaction between these factors in the majority of cells. The interaction was generally positive; that is, the neurons tended to respond exclusively when contrast polarity and side of figure were appropriate, as shown in Fig. 8.4. Furthermore, in 31 of 34 cases the preferred contrast polarity and the preferred figure side were combined in such a way that the cell's preferred color was the color of the figure; in only 3 cases was it the color of the ground. We discuss these findings later.

The Extent of Image Context Integration

Because the size of the square determines the region in which displays in Fig. 8.2, parts A and B (or C and D), are identical (Fig. 8.2E), any response difference indicates the use of image information from outside this region. Therefore, varying the size of the square can tell us about the extent of image context integration at the level of the recorded cell. We found that for most cells varying the square size only weakly affected the border ownership modulation, up to the largest sizes that we could test. Clear border ownership coding was found even with squares that measured 20° visual angle on a side, in which case only two corners of the squares were visible on the display (which subtended 21 by 17°). This shows that the cells use figural information from far outside their receptive fields (for the cells of V2, for example, the region outside which no response could be evoked by an edge was typically smaller than 1°).

Local and Global Mechanisms in Figure-Ground Processing

As theoretical studies have shown, figure-ground discrimination may be based, at least in part, on low-level mechanisms (i.e., mechanism that do not rely on object knowledge). A variety of cues can be used for this purpose. In the above experiment we excluded local cues.[2] We occasionally also tested edges of circular disks, in which case curvature is a local cue, and found strong modulation of responses depending on the side of the disk—the preferred side being the same as in the test with squares.

Edges in random-dot stereograms are another example of locally defined border ownership; these edges are invariably perceived as belonging to the nearer surface. Stereoscopic-edge-selective cells can be found in area V2 (von der Heydt, Zhou, & Friedman, 2000). Some of these cells also show border ownership modulation in the standard test (without the disparity cue). In these cells the preferred figure side nearly always corresponded to the side of the nearer plane of the preferred stereoscopic edge (Qiu, Macuda, & von der Heydt, 2001). Thus, displays in which border ownership depends on monocular form cues (and requires integration of image context) and stereoscopic displays in which the surface disparities dictate border ownership produced consistent results in the neurons of V2.

This finding helps in interpreting the phenomenon of figure side selectivity. The standard test (Fig. 8.3 and 8.4) suggests that side selectivity might be related to border ownership perception, but the link is speculative and may be questioned because perception of border ownership in those displays is somewhat ambiguous (with effort the square can also be perceived as a window). The comparison with the responses to random-dot stereograms is the crucial test because in this case perception of border ownership is not ambiguous. Thus, the finding of consistent stereoscopic-edge preference is strong support for the border ownership coding interpretation.

---

[2]Local cues are available if an image operation can be conceived that uses only a neighborhood of radius R around the receptive field to produce the correct response and if there is no principal lower limit to R. Thus, curvature is a local cue because it can in principle be determined from any small neighborhood. However, the straight edges of squares are locally ambiguous because no operation with R smaller than half the square size can determine the side of the figure (see Fig. 8.2).

How could border ownership be determined in the absence of local cues? For a single square figure on a uniform background relatively simple algorithms would be able to discriminate figure and ground. The convexity of the figure area could be used, or simply the orientation of the L junctions (corners) next to the receptive field, or that the figure is a region of one color enclosed by a region of a different color (surroundedness). Any of these strategies would work for the isolated square. However, for other displays in which border ownership is also perceptually clear, mechanisms based on one simple strategy would fail to produce the right answer. We used two other configurations besides squares to see how well the neural responses correlated with perception, a C-shaped figure as shown in panels 3 and 4 of Fig. 8.6 and a pair of overlapping squares as shown in panels 5 and 6 of the same figure. For the C-shape, the convexity is not valid, and the L junctions next to the receptive field are reflected to the other side in comparison with the square, but surroundedness would still be a valid cue. For the overlapping squares,

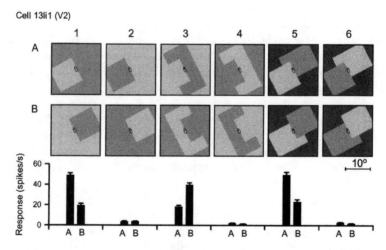

FIG. 8.6. Example of a V2 cell tested with single squares, C-shaped figures, and overlapping figures. The cell was color selective with a preference for violet (depicted here as light gray). In the standard test (1–2) the cell was found to be selective for border ownership and local contrast polarity, responding best to the edge of a violet square located on the lower lefthand side of the receptive field (A1). With C-shape figures (3–4), the cell responded better to B3 than A3, pointing to the lower left as the figure side, in agreement with perception. With overlapping figures (5–6), the cell responded better to A5 than B5, assigning the edge to the figure that is perceived as overlaying. From "Coding of Border Ownership in Monkey Visual Cortex," by H. Zhou, H. S. Friedman, and R. von der Heydt, 2000, *Journal of Neuroscience, 20*, p. 6594–6611. Copyright 2000 by Society for Neuroscience. Reprinted with permission.

surroundedness is violated, whereas convexity and orientation of L junctions are valid.

Fig. 8.6 shows an example of a cell of V2. The test displays are shown at the top, and the strength of the corresponding responses are represented at the bottom. Columns 1 and 2 show the standard test previously described. Besides being contrast selective, the cell preferred figure location on the lower left side of the receptive field (display A1). Columns 3 and 4 show the test with the C-shaped figure. It can be seen that the cell correctly preferred the display in which the C-shaped figure was located on the lower left (Fig. 8.6, part B3), although the L junctions next to the receptive field rather suggest a figure on the opposite side.

Columns 5 and 6 show the test with two overlapping figures. These displays are fairly symmetric about the receptive field as far as size of regions and distribution of colors are concerned, and neither of the figures is surrounded by uniform color. Nevertheless, the cell showed preference for Fig. 8.6, part A5, in which the border in the receptive field belongs to the bottom left figure. In this case the T junctions might account for the emergence of the occluding square as a figure, but convexity might also contribute because the overlapped region has a concavity, whereas the overlapping region does not.

The example of Fig. 8.6 and several other cells that we recorded showed a surprising degree of invariance of the border ownership signal. However, complete invariance was not the rule. Fig. 8.7 summarizes the results obtained with overlapping squares and C-shaped figures. Each dot represents a cell tested. The left and right columns represent the absence/presence of border ownership effects as determined with single squares. For the purpose of comparison, figure-right preference is assumed, as depicted at the top. The rows represent the results obtained with overlapping figures and C-shaped figures, as illustrated on the left, based on a significance criterion of $p < 0.01$. It can be seen that cells that exhibited border ownership selectivity with the single square (right column) nearly always preferred the same side of ownership with the other displays, if they showed any preference at all. However, many cells did not produce a significant signal for these more complex displays. In the case of overlapping figures, about half the cells were undecided, in the case of the C-figures more than half of them. Note also that 4 of 22 cells that did not differentiate sides with the single square (left column) did so with overlapping figures. Thus, we see that the outcome of different tests is not always the same in every cell, as if only some of the available cues were used in each case. On the other hand, contradictory results were rare (one cell, with overlapping figures).

Because the evaluation of different cues such as convexity, junctions, surroundedness, and so forth obviously requires different computational strategies, these results can be interpreted as evidence for a variety of mechanisms, each of which is specialized for certain cues and whose outputs are then combined successively to achieve cue invariance. Recording from randomly selected lines in such a network

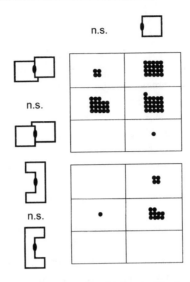

FIG. 8.7.   Summary of the results obtained with single squares, over-lapping figures, and C-shaped figures. Each dot represents a cell tested (9 of V1, 25 of V2, 25 of V4, and 5 of V1 or V2). The right column represents cells with significant side preference for single squares, and the left column represents cells with no significant pref-erence. The rows show the side preferences in the other tests, as in-dicated on the left. The top right box in each 2 × 3 frame represents cases in which a neuron showed a significant preference in both tests and the preferred side was the same, whereas the bottom right box represents cases of significant but opposite preference. There was only one such case. The four cells that exhibited the same preference for C shape and single square also showed the corresponding prefer-ence for overlapping figures, but one did not reach the criterion. Note also that many cells with significant side preference for single squares failed to differentiate border ownership for borders between overlap-ping figures or the inner contour of the C, indicating incomplete use of the available cues. From "Coding of Border Ownership in Monkey Visual Cortex," by H. Zhou, H. S. Friedman, and R. von der Heydt, 2000, *Journal of Neuroscience, 20,* p. 6594–6611. Copyright 2000 by Society for Neuroscience. Adapted with permission.

would show signals in which cues are integrated to various extents, and this is what our results show.

Time Course of Border Ownership Coding

A question that is of particular interest here is the time course of the border own-ership effect. If the response difference is due to central processes that influence low-level representations by means of back projections, then the difference should

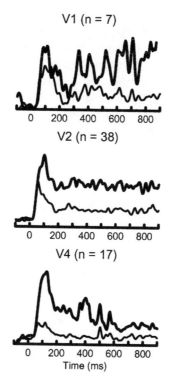

FIG. 8.8. The time course of border ownership modulation. The figure shows the average responses of neurons with significant border ownership modulation in the three areas. The responses of each cell were smoothed and normalized by its mean firing rate during the 1st second of fixation and averaged. Zero on the time scale refers to the onset of the figure-ground display. Thick and thin lines represent responses to preferred and nonpreferred sides, averaged over both contrast polarities. A differentiation was evident shortly after the response onset for cells in all three cortical areas. From "Coding of Border Ownership in Monkey Visual Cortex," by H. Zhou, H. S. Friedman, and R. von der Heydt, 2000, *Journal of Neuroscience, 20,* p. 6594–6611. Copyright 2000 by Society for Neuroscience. Reprinted with permission.

appear with some delay after the onset of responses. Fig. 8.8 shows the smoothed average time course of responses of cells with significant border ownership selectivity in the three areas. For these experiments, each trial started with a uniform display of the color midway between those of figure and ground, which was then replaced by one of the displays of Fig. 8.2. As always, stimulation in and around the receptive field was identical for the conditions to be compared. Thick lines represent responses for the preferred side; thin lines represent the responses for the non preferred side. It can be seen that the differentiation starts almost immediately after the onset of responses. By calculating the sum and the difference of the responses and determining the time when these signals reached half their maximal amplitude, we find delays of 12 ms for V1, 25 ms for V2, and 10 ms for V4. These intervals would probably be too short for a central-processing loop and therefore suggest low-level mechanisms as the source of border ownership selectivity. It is not clear at this point how the fast integration of large image contexts is achieved in these retinotopic representations.

DISCUSSION

We studied the neural representation of border ownership. Recordings from the monkey visual cortex showed that about half of the cells of V2 and V4 and even some cells of V1 signaled this aspect of contours by significant modulation of their responses. The responses depended on the side of the figure despite the stimuli in and around the receptive field being identical. The side preference seemed to be an invariant property of the neurons. In terms of the strength of response modulation and the proportion of cells involved, this border ownership effect was comparable to the well-known selectivity of cortical neurons to orientation, color, disparity, or direction of motion. For instance, the ratio of the responses to preferred and nonpreferred side of figure was greater than 2 in 32% of the cells of V2. For opposite directions of motion, such response ratios were found in 29% of the cells of V1 (De Valois, Yund, & Hepler, 1982) and for preferred and opponent color, in slightly less than 50% of the cells of upper layer V1 (based on Fig. 8.9 of Leventhal, Thompson, Liu, Zhou, & Ault, 1995). Thus, border ownership modulation is not a marginal effect.

The finding that neural responses depend on the side of the figure is not altogether surprising because, as psychophysical studies have shown, border ownership discrimination is fundamental to visual perception and must have its neural representation. What is surprising, perhaps, is to find this information represented explicitly at levels as low as V2 and V1 and as early as 10–25 ms after response onset, which suggests that low-level mechanisms might be responsible. Because border ownership assignment generally cannot be done by local processing but involves an image context, it might be expected to occur only at higher levels, such as infero-temporal cortex, where neurons have large receptive fields. That V1 and V2 neurons have tiny minimum response fields indicates that their responses indeed signal local features. Our results show that these cells, specifically those of V2, not only code location and orientation of contrast borders but also code how these borders belong to the adjacent regions. Each piece of border seems to be represented by two pools of cells, one that is active when the border belongs to an object on one side and the other when it belongs to an object on the other side. This is shown schematically for a pair of overlapping figures in Fig. 8.9, where

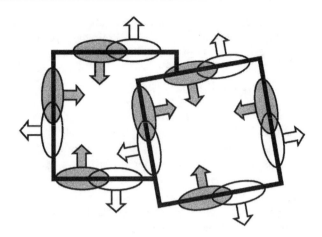

FIG. 8.9. Schematic illustration of the cortical representation of contrast borders for a display of two overlapping squares. Ellipses represent location and orientation of receptive fields, arrows represent preferred side of ownership, and shading indicates activation of neuron. Each border is represented by two populations of orientation selective cells whose relative activation codes the side of ownership. Thus, information about the location and orientation of borders, the color and luminance gradient at the border, and the side to which it belongs, is multiplexed in the responses of cortical neurons. From "Coding of Border Ownership in Monkey Visual Cortex," by H. Zhou, H. S. Friedman, and R. von der Heydt, 2000, *Journal of Neuroscience, 20*, p. 6594–6611. Copyright 2000 by Society for Neuroscience. Reprinted with permission.

ellipses represent the receptive fields and arrows the preferred side for each cell, and the active pool is indicated by shading.

That area V2 plays a key role in figure-ground organization was originally suggested by studies on the representation of illusory contours. The perception of illusory contours is generally associated with displays that imply spatial occlusion and stratification in different depth planes (Kanizsa, 1955). In V2, many cells respond to illusory contour displays as if these contours were contrast borders, signaling orientation (Peterhans & von der Heydt, 1989; von der Heydt & Peterhans, 1989) and the implied direction of occlusion (Baumann, van der Zwan, & Peterhans, 1997; von der Heydt, Heitger, & Peterhans, 1993). Integration of signals of end-stopped cells, which are activated by occlusion cues such as line terminations and *L* junctions, has been suggested as the mechanism of illusory contour generation (Heitger, Rosenthaler, von der Heydt, Peterhans, & Kübler, 1992; Heitger, von der Heydt, Peterhans, Rosenthaler, & Kübler, 1998; Peterhans & von der Heydt, 1989). The results discussed previousely and recent studies on the representation of three-dimensional edges and surfaces (Bakin, Nakayama, &

Gilbert, 2000; von der Heydt et al., 2000) confirm this role of V2. The findings on border ownership coding specifically demonstrate the linking of contour and surface attributes as we discuss in the following section.

Contour and Surface Coding

We found that many orientation selective cells also code color and brightness aspects of the stimulus and that these neurons are often selective for the contrast polarity of edges (see example in Fig. 8.4). To see how this fits in the broad picture of cortical visual coding it is important to realize that, contrary to common belief, color is represented to a large extent by orientation selective cells. Recent quantitative studies found virtually no correlation (or anticorrelation) of color and orientation selectivity (see Leventhal et al., 1995, for upper layer V1; Levitt, Kiper, & Movshon, 1994, and Gegenfurtner, Kiper, & Fenstemaker, 1996, for V2). Analyzing quantitatively a large sample of cells recorded in the awake monkey, Friedman, Zhou, & von der Heydt (2003) found the proportion of color selective cells to be exactly the same among the oriented and the unoriented populations of cells (about 50% in upper layer V1, 40% in V2). As a consequence, because more than 80% of the cells of V2 are strongly orientation selective, the vast majority of the color-coding cells are orientation selective.

When tested with large uniform figures more than half of these cells are sensitive to the polarity of border contrast (Fig. 8.5, sectors labeled "contrast" and "ownership and contrast"). These neurons signal the direction of the chromatic or luminance change at the border rather than the local color value at the receptive field. Many phenomena of visual perception, from the Cornsweet illusion to the filling-in under retinal image stabilization, indicate that surface color and brightness are generated from border signals, and this requires information about the direction of border contrast. Thus, the finding that oriented and contrast-polarity selectivity cells are common not only in V1 but also in extrastriate areas suggests that these kinds of border signals are used in perception of surface color.

The finding of border ownership coding shows that the color border signal generally refers to one side, the figure side, of the border. The activity of the cell of Fig. 8.4, for example, signals the presence of a horizontal edge in the receptive field and specifies that the edge belongs to an object below, whose surface is dark and reddish.[3] Thus, our results indicate that brightness and color of regions are coded in terms of directional border signals.

---

[3]"The cell signals" is abbreviated language often used by physiologists. We do not assume that the message is encoded in the response of a single neuron. Rather, we refer to an assembly of several different cells whose responses we infer from the responses of one cell to the different stimuli. The specification of orientation and color requires gamuts of cells with the same receptive field location tuned to different values in each of these dimensions. Similarly, pairs of related cells can code for contrast polarity and border ownership (see Zhou et al., 2000.) Because the combinations of these various dimensions have to be represented, an ensemble of dozens, perhaps hundreds, of cells is required to represent this message.

A similar argument can be made for depth, which is also a surface quality. Stereoscopic-edge-selective cells signal not only the presence and orientation of a three-dimensional edge but also its polarity, that is, the foreground-background direction (von der Heydt et al., 2000). Some of these cells are narrowly tuned to disparity. In these cells the tuning refers to the disparity on the foreground side; the disparity on the background side has to be farther, but its value does not matter. Cell 2 of Fig. 8.7 in von der Heydt et al. (2000) shows an example. Thus, depth of regions seems to be coded also by directional border signals. As previously mentioned, when stereoscopic-edge selectivity and selectivity for monocular form cues (as revealed by the test of Fig. 8.2) were combined in a single cell, the figure-ground directions were generally consistent; that is, the nearer side of the preferred stereo edge was the same as the preferred figure side (Qiu et al., 2001).

In the case of color and brightness as well as in the case of depth the same signals also carry orientation information. Thus, contour and surface attributes are represented by the same neurons. These findings support our conclusion that we are dealing with a mechanism for linking contours to regions. It is tempting to identify the hypothetical representation of visual surface structure postulated on the basis of human psychophysics (He & Nakayama, 1995; He & Ooi, 2000; Nakayama, He, & Shimojo, 1995) with the neural signals of area V2.

Cognitive Versus Low-Level Mechanisms in Figure-Ground Organization

We have seen that neurons can signal border ownership based on stimulus features that are far from the location of their receptive fields. It is not clear how the visual cortex performs such global context processing. In this section we discuss the neurophysiological results in the light of current theories of perceptual figure-ground segregation, assuming that the basic mechanisms are similar in the human and macaque visual systems.

Theoretical studies have proposed distributed cortical network mechanisms in which processing is not a unidirectional sequence of stages but involves interaction between different levels of representation (e.g., Finkel & Edelman, 1989; Finkel & Sajda, 1992; Grossberg, 1994; Tononi, Sporns, & Edelman, 1992). The various levels interact in an iterative process that generally converges to a final state, which is assumed to underlie perception. We refer to these models as low-level iterative models because they do not use object memory for figure-ground segregation.

Interaction with some form of object shape memory is postulated in cognitive theories, which conceive perception as a problem-solving task (the problem to find a configuration of objects in three-dimensional space that is compatible with the given sensory data; Gregory, 1972; Rock, 1983). The system is thought to compare several perceptual hypotheses with the given sensory representation and determine the one that is most likely.

The anatomical pattern of connectivity, showing that the projections fanning out from V1 to the extrastriate areas are matched by equally powerful feedback projections, would be compatible with both kinds of theories. The low-level feedback models would probably involve areas such as V2, V3, V3A, V4, and MT; the cognitive model would also include higher levels, such as IT cortex. Low-level mechanisms may also be combined with cognitive feedback. Grossberg (1994) and Vecera and O'Reilly (1998) specifically addressed the question of how object specific memory would interact with low-level figure-ground organization.

A third alternative is the classical hierarchical model, which has received little attention from theorists (but see Heitger et al., 1998; Peterhans & Heitger, 2001). This simple scheme does not involve back projections or iterative computations.

Recent neurophysiological studies showing figure enhancement in texture-evoked responses of V1 neurons concluded that figure-ground modulation in V1 reflects feedback from higher order cortical areas (Lamme, 1995; Lamme, Zipser, & Spekreijse, 1998; Lee, Mumford, Romero, & Lamme, 1998; Zipser, Lamme, & Schiller, 1996). However, it is not clear whether these signals come from higher centers, such as IT cortex, or lower order extrastriate areas. The enhancement seems to reflect the labeling of figure regions for the purpose of reading out information from the V1 representation (Lee et al., 1998; see also Mumford, 1992). Because it starts later than the onset of border ownership selectivity, it seems to be a consequence rather than the origin of figure-ground segregation.

In our results, the early appearance of border ownership signals and the varying degree of figure-ground cue invariance suggest hierarchical processing. First, a time difference of 10–25 ms between the onset of stimulus-evoked activity and the onset of the border ownership signal would probably not be enough for a network to complete the number of cycles that an iterative process requires for convergence (50 or more in Vecera & O'Reilly, 1998) if it involves a loop through IT cortex. Second, the iterative-processing models imply that the network reaches a final state of figure-ground organization. This is not a technical consequence of using feedback circuits but the main principle of design (and the beauty) of these models: The algorithm converges on a representation that takes into account all the available figure-ground cues. This final state is thought to correspond to perception. However, finding cells, for example, that signal border ownership for overlapping squares, but not for squares on uniform background, and others that show the converse, does not fit in this theory. We found that, if a border ownership signal was not detectable at the beginning of the responses, it failed to emerge also after continued stimulation. (We later come back to the question of how to interpret this diversity.) Thus, the border ownership signals of different cells did not converge over time. A similar conclusion can be drawn from a recent study on the contribution of depth information to contour integration and surface segmentation (Bakin et al., 2000). Depth cues outside the minimum response field produced facilitation of responses in cells of V2 but no latency differences. These and our results suggest that the emergence of contour and surface representations in V2 is a fast process rather than a gradually converging iteration. In conclusion, the time course of responses seems to rule out cognitive contributions to neural border ownership selectivity, whereas the diversity of patterns of cue integration among cells argues against iterative models with global convergence.

Proponents of the problem-solving theory argue that figure-ground segregation cannot rely entirely or mainly on low-level mechanisms because figure-ground cues are often ambiguous, which means that trying to identify the figure side of a contrast border by low-level mechanisms will often be inconclusive or even produce the wrong result. Why, then, would the visual system use low-level mechanisms at all to resolve figure-ground relationships? Because memory information will eventually be used to recognize objects, one may wonder what the advantage of low-level mechanisms is.

In the case of a single border, as in Fig. 8.9, assigning figure-ground direction reduces the number of shapes that have to be compared with memory from two to one (by eliminating the inverted L shape created by occlusion), which may not appear as a great saving. However, it is important to recognize that the problem is generally more complex. As an example, consider the display of Fig. 8.10, part A, which might be perceived as two elongated objects occluding one another, or, in keeping with the macaque perspective, a branch in front of a tree stem. Contrast borders divide the display into seven regions of different shapes. Because the contrast borders may be occluding contours, most of these shapes are meaningless because they are surfaces of partly occluded objects, that is, regions that do not own their borders. There are 10 segments of borders (not counting the frame), each of which could be owned by one of the adjacent regions, creating a total of

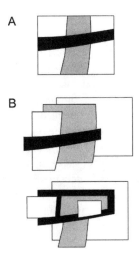

FIG. 8.10. The interpretation of the overlay structure of images is highly ambiguous. (A) Example of a display that would generally be perceived as two elongated objects occluding one another. (B) Two of about 1,000 possible interpretations of A.

$2^{10} = 1,024$ possible depth configurations. Each depth configuration defines a different set of shapes. To help the reader to see this, we illustrate two of the possible three-dimensional decompositions in Fig. 8.10B. Most of the configurations are generally not perceived. The point is that a large number of shapes could give rise to an image like that of Fig. 8.10A. All of these have to be searched in memory if the system is not able to assign the borders beforehand. If borders are assigned, only the two bars in front of a white background will be processed further. Thus, low-level border assignment reduces the load on the memory-matching process enormously in this example, and this is probably similar in images of natural scenes, which are generally complex.

How can our results be reconciled with evidence for top-down processing? It is a common observation that perception of ambiguous displays can be influenced voluntarily. For example, in Rubin's figure, subjects can voluntarily hold the percept of faces and thereby prolong its duration and similarly for the vase. Object familiarity has also been shown to affect the probability of perceptual border assignment. Thus, object memory can influence figure-ground perception (Peterson, Harvey, & Weidenbacher, 1991). Attention was probably not a factor in creating border ownership selectivity in our experiments because this selectivity was observed in responses to stimuli that were not attended (attention was engaged in the fixation task, Zhou et al., 2000). However, the influence of top-down attention on the responses of neurons in visual cortex is well documented for other experimental conditions (Moran & Desimone, 1985; Motter, 1994a, 1994b; see Desimone, 1998, for a review).

We argue that figure-ground organization is essentially a low-level operation (involving V1, V2 and V4 and perhaps other areas, such as V3 and MT) and that this process provides a structure on which attentional selection operates. Thus, we conceive perceptual organization and attentional selection as two orthogonal processes that interact in the visual cortex. As to the effects of attention and familiarity on perceptual border assignment, we point out that none of the areas that we have studied seems to represent border ownership unanimously (Fig. 8.7). A border may be given a strong assignment by a major group of cells but none by others, and some cells may even give it the opposite assignment. Contradictory votes were rare, but they clearly existed (we illustrated only the majority vote in Fig. 8.9). This means that these areas do not make the final decision that we experience in perception. Rather, several three-dimensional interpretations are carried along in parallel with different weights, given by strength of signals and number of cells. This is fundamentally different from an image representation, where each point has a single color value. The coding in the visual cortex is more complex; multiple orientations can be represented for each point, and borders can be assigned in two ways for each orientation. The output of this stage of processing is a representation of multiple solutions. Compared with a raw representation of local features the number of solutions is greatly reduced, and each is represented with a weighting coefficient indicating its likelihood, as defined by those mechanisms.

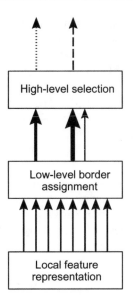

FIG. 8.11. Low-level and high-level processes in a hypothetical hierarchical system. Low-level border assignment mechanisms reduce the number of possible interpretations to three alternatives, which the system represents with different weights (e.g., given by level of activity and number of cells). Central control of attention and recognition processes can select among these. Thus, evidence for involvement of object specific memory in perception does not necessarily mean that low-level representations are modified by top-down projections.

Fig. 8.11 illustrates this idea. The local feature representation is highly ambiguous, leaving many possibilities for figure-ground organization. The possible solutions are symbolized by arrows. Low-level border ownership mechanisms make a few of these explicit and represent them with variable strength, as indicated by thickness of arrows. Finally, of these explicit representations one is selected by the high-level process (selected meaning that the corresponding information is routed to other centers for further processing).

In this scheme, attentional processes and memory matching will still be able to select between alternatives and will therefore influence perception and behavioral response. The influence of the central processes will be most obvious in situations in which figure-ground cues are balanced so that the low-level processes produce two solutions with approximately equal weights, as in Rubin's figure. Thus, observations that regions of familiar shape are perceived more often as figure than regions of unfamiliar shape are compatible with the existence of low-level mechanisms of border ownership coding. Depending on the given information, the border assignment stage is more or less effective in weeding out multiple interpretations. If the figure-ground cues lead to a single strong representation at this stage (e.g., as in the case of random-dot stereograms), this will be automatically perceived, but in cases in which two low-level solutions come out with approximately equal strengths, the high-level process will determine which is perceived (dotted and dashed arrows). Thus, low-level and high-level processes naturally combine to a complementary strategy.

The influences of attentional selection and object memory in perception are often conceived as involving back projections that modulate signals at the level of local feature representations. Indeed, this is how the system appears to work. In Rubin's figure, the border appears to switch from the vase to the faces when we direct our attention to the face interpretation, and once we have seen the dalmation dog[4] in the picture of black and white spots, it pops out immediately every time we see the picture. However, it is important to see that evidence for involvement of both low-level and high-level processes is also compatible with a hierarchical processing scheme with no back projections involved at all. Fig. 8.11 is meant to illustrate this possibility (not to draw a conclusion).

ACKNOWLEDGMENTS

We wish to thank Zijiang He, Carl R. Olson, and Mary A. Peterson for critical comments and suggestions. This work was supported by National Institutes of Health grants EY02966 and NS38034. H. S. Friedman was supported by the Whitaker Foundation.

REFERENCES

Bakin, J. S., Nakayama, K., & Gilbert, C. D. (2000). Visual responses in monkey areas V1 and V2 to three-dimensional surface configurations. *Journal of Neuroscience, 20,* 8188–8198.

Barlow, H. B., Blakemore, C., & Pettigrew, J. D. (1967). The neural mechanism of binocular depth discrimination. *Journal of Physiology, 193,* 327–342.

Baumann, R., van der Zwan, R., & Peterhans, E. (1997). Figure-ground segregation at contours: A neural mechanism in the visual cortex of the alert monkey. *European Journal of Neuroscience, 9,* 1290–1303.

De Valois, R. L., Yund, E. W., & Hepler, N. (1982). The orientation and direction selectivity of cells in macaque visual cortex. *Vision Research, 22,* 531–544.

Desimone, R. (1998). Visual attention mediated by biased competition in extrastriate visual cortex. *Philosophical Transactions of the Royal Society of London B Biological Sciences, 353,* 1245–1255.

Finkel, L. H., & Edelman, G. M. (1989). Integration of distributed cortical systems by reentry: A computer simulation of interactive functionally segregated visual areas. *Journal of Neuroscience, 9,* 3188–3208.

Finkel, L. H., & Sajda, P. (1992). Object discrimination based on depth-from-occlusion. *Neural Computation, 4,* 901–921.

---

[4]An image often used in textbooks to demonstrate the effect of experience on perception (see Fig. 8.3-1 of Marr, 1982).

Friedman, H. S., Zhou, H., & von der Heydt, R. (2003). The coding of uniform color figures in monkey visual cortex. *Journal of Physiology*, in press.

Gegenfurtner, K. R., Kiper, D. C., & Fenstemaker, S. B. (1996). Processing of color, form, and motion in macaque area V2. *Visual Neuroscience, 13*, 161–172.

Gregory, R. L. (1972). Cognitive contours. *Nature, 238*, 51–52.

Grossberg, S. (1994). Three-dimensional vision and figure-ground separation by visual cortex. *Perception and Psychophysics, 55*, 48–120.

He, Z. J., & Nakayama, K. (1995). Visual attention to surfaces in three-dimensional space. *Proceedings of the National Academy of Sciences of the United States of America, 92*, 11155–11159.

He, Z. J., & Ooi, T. L. (2000). Perceiving binocular depth with reference to a common surface. *Perception, 29*, 1313–1334.

Heitger, F., Rosenthaler, L., von der Heydt, R., Peterhans, E., & Kübler, O. (1992). Simulation of neuronal contour mechanisms: From simple to endstopped cells. *Vision Research, 32*, 963–981.

Heitger, F., von der Heydt, R., Peterhans, E., Rosenthaler, L., & Kübler, O. (1998). Simulation of neural contour mechanisms: Representing anomalous contours. *Image and Vision Computing, 16*, 409–423.

Kanizsa, G. (1955). Margini quasi-percettivi in campi con stimulazione omogenea. *Rivista di Psicologia, 49*, 7–30.

Kanizsa, G. (1987). Quasi-perceptual margins in homogeneously stimulated fields. In S. Petry & G. E. Meyer (Eds.), *The Perception of Illusory Contours* (pp. 40–49). New York: Springer.

Koffka, K. (1935). *Principles of Gestalt psychology*. New York: Harcourt, Brace.

Lamme, V. A. F. (1995). The neurophysiology of figure-ground segregation in primary visual cortex. *Journal of Neuroscience, 15*, 1605–1615.

Lamme, V. A. F., Zipser, K., & Spekreijse, H. (1998). Figure-ground activity in primary visual cortex is suppressed by anesthesia. *Proceedings of the National Academy of Sciences of the United States of America, 95*, 3263–3268.

Lee, T. S., Mumford, D., Romero, R., & Lamme, V. A. F. (1998). The role of the primary visual cortex in higher level vision. *Vision Research, 38*, 2429–2454.

Leventhal, A. G., Thompson, K. G., Liu, D., Zhou, Y., & Ault, S. J. (1995). Concomitant sensitivity to orientation, direction, and color of cells in layers 2, 3, and 4 of monkey striate cortex. *Journal of Neuroscience, 15*, 1808–1818.

Levitt, J. B., Kiper, D. C., & Movshon, J. A. (1994). Receptive fields and functional architecture of macaque V2. *Journal of Neurophysiology, 71*, 2517–2542.

Marr, D. (1982). *Vision. A computational investigation into the human representation and processing of visual information*. San Francisco: Freeman.

Metzger, W. (1953). Gesetze des Sehens (Laws of Vision) (2nd ed.). Frankfurt: W. Kramer.

Moran, J., & Desimone, R. (1985). Selective attention gates visual processing in the extrastriate cortex. *Science, 229*, 782–784.

Motter, B. C. (1994a). Neural correlates of attentive selection for color or luminance in extrastriate area V4. *Journal of Neuroscience, 14*, 2178–2189.

Motter, B. C. (1994b). Neural correlates of feature selective memory and pop-out in extrastriate area V4. *Journal of Neuroscience, 14*, 2190–2199.

Mumford, D. (1992). On the computational architecture of the neocortex II. *Biological Cybernetics, 66*, 241–251.

Nakayama, K., He, Z. J., & Shimojo, S. (1995). Visual surface representation: A critical link between lower-level and higher-level vision. In S. M. Kosslyn & D. N. Osherson (Eds.), *Invitation to Cognitive Science* (pp. 1–70). Cambridge, MA: MIT.

Peterhans, E., & Heitger, F. (2001). Simulation of neuronal responses defining depth order and contrast polarity at illusory contours in monkey area V2. *Journal of Computational Neuroscience, 10*, 195–211.

Peterhans, E., & von der Heydt, R. (1989). Mechanisms of contour perception in monkey visual cortex. II. Contours bridging gaps. *Journal of Neuroscience, 9,* 1749–1763.

Peterson, M. A., Harvey, E. M., & Weidenbacher, H. J. (1991). Shape recognition contributions to figure-ground reversal: Which route counts? *Journal of Experimental Psychology: Human Perception and Performance, 17,* 1075–1089.

Qiu, F. T., Macuda, T. J., & von der Heydt, R. (2001). Neural coding of border ownership: Figural and stereoscopic cues. *Society of Neuroscience Abstracts, 27,* (165.6).

Rock, I. (1983). *The Logic of Perception.* Cambridge, MA: The MIT Press.

Schiller, P. H., Finlay, B. L., & Volman, S. F. (1976). Quantitative studies of single-cell properties in monkey striate cortex. I. Spatiotemporal organization of receptive fields. *Journal of Neurophysiology, 39,* 1288–1319.

Tononi, G., Sporns, O., & Edelman, G. M. (1992). Reentry and the problem of integrating multiple cortical areas: Simulation of dynamic integration in the visual system. *Cerebral Cortex, 2,* 310–335.

Vecera, S. P., & O'Reilly, R. C. (1998). Figure-ground organization and object recognition processes: An interactive account. *Journal of Experimental Psychology: Human Perception and Performance, 24,* 441–462.

von der Heydt, R., Heitger, F., & Peterhans, E. (1993). Perception of occluding contours: Neural mechanisms and a computational model. *Biomedical Research, 14,* (Suppl. 4) 1–6.

von der Heydt, R., & Peterhans, E. (1989). Mechanisms of contour perception in monkey visual cortex. I. Lines of pattern discontinuity. *Journal of Neuroscience, 9,* 1731–1748.

von der Heydt, R., Zhou, H., & Friedman, H. S. (2000). Representation of stereoscopic edges in monkey visual cortex. *Vision Research, 40,* 1955–1967.

Zhou, H., Friedman, H. S., & von der Heydt, R. (2000). Coding of border ownership in monkey visual cortex. *Journal of Neuroscience, 20,* 6594–6611.

Zipser, K., Lamme, V. A. F., & Schiller, P. H. (1996). Contextual modulation in primary visual cortex. *Journal of Neuroscience, 16,* 7376–7389.

9 Neuronal Correlates of Perceptual Organization in the Primate Visual System

Thomas D. Albright
Howard Hughes Medical Institute
Salk Institute for Biological Studies
Lisa J. Croner
Robert O. Duncan
Gene R. Stoner
Salk Institute for Biological Studies

The primate visual system has been studied by neurobiologists for nearly 4 decades. As a result, we know a great deal about how neurons at early levels of visual processing represent basic features of the retinal image, such as the orientation of a contour or the color of a patch of light. Nevertheless, we know very little about how such cells give rise to our perceptual experience of the world. One reason for this limited knowledge is that perception is context dependent. Just as the meaning of a word depends on the sentence in which the word is embedded, the perceptual interpretation of a retinal image feature depends on the spatial and temporal context in which the feature appears. Until recently, contextual manipulations have been largely excluded from studies of the response properties of visual neurons, primarily as a matter of investigative convenience.

To appreciate the importance of the contextual influence on perception, consider Fig. 9.1. Panels A–C each contain an identical, horizontally oriented bar. The perceptual interpretations of the three bars are very different: Human observers typically report that the bar in Panel A appears to be a region of overlap between two light gray rectangular surfaces, one of which is transparent. The bar in Panel B appears as a variation in surface reflectance, as though a dark gray stripe has been painted horizontally across a larger light gray planar surface. The bar in Panel C appears to be a shaded portion of a larger object that is folded in three dimensions.

A   B   C

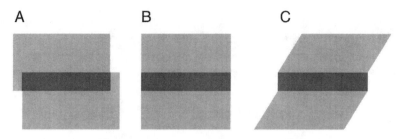

FIG. 9.1. Illustration of the influence of visual context on perception. Each of the three images displayed here contains a horizontal dark gray rectangle. Although these rectangles are physically identical, the surrounding features (the contexts) differ in the three images. As a result, the rectangle is perceptually attributed to different environmental causes in the three instances. (A) The rectangle appears to result from the overlap of two surfaces, one of which is transparent (e.g., a piece of tinted glass). (B) The rectangle appears to result from a variation in surface reflectance (e.g., a stripe painted across a large flat canvas). (C) The rectangle appears to result from partial shading of a surface (i.e., variation in the angle of the surface with respect to the source of illumination). These markedly different perceptual interpretations argue for the existence of different neuronal representations of the rectangle. These representations can only be identified in neurophysiological experiments if appropriate contextual cues are used for visual stimulation.

The different perceptual interpretations of the dark gray bars in Fig. 9.1, Panels A–C, follow from the different spatial contexts in which the bars appear. Such contextual influences, which are ubiquitous in normal visual experience, raise two important questions for neurobiologists: (1) At what stage of visual processing is contextual information incorporated to achieve neuronal representations of things perceived (scene-based representations), rather than local features of the retinal image (image-based representations)? (2) What neuronal mechanisms underlie the transformation from image-based to scene-based representations?

Our laboratory spent much of the past decade addressing these questions, primarily in the domain of visual motion processing (for review see Albright, 1993; Croner & Albright, 1999b; Stoner & Albright, 1993). In this review, we summarize two recent experiments from our laboratory. These experiments address the phenomenology and neuronal bases of two key elements of perceptual organization: feature interpretation and feature grouping.

FEATURE INTERPRETATION

When viewing any natural scene, the visual system interprets each feature—such as a corner, edge, patch, and so on—as belonging to a particular object. Fig. 9.2 illustrates the relevance of feature interpretation to motion processing. The scene in

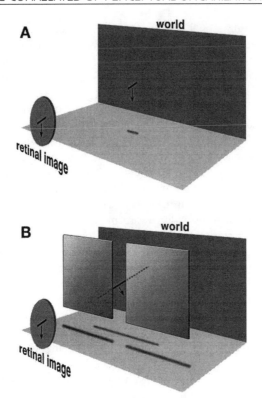

FIG. 9.2. Illustration of the contextual dependence of motion perception. Two simple visual scenes are shown, along with the retinal image motions that they give rise to. (A) This visual scene contains a single moving object (an elongated bar), which is oriented obliquely and moving directly down. The retinal image motion directly reflects the object motion. (B) This visual scene contains a single obliquely oriented bar, but in this case the bar is moving to the lower right (in a direction orthogonal to its orientation). The scene also contains two static opaque occluders, which block the observer's view of the two ends of the moving bar. The resulting retinal image motion in Panel B is identical to that caused by the scene in Panel A, although the visual scene motions are clearly different. The different contexts present in the two scenes—no surrounding features in Panel A, occluding panels present in Panel B—allow the different visual scenes to be perceived veridically.

Fig. 9.2A contains a single moving object—a sticklike figure—oriented obliquely and moving directly downward. The left-hand side of the figure illustrates the retinal image rendered by this simple scene. The scene in Fig. 9.2B also contains a single moving object—once again, a sticklike figure—obliquely oriented but moving toward the lower right corner of the scene. Unlike the scene in Fig. 9.2A, this scene also contains two opaque surfaces, each occluding one end of the moving object. The resulting retinal image of the moving object, shown at left, is an obliquely oriented line moving directly downward. Importantly, the retinal image motion rendered by the bar in the second scene (Fig. 9.2B) is physically identical to that rendered by the bar in the first scene (Fig. 9.2A), although the object motions are clearly different.

Human observers perceive the different object motions correctly in the two cases, and they do so because of the two different spatial contexts (with occluding panels in Fig. 9.2B; without panels in Fig. 9.2A), in which the image motions appear. In particular, the two contexts lead to different interpretations of the terminations of the moving line in the retinal image (Shimojo, Silverman, & Nakayama, 1989). In Fig. 9.2A, the line terminators of the retinal image are interpreted as the ends of an elongated object in the visual scene (i.e., they are intrinsic features of that object). As such, their downward motions reflect the motion of the object itself. By contrast, the line terminators of the retinal image in Fig. 9.2B are accidents of occlusion and thus extrinsic to the moving object. Unlike the intrinsic features of Fig. 9.2A, the downward retinal image motions of the extrinsic features in Fig. 9.2B do not reflect the motion of the object and hence do not figure into the computation of object motion. Thus, the manner in which the terminator features are interpreted determines how the retinal image motions are perceived.

These perceptual phenomena prompt us to ask whether visual neurons respond differently to the motions represented in Fig. 9.2A versus Fig. 9.2B, thereby encoding object motion rather than image motion. Experiments conducted over the past 40 years yielded a wealth of information regarding the response properties of motion-sensitive neurons in the primate visual system. Consider, for example, the responses illustrated in Fig. 9.3. These data, which were published by Hubel and Wiesel in 1968, document a property known as directional selectivity, which is now known to be common among visual cortical neurons (Albright, 1993). The data illustrated were recorded from a single neuron in the primary visual cortex (area V1) of a rhesus monkey. The visual stimulus was an oriented bar of light (oriented lines in left column of Fig. 9.3) that was swept through the receptive field (dashed rectangles) of the neuron under study. Neuronal responses to these stimuli are shown on the right-hand side of the figure as spike trains, in which action potentials (vertical lines) are plotted as a function of time. The stimulus that elicited the largest number of action potentials was oriented diagonally and drifted to the upper right through the receptive field. Response magnitude waned as the motion deviated from this preferred direction.

Observations of this sort have been made repeatedly since the discovery of neuronal directional selectivity, and they have revealed much about the way in which cortical neurons encode image motion. Do these findings enable us to predict how motion sensitive neurons will behave when presented with stimuli such as those in Fig. 9.2 or under other stimulus conditions that approximate the richness of normal perceptual experience? If such cells were sensitive only to light within their

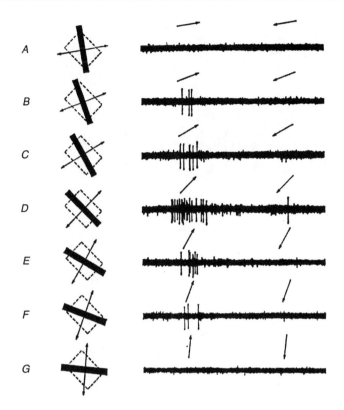

FIG. 9.3. Directional selectivity of one neuron, as first observed by Hubel and Wiesel (1968) in primary visual cortex (area V1) of rhesus monkey. The neuronal receptive field is indicated by broken rectangles in the left column. The visual stimulus was a bar of light moved in each of 14 directions (rows A–G, opposing directions indicated by arrows) through the receptive field. Recorded traces of cellular activity are shown at right, where the horizontal axis represents time (2s/trace) and each vertical line represents an action potential. This neuron responds most strongly to motion up and to the right (row D). From "Receptive Fields and Functional Architecture of Monkey Striate Cortex," by D. H. Hubel and T. N. Wiesel, 1968, *Journal of Physiology, 195*, p. 214. Copyright 1968 by The Physiological Society. Reprinted with permission.

receptive fields, their responses would be a simple function of the receptive field profile and the spatiotemporal pattern of light falling in the receptive field. Evidence suggests, on the contrary, that some modulatory effects arise from stimulation outside of the classically defined receptive field (CRF). It is therefore impossible to predict how these neurons will respond to a stimulus that is more complex than that used to characterize its CRF.

Barber-Diamond

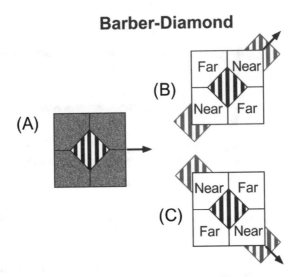

FIG. 9.4. Schematic depiction of barber-diamond stimuli used to study the influence of context on perceived motion and on its neuronal correlates (a demonstration can be seen at http://www.cnl. salk.edu/~gene/). (A) Stimuli consisted of a moving square-wave grating framed by a static, diamond-shaped aperture. The grating itself was placed in the plane of occular fixation, and four textured panels that defined the aperture were independently positioned in depth using binocular disparity cues. The grating was moved either leftward or rightward on each trial. Each of the four stimulus conditions used was a unique conjunction of direction of grating motion (right vs. left) and depth-ordering configuration. The two conditions illustrated (B and C) were created using rightward moving gratings; two additional conditions (not shown) were created using leftward moving gratings. Near and Far identify the depth ordering of the textured panels relative to the plane of the grating. For the condition shown in B, the upper right and lower left panels were placed in the near depth plane, whereas the upper left and lower right panels were in the far depth plane. The line terminators formed at the boundary of the near surfaces and the grating are classified as extrinsic features resulting from occlusion, and the grating appears to extend behind the near surface. (Note that gray stripes are not part of the stimulus and are used solely to illustrate perceptual completion of the partially occluded grating.) Conversely, line terminators formed at the boundary of the far surfaces and the grating are classified as intrinsic (i.e., they appear to result from the physical termination of the surface on which the stripes are painted). As a result of this depth-ordering manipulation and ensuing feature interpretation, observers typically perceive the moving grating in B as belonging to a surface that slides behind the near panels and across the far panels (i.e., to the upper right). This direction is identified with motions of intrinsic terminators. The condition shown in C contains the same rightward grating motion but employs the depth-ordering configuration that is complementary to B. In this case, observers

310

Most neurophysiological studies to date have not manipulated visual context; hence, there are no existing data that enable us to determine whether visual neurons will respond similarly or differently to the two configurations in Fig. 9.2. We hypothesize, however, that the visual system first extracts simple features within an image and then integrates the neural representations of these features—using context as a guide—to create a new scene-based representation that reflects the structure and properties of the scene. If this were the case, then there should be a population of neurons whose responses are sensitive to the context surrounding their CRFs. We undertook studies to locate such neurons, hypothesizing that they would (1) be differentially sensitive to the motions of intrinsic vs. extrinsic image features, and (2) represent the motions of visual scene elements (i.e., objects and their surfaces) rather than simply the motions of retinal image features.

Barber-Diamond Stimuli

To identify neurons sensitive to visual scene motion, we developed visual stimuli in which a simple contextual manipulation dramatically affects feature interpretation and motion perception (Duncan, Albright, & Stoner, 2000). That stimulus, which we have termed the barber-diamond because of its close relationship to the classic barber-pole illusion (Wallach, 1935), is illustrated schematically in Fig. 9.4. As shown in Fig. 9.4A, the barber-diamond is composed of a pattern of vertically oriented stripes viewed through a diamond-shaped window. The stripes can be moved leftward or rightward within the stationary window. The window is surrounded by a randomly textured field composed of four adjacent panels that could be independently placed in either near or far depth planes (relative to the plane of ocular fixation) using binocular disparity cues.

In our experiments, we manipulated two independent variables: the direction of motion of the stripes (rightward or leftward) and the relative placement of the textured panels in different depth planes. Two depth configurations, shown in Fig. 9.4B and 9.4C, were used. In one case (Fig. 9.4B), the upper left and lower right textured panels were placed in a far depth plane relative to the stripes/fixation point, and the upper right and lower left panels were placed in a near depth plane. In the other case (Fig. 9.4C), the upper left and lower right textured panels were placed in a near depth plane, and the upper right and lower left panels were placed in a far depth plane. The conjunction of two directions of stripe motion and the two depth configurations yielded four distinct stimulus conditions.

←———

FIG. 9.4. (continued) typically perceive the grating belonging to a surface that is drifting to the lower right. See text for details. From "Occlusion and the Interpretation of Visual Motion: Perceptual and Neuronal Effects of Context," by R. O. Duncan, T. D. Albright, and G. R. Stoner, 2000, *Journal of Neuroscience, 20*, p. 5890. Copyright 2000 by The Society for Neuroscience.

The two different depth configurations were expected to elicit different intrinsic versus extrinsic feature interpretations for the terminators of the vertical stripes. Specifically, line terminators lying adjacent to far panels were expected to be interpreted as intrinsic to the stripe because the depth edge provides evidence that these terminators lie at the edge of a striped surface. By contrast, line terminators lying adjacent to near panels were expected to be interpreted as extrinsic features because the depth edge here suggests that their termination by occlusion is a more likely possibility. Following this logic outlined, we predicted that motion of the vertical stripes—which was, we emphasize, always physically leftward or rightward along the horizontal axis—would be perceived to follow the motions of the intrinsic terminators (thereby ignoring extrinsic terminator motion). Thus, for the example illustrated in Fig. 9.4B, perceived motion should be toward the upper right corner. Likewise, for the example shown in Fig. 9.4C, perceived motion should be toward the lower right corner.

Feature Interpretation Influences Perceived Motion

We first investigated how the barber-diamond stimuli (Duncan et al., 2000) were perceived by human subjects. For each trial, the subject fixated a small 0-disparity fixation target at the center of the stimulus, while the vertical bars of the barber-diamond moved for 1.5s. After each trial, the subject indicated the perceived direction of motion by orienting a bar displayed on the display monitor. The results for each of the four stimulus conditions are plotted in Fig. 9.5 as frequency distributions of directional reports. Data are summed over all seven subjects studied. Subjects overwhelmingly reported that perceived direction of motion was in the direction of intrinsic terminator motion. These findings support our hypothesis that feature interpretation, derived from contextual cues unrelated to motion, has a marked influence on perceived motion. A demonstration of this perceptual effect can be seen at http://www.cnl.salk.edu/~gene/.

Cortical Motion-Sensitive Neurons Encode Object Motion Using Intrinsic Features

Having confirmed that perceived motion direction depends on contextual cues for depth ordering, we next sought to identify the neuronal bases of these effects. Fig. 9.6A provides a partial summary of the organization of the visual cortex in nonhuman primates (rhesus monkeys), based on a large number of neurophysiological, neuroanatomical, and neuropsychological studies conducted over the past 30 years. Some of the major sulci in the posterior portion of the brain have been partially opened to illustrate the visual areas lying within these sulci. Approximate boundaries between visual areas are identified by broken lines. Fig. 9.6B diagrams the main anatomical connections extending from the retina through several stages

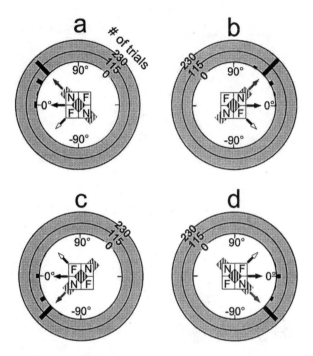

FIG. 9.5. Perceptual reports to centrally presented barber-diamonds. Stimuli were viewed within 11° apertures and possessed gratings of 0.59 cycles/deg. Data were obtained from seven human subjects. Each panel (A, B, C, and D) depicts responses to a particular barber-diamond condition as indicated by the central icons. Black arrows indicate direction of grating motion for each condition. N and F indicate crossed- and uncrossed-disparity regions that make up each depth-ordering configuration. Each barber-diamond condition consisted of a different combination of grating motion (left: A and C, right: B and D) and depthordering configuration (A and D or B and C). The implied direction of surface motion (intrinsic terminator motion) that results from these combinations is indicated by gray arrows. White arrows indicate the direction of extrinsic terminator motion. For each graph, the direction of motion reported is plotted on the polar axis, and the frequency of responses for each direction is plotted on the radial axis, (black bars). Left/right perceived motion is indicated on the horizontal axis, and up/down motion is represented on the vertical axis. Each subject participated in 40 trials per condition ($N = 1120$). Most of the reports for each condition were biased in the direction of the intrinsic terminators. From "Occlusion and the Interpretation of Visual Motion: Perceptual and Neuronal Effects of Context," by R. O. Duncan, T. D. Albright, and G. R. Stoner, 2000, *Journal of Neuroscience, 20*, p. 5890. Copyright 2000 by The Society for Neuroscience. Adapted with permission.

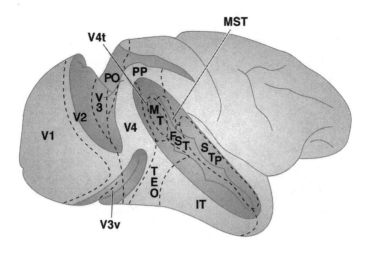

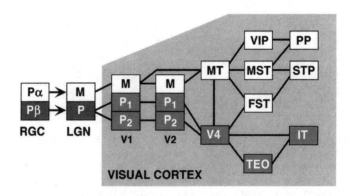

FIG. 9.6. (A) Lateral view of macaque brain showing location of striate cortex (V1) and some extrastriate visual areas. Sulci have been partially opened (shaded regions). Indicated borders of visual areas (dashed lines) are approximate. (EC, external calcarine sulcus; IO, inferior occipital sulcus; IP, intraparietal sulcus; LA, lateral sulcus; LU, lunate sulcus; PO, parieto-occipital sulcus; ST, superior temporal sulcus.) (B) Diagram of anatomical connectivity, emphasizing hierarchical organization and parallel processing streams along the geniculo-striate-extrastriate pathway. Except where indicated by arrows, connections are known to be reciprocal. Not all known components of magnocellular (unshaded) and parvocellular (shaded) pathways are shown. (RGC, retinal ganglion cell layer; LGN, lateral geniculate nucleus of the thalamus; M, magnocellular subdivisions; P_1 & P_2, parvocellular subdivisions; MT, middle temporal; MST, medial superior temporal; FST, fundus superior temporal; PP, posterior parietal cortex; VIP, ventral intraparietal; STP, superior temporal polysensory). From "Cortical Processing of Visual Motion," by T. D. Albright, 1993, In: J Wallman and FA Miles (eds.) *Visual Motion and Its Role in the Stabilization of Gaze. 5*, p. 178. Copyright 1993 by Elsevier Science. Reprinted with permission.

of cortical visual processing. As previously noted, many neurons in V1 exhibit selectivity for the direction of stimulus motion (Albright, 1984; Hubel & Wiesel, 1968), but this property is particularly prominent in the middle temporal visual area (Albright, 1984), which is commonly known as area MT. Area MT is a relatively small visual area in the lower bank of the superior temporal sulcus and receives direct input from V1 (Gattass & Gross, 1981; Ungerleider & Mishkin, 1979; Van Essen, Maunsell, & Bixby, 1981). MT is thus at an early level of processing in the cortical visual hierarchy. Approximately 90% of MT neurons are selective for the direction of stimulus motion (Albright, 1984; Allman & Kaas, 1971; Maunsell & Van Essen, 1983; Zeki, 1974).

Directional responses from one such neuron are shown in Fig. 9.7. On the basis of this striking selectivity, as well as related findings (e.g., Albright, 1992; Albright,

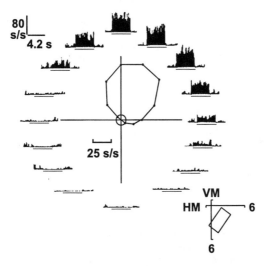

FIG. 9.7. Example of direction tuning of a typical MT neuron. Individual histograms represent responses summed over five trials to each of 16 directions of motion of a random-dot pattern moving at 20°/s. The line beneath each histogram indicates period of time during which stimulus was moving through the receptive field (shown at lower right). In the center, response to each direction is plotted on a polar graph. The polar axis represents direction of stimulus motion, the radial axis represents response (measured as spikes per second), and the small circle represents the level of spontaneous activity. The marked suppression of activity seen when the stimulus moved 180° from the optimal direction is characteristic of many MT neurons. VM, vertical meridian; HM, horizontal meridian. From "Direction and Orientation Selectivity of Neurons in Visual Area MT of the Macaque," by T. D. Albright, 1984, *Journal of Neurophysiology, 52,* p. 1109. Copyright 1984 by The American Physiological Society. Reprinted with permission.

(A) CIRCULAR GRATING RESPONSES

(B) ACTUAL RESPONSES TO BARBER-DIAMONDS

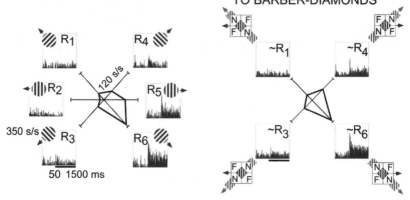

PREDICTED RESPONSES TO BARBER-DIAMONDS

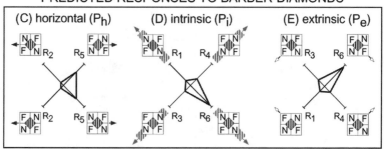

FIG. 9.8. Influence of depth ordering on direction selectivity of an MT neuron. The receptive field of this neuron was located 4° eccentric to the center of gaze and was 4.5° in diameter. (A) Peristimulus time histograms (PSTHs) illustrate neuronal responses to circular gratings moved in each of six directions. Average responses are indicated on the polar plot at center, in which polar angle corresponds to direction of stimulus motion and radial amplitude corresponds to response in spikes/second. These responses ($R1$–$R6$) were used to form three different predictions for barber-diamond stimuli (C, D, and E). (B) Actual responses to barber-diamond stimuli. PSTHs for each of the four barber-diamond conditions are presented. The average responses to moving barber-diamonds are plotted in polar coordinates at center. The bars under the lower left histograms in A and B indicate the period of stimulus movement (C) Horizontal motion prediction (P_h). Icons illustrate the stimulus configuration for each of four experimental conditions. Predicted neuronal responses to each condition are shown on the polar plot at center. This prediction holds that neuronal responses are influenced solely by the direction of grating motion (black arrows) and, hence, are of the same relative magnitude as responses to circular gratings moved leftward (R2) and rightward (R5), regardless of depth-ordering configuration. (D) Intrinsic motion prediction (P_i). This prediction holds that responses are associated with the direction of

316

Desimone, & Gross, 1984; Dobkins & Albright, 1994; Movshon, Adelson, Gizzi, & Newsome, 1985; Newsome, Britten, & Movshon, 1989; Newsome & Pare, 1988; Rodman & Albright, 1987; Rodman & Albright, 1989; Stoner & Albright, 1992), area MT is widely regarded as a primary component of the neural substrate for visual motion perception. For this reason, we began our investigation of the neuronal bases of contextual influences on motion perception by recording activity from isolated neurons in area MT while rhesus monkeys viewed barber-diamond stimuli (Duncan et al., 2000).

Stimuli were configured precisely as they had been for the psychophysical experiments previously described and were positioned so that the vertical bars covered the CRF of each neuron studied. We predicted that MT neurons would exhibit selectivity for the direction in which the intrinsic terminators moved, consistent with perception. An illustration of this prediction for one MT neuron is shown in Fig. 9.8. Fig. 9.8A illustrates the direction tuning of the neuron, assessed using a drifting pattern of stripes (grating) presented within a circular aperture over the classical receptive field. Average responses for gratings moved in each of six different directions and are plotted in polar coordinates at the center of Fig. 9.8A, with angle corresponding to the direction of stimulus motion. Peristimulus histograms around the perimeter of the plot show summed responses as a function of time. This cell responded most strongly to motion downward and rightward.

From the data in Fig. 9.8A, we considered three different predictions for the responses of this neuron to barber-diamonds. For each prediction (illustrated in Fig. 9.8C, 9.8D, and 9.8E), the expected responses to the four barber-diamond conditions are shown. The simplest prediction, shown in Fig. 9.8C, is that of the null hypothesis, which assumes that the depth configuration (i.e., the context) has no influence over the directional selectivity of the cell. If true, the neuronal response would be determined exclusively by the leftward or rightward direction of motion of the barber-diamond stripes. The predicted responses to both leftward

---

FIG. 9.8. (*continued*) intrinsic terminator motion (gray arrows), and hence are of the same relative magnitude as responses to circular grating moving in the corresponding oblique directions (R1, R3, R4, and R6). (E) Extrinsic motion prediction (P_e). This prediction holds that responses will be associated with the direction of extrinsic terminator motion (white arrows), and hence be of the same relative magnitude as the intrinsic motion prediction but reflected about the horizontal axis. Observed responses (panel B) of this neuron to barber-diamond stimuli ($R_{i|h} = 0.85$) were more closely correlated with the intrinsic motion prediction than with either the horizontal or extrinsic motion prediction. From "Occlusion and the Interpretation of Visual Motion: Perceptual and Neuronal Effects of Context," by R. O. Duncan, T. D. Albright, and G. R. Stoner, 2000, *Journal of Neuroscience, 20*, p. 5889. Copyright 2000 by The Society for Neuroscience. Adapted with permission.

motion conditions are thus equal to the responses to the corresponding leftward motion ($R2$) seen in Fig. 9.8A. Similarly, the predicted responses to rightward motion conditions are equal to $R5$.

The intrinsic motion prediction is shown in Fig. 9.8D. According to this prediction, neuronal responses to the four barber-diamond conditions reflect the four directions of intrinsic terminator motion and, hence, will match the pattern of responses seen for the gratings moving in those four directions. Specifically, the four predicted responses are equal to the responses measured for the corresponding directions ($R1$, $R3$, $R4$, and $R6$) seen in Fig. 9.8A. To cover all possibilities, we also considered the extrinsic motion prediction shown in Fig. 9.8E. Because the extrinsic terminators always move orthogonally to the intrinsic terminators in the barber-diamond, the extrinsic prediction is simply the intrinsic prediction reflected about the horizontal axis.

The responses of this neuron to the barber-diamond stimuli are shown in Fig. 9.8B. The pattern of selectivity clearly violated the null hypothesis because the responses were not independent of the depth-ordering configuration (e.g., the response to the upper right barber-diamond condition was much smaller than that elicited by the lower right stimulus). Moreover, as predicted, the largest response occurred when the intrinsic terminators moved in the preferred direction for the cell (downward and rightward, see Fig. 9.8A). Indeed, the shape of the direction tuning curve obtained with barber-diamond stimulation more closely matched that of the intrinsic prediction (Fig. 9.8D), than it did either the horizontal (Figure 9.8C) or extrinsic (Figure 9.8E) prediction. To quantify the accuracy of our predictions, we computed a measure of the correlation between the intrinsic prediction and the actual barber-diamond data ($R_{i|h}$).[1] $R_{i|h}$ varies between -1 and $+1$, with larger positive values reflecting increased correlation with the intrinsic predictor. The value of the coefficient $R_{i|h}$ for the cell documented in Fig. 9.8 is 0.85.

Several additional examples of the effect of barber-diamond stimulation are shown in Fig. 9.9. For five of the six cases shown, responses to the barber-diamonds (gray lines) were positively correlated with the intrinsic predictor (black lines) (values of $R_{i|h}$ range from 0.54 to 0.87). The sixth case (lower right) illustrates that, although it may be common, this phenomenon is not universal: Here the barber-diamond response was negatively correlated with the intrinsic prediction (and thus positively correlated with the extrinsic prediction).

Fig. 9.10 shows the distribution of correlation coefficients ($R_{i|h}$). Plotted are the values of $R_{i|h}$ for all of the MT neurons studied ($n = 265$; white bars), as well as for the subset of sampled neurons for which the values of $R_{i|h}$ were significantly different from 0 ($n = 90$; gray bars). The distribution as a whole is shifted toward positive coefficients, with the average $R_{i|h}$ (0.10) being significantly different

---

[1] Because the horizontal motion prediction is itself correlated with the intrinsic prediction, we computed a partial correlation coefficient for the intrinsic predictor with the horizontal predictor partialed out. Conveniently, the partial correlation coefficient for the extrinsic predictor is equal in magnitude to that for the intrinsic predictor but of opposite sign. See Duncan et al. (2000) for details.

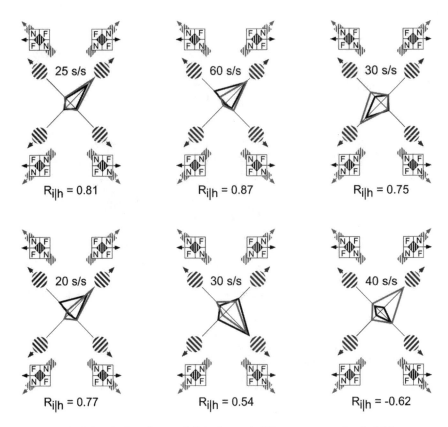

$R_{i|h} = 0.81$ $R_{i|h} = 0.87$ $R_{i|h} = 0.75$

$R_{i|h} = 0.77$ $R_{i|h} = 0.54$ $R_{i|h} = -0.62$

FIG. 9.9. Barber-diamond data from six MT neurons, each of which demonstrated significant influences of depth ordering on directional responses. Five of these neurons had positive intrinsic correlation coefficients and one neuron had a negative coefficient (*lower right*). Responses to circular gratings were averaged across five trials and plotted in polar coordinates (black lines). The direction of motion for each grating condition is indicated by the icons along the polar axis and the mean response to each condition is plotted along the radial axis. Responses to each barber-diamond condition were averaged across 10 trials and plotted along with corresponding icons on the same graphs (gray lines). Each of these neurons demonstrated individually significant responses to barber-diamonds that were configured to elicit upward versus downward motion (ANOVA; all $p < 0.0004$). Neurons with positive coefficients ($R_{i|h}$) have directionally selective responses consistent with the direction of motion of the intrinsic terminators. See also caption to Fig. 9.8. From "Occlusion and the Interpretation of Visual Motion: Perceptual and Neuronal Effects of Context," by R. O. Duncan, T. D. Albright, and G. R. Stoner, 2000 *Journal of Neuroscience, 20*, p. 5891. Copyright 2000, by The Society for Neuroscience. Adapted with permission.

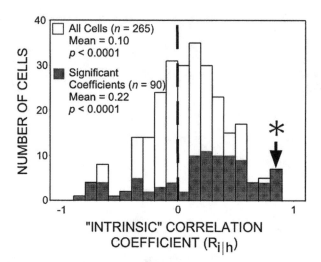

**"INTRINSIC" CORRELATION
COEFFICIENT ($R_{i|h}$)**

FIG. 9.10. Neuronal population data from barber-diamond studies. Distribution of intrinsic correlation coefficients ($R_{i|h}$) for the sample of 265 MT neurons studied (unfilled bars). The subset of cells for which coefficients reached statistical significance (ANOVA; all $p < 0.05$) is indicated by the gray bars. Positive coefficients reflect a positive correlation with the motion of intrinsic terminators. The population displays a significant positive shift of the mean (0.10) for intrinsic correlation coefficients (t test; $p < 0.0001$). The population of individually significant cells displays a larger number of positive coefficients ($n = 67$) relative to negative ones ($n = 23$). Asterisk denotes coefficient for neuron illustrated in Fig. 9.7. For the entire sample of 265 neurons, mean eccentricity of receptive field centers was 5.5°, and mean receptive field diameter was 5.4°. From "Occlusion and the Interpretation of Visual Motion: Perceptual and Neuronal Effects of Context," by R. O. Duncan, T. D. Albright, and G. R. Stoner, 2000, *Journal of Neuroscience, 20*, p. 5892. Copyright 2000 by The Society for Neuroscience. Adapted with permission.

from 0. Moreover, the distribution of individually significant coefficients is skewed toward positive values (mean $R_{i|h} = 0.22$). Thus, for at least a subset of MT neurons, we observed a high degree of correspondence between the intrinsic predictor and barber-diamond responses (Duncan et al., 2000), supporting our hypothesis that context and feature interpretation influence the signals produced by cortical neurons (Stoner & Albright, 1993). More generally, these data provide striking evidence that some MT neurons encode the perceived motions of surfaces, rather than indiscriminately representing the motions of isolated retinal image features.

It is reassuring to find that the signals of neurons at relatively early stages of visual processing represent the structure of the world—the things perceived—as opposed to undifferentiated retinal image features. These findings encourage us to search for the mechanisms by which the representational transformation comes about. This will be a major focus of research in coming years.

Feature Grouping

The experiments previously described addressed how motion processing is influenced by the assignment of features to particular objects in a scene. We now turn to a related problem: how motion processing is influenced by the perceptual grouping of image features that are visually related to each other—for example, the grouping of features that have the same color.

To appreciate how grouping influences motion processing, consider the following real-world problem. You are standing on the balcony of Grand Central Station during a busy rush hour looking down on the concourse, upon which hundreds (if not thousands) of people are moving in many different directions. Through this crowd moves a scattered group of schoolchildren, and you are hoping to identify the exit for which they are heading so that you can meet them there. Under normal circumstances, owing to the density of people, their lack of individual distinctiveness, and the complexity of their motions, it would be difficult to track the motion of the schoolchildren. The schoolchildren, however, wear distinctive red hats, making them easy to detect. Moreover, you find that even in the presence of abundant dynamic visual noise (the other travelers, slight direction changes by the individual children as they navigate through the crowd), it is a simple matter to determine the average direction of the children as they move through the crowd. Intuitively, it seems that the chromatic distinctiveness of signal and noise elements in the scene enables them to be grouped independently and facilitates the processing of their motion. Moreover, context is a critical parameter. In this case, the relevant context is the color of the signal elements relative to that of the noise.

Although this contextual effect on motion processing is easy to understand intuitively, it poses a problem for visual neurophysiology because for many years it has been thought that motion-sensitive neurons are blind to chromatic information. Earlier experiments on color selectivity and motion processing have not, however, manipulated the chromatic context in which stimuli are moved: hence, they are irrelevant to the phenomenon exemplified in the real-world example. To elucidate the neuronal bases of the contextual effect of color on motion processing, we therefore performed a series of studies that included psychophysical experiments with human subjects and paired neurophysiological/psychophysical experiments with rhesus monkeys.

The Stochastic Motion Stimulus

For these experiments we used a visual stimulus that both captures essential features of the real-world problem previously described and can be manipulated parametrically. This stimulus (Fig. 9.11) is based on one used in previous studies

Homochromatic

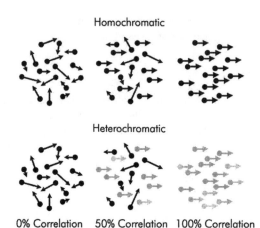

Heterochromatic

0% Correlation   50% Correlation   100% Correlation

FIG. 9.11. Schematic depiction of the stimulus used to study the influence of chromatic context on perceived motion and its neural correlates. Each stimulus consisted of a sequence of frames of randomly positioned bright dots appearing against a dark background on a CRT screen. Dots in each of the six circular apertures of the figure represent dots in six different stimuli. Arrows indicate velocity (direction and speed). The proportion of dots moving in the same direction at the same speed, expressed as a percentage and termed the motion coherence describes the strength of the motion signal. At 0% motion coherence, all of the dots move randomly. At 50% motion coherence, half the dots have the same velocity. At 100% motion coherence, all of the dots have the same velocity. In the homochromatic condition, all of the dots have the same color. In the heterochromatic condition, the signal dots are a different color from the noise dots. From "Segmentation by Color Influences Responses of Motion-Sensitive Neurons in the Cortical Middle Temporal Visual Area," by L. J. Croner and T. D. Albright, 1999, *Journal of Neuroscience, 19*, p. 3936. Copyright 1999 by The Society for Neuroscience. Reprinted with permission.

by Newsome and colleagues (e.g., Newsome et al., 1989; Newsome & Pare, 1988; Salzman, Britten, & Newsome, 1990), designed to quantify the motion sensitivity of primate observers and cortical neurons. Details of stimulus construction and display are provided in Croner and Albright (1997, 1999a). Briefly, the stimulus (Fig. 9.11A) used in previous studies consisted of a patch of randomly positioned dots that were displaced on each temporal frame. A variable fraction of these dots— the signal—as displaced by a common motion vector. The remaining dots—the noise—were displaced randomly and with uncorrelated motion vectors. Motion signal strength is the proportion of correlated motions in the stimulus and could be varied continuously from 0% (the motion of each dot is independent of the motions of all other dots) to 100% (the motion of all dots is in the same direction and speed). Because signal and noise dots were otherwise identical (i.e., the same color), we refer to this traditional stochastic motion stimulus as homochromatic. Using this stimulus, Newsome and colleagues showed that the ability of human and nonhuman primate observers to discriminate direction of motion exhibits a reliable dependence on motion signal strength (Newsome & Pare, 1988). In addition, these investigators demonstrated that the directionally selective responses of individual MT neurons exhibit a similar dependence on motion signal strength (Newsome et al., 1989).

Our adaptation of the traditional stochastic motion stimulus was composed of signal dots of one color (e.g., red) and noise dots of a different color (e.g., green) (Fig. 9.11B). This heterochromatic version is identical to the homochromatic version in all respects, save the chromatic difference between signal and noise dots.

Feature Grouping by Color Improves Perceptual Discrimination of Motion in Visual Noise

The analogy between our heterochromatic stimulus and the real-world example previously described needs little explication. Tracking the global motion of the schoolchildren was simplified because of their red hats. Similarly, we predicted that it would be easier to discern the direction of signal motion in the heterochromatic condition relative to the homochromatic condition. Specifically, we predicted that for a given motion signal strength, direction discriminability would improve (provided it was not already at ceiling), and the discriminability threshold for heterochromatic stimuli would be markedly lower than for homochromatic stimuli (Croner & Albright, 1997).

Five human subjects viewed both homo- and heterochromatic motion stimuli (Fig. 9.11), which were randomly interleaved from trial to trial. Both stimulus types were presented at a number of different motion signal strengths, spanning the extremes of behavioral performance including threshold. Color (red vs. green) assignments for signal and noise dots in heterochromatic stimuli were randomized across trials. Subjects fixated a small target while each stimulus was presented at the center of gaze for 2s. Signal motion was either leftward or rightward on each trial, following a pseudorandom schedule. At the conclusion of each presentation, subjects indicated the perceived direction of signal motion (2-Alternative Forced-Choice; left vs. right).

Data from one human subject are shown in Fig. 9.12. Task performance (proportion of correct direction judgments) is plotted as a function of motion signal strength for homochromatic (open triangles) and heterochromatic (filled circles) stimuli. Consistent with previous findings (Newsome et al., 1989), directional discriminability increased with motion signal strength, as revealed by the sigmoidal psychometric functions. The effect of the heterochromatic manipulation manifested as a pronounced leftward shift of the psychometric function. This reflects

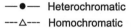

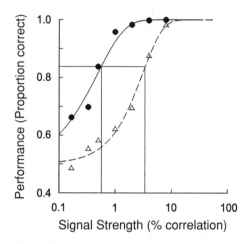

FIG. 9.12. Performance functions measured for a representative human subject discriminating signal direction in homochromatic (open triangles) and heterochromatic (filled circles) stimuli. Also shown are curves fit to the homochromatic (dashed lines), and heterochromatic (solid lines) data. Threshold performance (0.82) is illustrated by a thin horizontal line. Where this line intersects each psychometric function, a thin vertical line is drawn to intersect the x-axis at the threshold motion coherence for the function. Threshold motion coherence for the homochromatic condition was 3.1%, and for the heterochromatic condition it was 0.5%, indicating an approximately sixfold decrease in threshold when signal and noise dots were distinguished by color. From "Image Segmentation Enhances Discrimination of Motion of Visual Noise," by L. J. Croner and T. D. Albright, 1997, *Vision Research, 37,* p. 1418. Copyright 1997 by Elsevier Science. Adapted with permission.

the predicted improved sensitivity to motion direction in hetero- versus homochromatic stimuli: The discriminability threshold was significantly reduced for hetero- (0.5%) versus homochromatic stimuli (3.1%). Although the magnitude of threshold reduction varied across human subjects, significant effects of chromatic context on thresholds for direction discrimination were observed in every case.

From these psychophysical findings we speculated that the effects of grouping by color cues on motion perception were implemented by a dynamic gating mechanism. Specifically, we hypothesized that, during each stimulus presentation, the visual system created a chromatic filter that blocked information about noise dots from reaching motion detection circuits in the visual cortex (Croner & Albright, 1997). This simple hypothesis, of course, begs important questions regarding the mechanism by which such a filter may be implemented. Answers to these questions must await additional research.

Feature Grouping by Color Improves Neuronal Discrimination of Motion in Visual Noise

Using the homochromatic version of the stochastic motion stimulus, Newsome and colleagues found that the discriminability of direction by individual MT neurons closely matched monkeys' performance on the direction discrimination task (Newsome et al., 1989). These investigators thus hypothesized that the monkeys' perceptual decisions were based on the signals provided by MT neurons. If this hypothesis were correct, we would expect that stimulus manipulations influencing psychophysical performance would also influence neuronal discriminability. Because we found that chromatic context influences direction discrimination performance by humans, it follows that there may be parallel changes in the sensitivity of MT neurons. To test this, we trained monkeys to discriminate direction using both homo- and heterochromatic stochastic motion stimuli and then recorded from individual MT neurons while animals performed the task. Aside from the key stimulus differences, our behavioral paradigm was identical to that used by Newsome and colleagues (Newsome et al., 1989; Newsome & Pare, 1988) and is summarized schematically in Fig. 9.13.

The first goal of these experiments was to determine whether chromatic context improves motion discrimination thresholds in monkeys as it does in humans. Fig. 9.14 illustrates that not only did monkeys exhibit a consistent decrease in psychometric threshold for hetero- versus homochromatic stimuli, but also the effect generalized across a range of visual field eccentricities and axes of motion. This generalization was critical because it subsequently enabled us to customize the stochastic motion stimuli to the receptive field position and direction preference of individual MT neurons. (For a more complete comparison of behavioral data from monkeys and humans, see Croner & Albright, 1999a.)

We next examined the effects of these manipulations on the directional selectivity of individual MT neurons (Croner & Albright, 1999a). Stimuli were centered on the CRF of each MT neuron studied, and the two directions of signal motion were aligned with the neuron's preferred and antipreferred directions. Color (red vs. green) assignments for signal and noise dots in heterochromatic stimuli were randomized across trials. To quantify each neuron's ability to discriminate motion direction, we adopted the methods of signal detection theory (Swets, Green, Getty, & Swets, 1978) previously used for similar purposes by Newsome and colleagues (Newsome et al., 1989). Briefly, we examined the distributions of responses elicited by preferred and antipreferred directions of each stimulus condition (each signal strength of homo- or heterochromatic stimuli) and performed an analysis of receiver operating characteristics (ROC) based on these responses. We then computed the probability that an ideal observer could correctly determine the direction

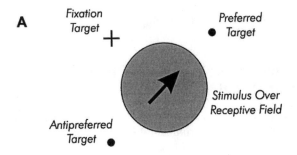

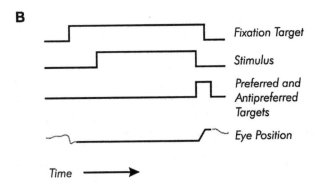

FIG. 9.13. Schematic depiction of paradigm developed by Newsome and colleagues (e.g., Newsome et al., 1989) and subsequently used by Croner and Albright (1999) to investigate influence of feature grouping on motion processing. (A) Example spatial configuration of the fixation target, stimulus aperture, and targets for direction choice. The stimulus aperture was superimposed on the receptive field of the neuron under study. Signal motion during each trial was in either the neuron's preferred or antipreferred direction; the targets for direction choice were positioned according to the neuron's preferred direction. (B) Diagram of the temporal sequence of events during one trial. The trial was initiated with the onset of the fixation target (Fixation Target). Five hundred ms after fixation was achieved (Eye Position), the motion stimulus was presented for 2 s (Stimulus). When the stimulus was extinguished, the Preferred and Antipreferred Targets appeared and remained on until the monkey indicated its direction choice by making a saccadic eye movement to one of them. From "Segmentation by Color Influences Responses of Motion-Sensitive Neurons in the Cortical Middle Temporal Visual Area," by L. J. Croner and T. D. Albright, 1999, *Journal of Neuroscience, 19,* p. 3938. Copyright 1999 by The Society for Neuroscience. Reprinted with permission.

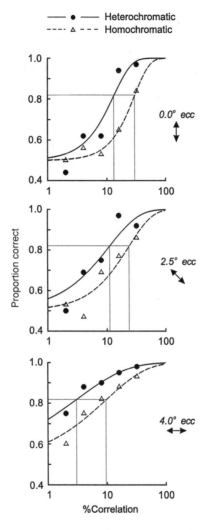

FIG. 9.14. Performance data obtained from monkeys discriminating signal direction in homochromatic (open triangles) and heterochromatic (filled circles) stimuli. Also shown are curves fit to the homochromatic (dashed lines) and heterochromatic (solid lines) data. The inset to the right of each plot gives the retinal eccentricity of the stimulus and the axis of signal direction used in each block. Thin straight lines indicate performance thresholds, as in Fig. 9.12. The homochromatic and heterochromatic psychophysical thresholds, respectively, were 29.7% and 13.2% (top), 23.5% and 10.9% (middle), and 9.5% and 2.9% (bottom). From "Segmentation by Color Influences Responses of Motion-Sensitive Neurons in the Cortical Middle Temporal Visual Area," by L. J. Croner and T. D. Albright, 1999, *Journal of Neuroscience, 19*, p. 3939. Copyright 1999 by The Society for Neuroscience. Reprinted with permission.

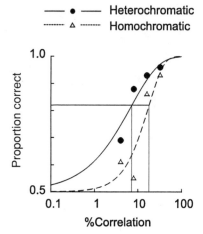

FIG. 9.15. Paired neurometric functions obtained from one neuron's responses to the homo- and heterochromatic stimuli. In this experiment, we measured significantly different neuronal thresholds for the two conditions. Thin straight lines illustrate thresholds, as in Fig. 9.12. The homochromatic and heterochromatic neurometric thresholds were, respectively, 17.6 and 7.0%. From "Segmentation by Color Influences Responses of Motion-Sensitive Neurons in the Cortical Middle Temporal Visual Area," by L. J. Croner and T. D. Albright, 1999, *Journal of Neuroscience, 19,* p. 3942. Copyright 1999 by The Society for Neuroscience. Reprinted with permission.

of stimulus motion given the observed responses for each condition. These probability estimates served as an index of neuronal directional discriminability and were used to generate a neurometric function relating discriminability to motion signal strength for each cell. Fig. 9.15 shows the neurometric functions for homo- (open triangles) and heterochromatic stimuli (filled circles) obtained from one MT neuron. This neuron exhibited a dramatic threshold reduction for heterochromatic stimuli, paralleling the typical psychophysical threshold reduction.

To convey the distribution of this effect on neuronal discriminability, we include Fig. 9.16, which contains a plot of homo- versus heterochromatic threshold for each neuron studied. Although the thresholds were significantly different—like the example in Fig. 9.15—in only a subset of cases (filled circles), the average ratio of hetero- to homochromatic threshold (0.74) was significantly less than 1.0 (see diagonal plot), and the ratio for the subset of individually significant neurons (0.35, black bars) revealed a strong effect of chromatic context.

Relative to the homochromatic stimulus, the heterochromatic stimulus thus elicited lower average psychophysical and neuronal thresholds for motion discriminability. These findings support the hypotheses that (1) MT neurons account for the perceptual discriminability of motion direction with chromatic grouping

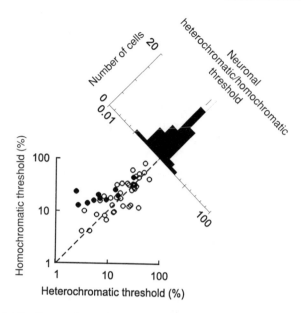

FIG. 9.16. Comparison of neuronal performance for homochromatic and heterochromatic conditions. The bottom panel shows a scatter-plot of the absolute thresholds obtained in experiments with single neurons. The black symbols signify neurons for which the two thresh-olds were significantly different from each other; the broken line illus-trates where points would fall if the thresholds were identical. The top right panel shows a frequency distribution of the ratios of heterochro-matic to homochromatic thresholds, formed by summing across the scatterplot within diagonally oriented bins. The dotted line indicates unity, and the solid line segment is aligned with the geometric mean. Ratios less than unity indicate that neuronal performance was better (threshold was lower) for the heterochromatic condition. The black bars show the threshold ratios for experiments in which the two thresholds were significantly different from each other. From "Seg-mentation by Color Influences Responses of Motion-Sensitive Neu-rons in the Cortical Middle Temporal Visual Area," by L. J. Croner and T. D. Albright, 1999, *Journal of Neuroscience, 19*, p. 3943. Copyright 1999 by The Society for Neuroscience. Reprinted with permission.

of signal versus noise and (2) these neurons have access to contextual (chromatic, in this case) information unrelated to motion per se. Because both psychophysical and neuronal data were obtained on each trial, however, we can address a still finer question: Do fluctuations in psychophysical performance correlate with fluctua-tions in neuronal discriminability? We approached this question by assessing the change in psychophysical threshold as a function of the change in the neuronal threshold for each block of trials. The results are plotted in Fig. 9.17. Here, each data set represents a complete experiment for one neuron, with the four relevant

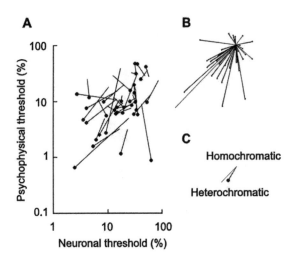

FIG. 9.17. Comparison of the change in absolute neuronal and behavioral thresholds afforded by color segmentation. (A) Vectors show
the change in thresholds measured in each experiment. The plain
end of each vector shows the relation between behavioral and neuronal thresholds for the homochromatic condition, and the end with
a black dot shows the same relation for the heterochromatic condition. Vectors with a downward component (from homochromatic
to heterochromatic) indicate enhanced behavioral sensitivity to the
heterochromatic condition; vectors with an upward component indicate the converse. Vectors with a leftward component indicate enhanced neuronal sensitivity to the heterochromatic condition; vectors
with a rightward component indicate the converse. (B) The vectors
are redrawn from the same origin, which represents the homochromatic thresholds. (C) The single vector is the average of the vectors
shown in B. In B and C the dotted line is the 45° diagonal, where vectors would lie if color segmentation influenced behavioral and neuronal thresholds equally. From "Segmentation by Color Influences Responses of Motion-Sensitive Neurons in the Cortical Middle Temporal
Visual Area," by L. J. Croner and T. D. Albright, 1999, *Journal of
Neuroscience, 19*, p. 3944. Copyright 1999 by The Society for Neuroscience. Reprinted with permission.

thresholds (psycho-hetero, psycho-homo, neuro-hetero, neuro-homo) represented
by a single vector in a two-dimensional space (Fig. 9.17A). In this figure, psychophysical threshold is plotted as a function of neuronal threshold. The plain end
of each vector shows the psychophysical/neuronal threshold pair obtained using the
homochromatic stimulus, and the end with the black dot shows the corresponding
threshold pair obtained using the heterochromatic stimulus. Vectors with vertical
and horizontal components of equal direction and magnitude indicate experiments
in which the stimulus manipulation had equivalent effects on the neuron and the
behavior. To facilitate inspection of these data, the vectors are plotted from a

common homochromatic origin in Fig. 9.17B. Clearly, not all neurons exhibit threshold shifts that match the perceptual change. However, from this plot, one can more fully appreciate the trend, which is toward neuronal and perceptual decreases of similar magnitude (though not identical; see Croner & Albright, 1999a). The point is further emphasized in Fig. 9.17C, where we have plotted the average data vector (solid line) and the neuronal-perceptual identity vector (dashed line). On average, the introduction of a chromatic context that enables feature grouping elicits comparable changes in simultaneously assessed indices of neuronal and perceptual sensitivity.

Sources of Enhanced Directional Discriminability by Cortical Neurons

To understand the mechanisms responsible for the context-dependent changes in neuronal thresholds, we evaluated the response changes underlying the observed threshold reduction. Neuronal directional discriminability, as we measured it, depends on the degree of overlap between the distributions of responses to preferred and antipreferred directions of motion. The degree of overlap is affected by two simple attributes of these distributions: average response and variance. All else being equal, divergence of the means (by preferred direction response increase, antipreferred direction response decrease, or both) leads to greater discriminability. Similarly, reduction of the variance (for either preferred or antipreferred responses, or both) leads to greater discriminability.

Britten and colleagues (Britten, Shadlen, Newsome, & Movshon, 1992) demonstrated that, for homochromatic stimuli, improvement of neuronal discriminability with increasing signal strength results from both an increase in the magnitude of the preferred direction response and a decrease in the magnitude of the antipreferred direction response. Analysis of our homochromatic data confirmed that finding. By contrast, we found that the improved discriminability for heterochromatic stimuli, relative to that for homochromatic stimuli of the same signal strength, was associated with altered responses only to the preferred direction stimuli. Specifically, heterochromatic preferred direction stimuli evoked both larger and less variable responses than did preferred direction homochromatic stimuli of the same signal strength. These findings are summarized schematically in Fig. 9.18A. To facilitate comparison of these response changes with those elicited by increases in signal strength, we have illustrated the latter schematically in Fig. 9.18B. This comparison reveals an important point: Although either the addition of chromatic context or an increase in signal strength can improve neuronal discriminability, the underlying mechanisms are very different.

Precisely what those mechanisms are remains unclear, but the reduction of variance associated with heterochromatic stimulation is provocative, suggesting that the neuron is driven more effectively for the heterochromatic stimuli. We propose that the observed response changes reflect a unique decision strategy being used by the monkey when features are grouped by chromatic cues (or any other

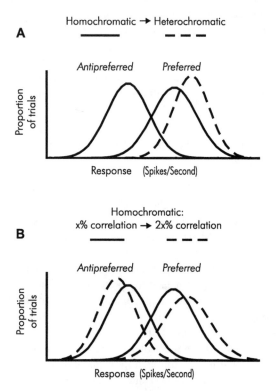

FIG. 9.18.   Schematic diagrams showing the response changes associated with enhanced discriminability by neurons with significantly different homochromatic and heterochromatic thresholds. (A) Hypothetical frequency distributions of the responses of a neuron to homochromatic stimuli (solid lines) and to heterochromatic stimuli (dashed lines) of one stimulus motion coherence. The horizontal axis in each graph represents response strength (spikes/s). Each curve represents a distribution of response strengths across multiple trials, in which motion was either in the preferred or antipreferred direction. (B) Hypothetical frequency distributions of the responses of a neuron to homochromatic stimuli of a low stimulus motion coherence (solid lines) and to homochromatic stimuli of twice that value (dashed lines). From "Segmentation by Color Influences Responses of Motion-Sensitive Neurons in the Cortical Middle Temporal Visual Area," by L. J. Croner and T. D. Albright, 1999, *Journal of Neuroscience, 19*, p. 3948. Copyright 1999 by The Society for Neuroscience. Reprinted with permission.

cues allowing feature grouping). One possibility is that the chromatic cue enables attention to be directed selectively to signal dots, thus freeing the discriminative apparatus from concern with the noise dots. A precedent for this general type of mechanism can be found in the fact that attentional selection by color has a gating effect on responses in area V4 (Motter, 1994).

CONCLUSIONS

We described two sets of experiments showing that the responses of some MT neurons are influenced by the spatial context in which moving stimuli appear. In both cases, nonmotion cues (depth ordering for the first set of experiments and color for the second set) clarify the evaluation of motion signals that would be ambiguous in the domain of image motion alone. Based on these findings, we conclude that nonmotion attributes allow the visual system to select relevant image motions—that of intrinsic line terminators in the first set of experiments and of signal dots in the second set—for further processing leading to perception.

Our experiments contribute to a growing body of evidence that the responses of neurons relatively early in the visual processing hierarchy underlie perceptual organization. What remains unknown are the mechanisms by which these responses arise. Detailed mechanistic studies face formidable technical challenges (consider, e.g., the problem of revealing local anatomical circuitry in the functioning visual cortex).

Nevertheless, some progress has been made. For example, that visual context affects scene perception in particular ways implies that visual neurons have ready access to specific contextual information, and this constrains the kind of information flow we should expect to find in the visual cortex. In some cases, the process of perceptual organization seems to invoke attentional mechanisms, the neuronal bases of which can be explored by direct manipulation of the observer's attentional focus (e.g. Reynolds, Chelazzi, & Desimone, 1999).

Regardless of the exact mechanisms involved, the insight that contextual information has specific influences over neuronal representation in the visual cortex significantly affects our understanding of how the visual system is organized. In addition, this insight signals that an important bridge has been crossed: Neurobiologists and psychologists have begun to speak in the same terms, value the same concepts, and target the same problems of perception. It is only a matter of time before we truly understand how the brain accomplishes visual perception.

ACKNOWLEDGMENTS

We thank J. Costanza for superb technical assistance and Carl Olson and Rudiger von der Heydt for comments on the manuscript. The work reviewed herein was supported, in part, by grants from the NEI (TDA, GRS), the NIMH (TDA), an individual NRSA (LJC), an award from the Fight for Sight research division of Prevent Blindness America (LJC), and a fellowship from the McDonnell-Pew Center for Cognitive Neuroscience at San Diego (GRS). T. D. Albright is an investigator of the Howard Hughes Medical Institute.

REFERENCES

Albright, T. D. (1984). Direction and orientation selectivity of neurons in visual area MT of the macaque. *Journal of Neurophysiology, 52*(6), 1106–1130.

Albright, T. D. (1992). Form-cue invariant motion processing in primate visual cortex. *Science, 255*(5048), 1141–1143.

Albright, T. D. (1993). Cortical processing of visual motion. *Reviews of Oculomotor Research, 5,* 177–201.

Albright, T. D., Desimone, R., & Gross, C. G. (1984). Columnar organization of directionally selective cells in visual area MT of the macaque. *Journal of Neurophysiology, 51,* 16–31.

Allman, J. M., & Kaas, J. H. (1971). Representation of the visual field in striate and adjoining cortex of the owl monkey (*Aotus Trivirgatus*). *Brain Resarch., 35,* 89–106.

Britten, K. H., Shadlen, M. N., Newsome, W. T., & Movshon, J. A. (1992). The analysis of visual motion: a comparison of neuronal and psychophysical performance. *Journal of Neuroscience, 12*(12), 4745–1465.

Croner, L. J., & Albright, T. D. (1997). Image segmentation enhances discrimination of motion in visual noise. *Vision Research, 37*(11), 1415–1427.

Croner, L. J., & Albright, T. D. (1999a). Segmentation by color influences responses of motion-sensitive neurons in the cortical middle temporal visual area. *Journal of Neuroscience, 19*(10), 3935–3951.

Croner, L. J., & Albright, T. D. (1999b). Seeing the big picture: integration of image cues in the primate visual system. *Neuron, 24*(4), 777–789.

Dobkins, K. R., & Albright, T. D. (1994). What happens if it changes color when it moves? The nature of chromatic input to macaque visual area MT. *Journal of Neuroscience, 14*(8), 4854–4870.

Duncan, R. O., Albright, T. D., & Stoner, G. R. (2000). Occlusion and the interpretation of visual motion: Perceptual and neuronal effects of context. *Journal of Neuroscience, 20*(15), 5885–5897.

Gattass, R., & Gross, C. G. (1981). Visual topography of striate projection zone (MT) in posterior superior temporal sulcus of the Macaque. *Journal of Neurophysiology, 46*(3), 621–638.

Hubel, D. H., & Wiesel, T. N. (1968). Receptive fields and functional architecture of monkey striate cortex. *The Journal of Physiology, 195,* 215–243.

Maunsell, J. H. R., & Van Essen, D. C. (1983). Functional properties of neurons in middle temporal visual area of the macaque monkey. I. Selectivity for stimulus direction, speed and orientation. *Journal of Neurophysiology, 49*(5), 1127–1147.

Motter, B. C. (1994). Neural correlates of attentive selection for color or luminance in extrastriate area V4. *Journal of Neuroscience, 14*(4), 2178–89.

Movshon, J. A., Adelson, E. A., Gizzi, M., & Newsome, W. T. (1985). The analysis of moving visual patterns. In C. Chagas, R. Gattass, & C. G. Gross (Eds.), *Study group on pattern recognition mechanisms* (pp. 117–151). Vatican City: Pontifica Academia Scientiarum.

Newsome, W. T., Britten, K. H., & Movshon, J. A. (1989). Neuronal correlates of a perceptual decision. *Nature, 341*(6237), 52–54.

Newsome, W. T., & Pare, E. B. (1988). A selective impairment of motion perception following lesions of the middle temporal visual area (MT). *Journal of Neuroscience, 8*(6), 2201–2211.

Reynolds, J. H., Chelazzi, L., & Desimone, R. (1999). Competitive mechanisms subserve attention in macaque areas V2 and V4. *Journal of Neuroscience, 19*(5), 1736–1753.

Rodman, H. R., & Albright, T. D. (1987). Coding of visual stimulus velocity in area MT of the macaque. *Vision Research, 27,* 2035–2048.

Rodman, H. R., & Albright, T. D. (1989). Single-unit analysis of pattern-motion selective properties in the middle temporal visual area (MT). *Experimental Brain Research, 75,* 53–64.

Salzman, C. D., Britten, K. H., & Newsome, W. T. (1990). Cortical microstimulation influences perceptual judgements of motion direction. *Nature, 346*(6280), 174–177.

Shimojo, S., Silverman, G. H., & Nakayama, K. (1989). Occlusion and the solution to the aperture problem for motion. *Vision Research, 29*(5), 619–626.

Stoner, G. R., & Albright, T. D. (1992). Neural correlates of perceptual motion coherence. *Nature, 358*(6385), 412–414.

Stoner, G. R., & Albright, T. D. (1993). Image segmentation cues in motion processing: Implications for modularity in vision. *Journal of Cognitive Neuroscience, 5,* 129–149.

Swets, J. A., Green, D. M., Getty, D. J., & Swets, J. B. (1978). Signal detection and identification at successive stages of observation. *Perception and Psychophysics, 23*(4), 275–89.

Ungerleider, L. G., & Mishkin, M. (1979). The striate projection zone in the superior temporal sulcus of macaca mulatta: Location and topographic organization. *The Journal of Comparative Neurology, 188,* 347–366.

Van Essen, D. C., Maunsell, J. H. R., & Bixby, J. L. (1981). The middle temporal visual area in the macaque: Myeloarchitecture, connections, functional properties and topographic connections. *The Journal of Comparative Neurology, 199,* 293–326.

Wallach, H. (1935). Über visuell wahrgenommenr Bewegungsrichtung. *Psychologische Forschung, 20.* [About Visually Perceived Direction of Motion, *Phychological Research, 20,* 325–380.

Zeki, S. M. (1974). Cells responding to changing image size and disparity in the cortex of the rhesus monkey. *The Journal of Physiology, 242,* 827–841.

10 Visual Perceptual Organization: Lessons From Lesions

Marlene Behrmann
Carnegie Mellon University

Ruth Kimchi
University of Haifa

The visual world consciously perceived is very different from the chaotic juxtaposition of different colors and shapes that stimulate the individual retinal receptors. Objects are seen as detached and separable from adjacent objects and surfaces despite the fact that parts of a single object may be spatially or temporally discontinuous, and have different colors or even transect several different depth planes. Additionally, because most surfaces are opaque, portions of objects are routinely hidden from view, and, as we move around, surfaces continually undergo occlusion and fragmentation. As is apparent from this description, the objects of phenomenal perception are not given in any direct way in the retinal image. Some internal processes of organization must clearly be responsible, then, for producing a single, coherent percept. Exactly what these processes are remains poorly understood despite the roughly 100 years since the Gestalt psychologists first articulated the principles of perceptual organization. Although the Gestalt work on perceptual organization has been widely accepted as identifying crucial phenomena of perception, there has been, until the last decade or so, relatively little theoretical and empirical emphasis on perceptual organization with a few exceptions. And, to the extent that progress has been made, there still remain many open questions. In this chapter, we explore some of these open issues in light of data we have obtained through a series of neuropsychological investigations with individuals who are impaired in perceptual organization following brain damage, hence the title of this chapter.

PERCEPTUAL ORGANIZATION: MONOLITHIC ENTITY?

A traditional view of most, although not all, theories of visual perception is that perceptual organization is a unitary phenomenon that operates at a single, early, preattentive stage, in a bottom-up fashion, to create units that then serve as candidate objects for later and more elaborated processing, including object recognition and identification (Marr, 1982; Neisser, 1967; Treisman, 1982, 1983). Implicit in this view is the idea that perceptual organization processes are not really differentiable in their attentional demands, time course, and relative contribution to object recognition. Several recent studies, however, challenged this view from a variety of perspectives. First, some researchers argued that grouping does not occur as early as had been widely assumed (Palmer, Neff, & Beck, 1996; Palmer, this volume; Rock & Brosgole, 1964; Rock, Nijhawan, Plamer, & Tudor, 1992). Second, in contrast to the standard view that assumes that grouping occurs preattentively (e.g., Neisser, 1967; Treisman, 1982, 1983), recent studies showed that grouping does, in fact, require attention (Mack, Tang, Tuma, Kahn, & Rock, 1992), though other recent studies suggest that certain forms of grouping can occur under conditions of inattention (Driver, Davis, Russell, Turatto, & Freeman, 2001; Moore & Egeth, 1997; Kimchi & Razpurker-Apfeld, 2001). Finally, the monolithic quality of grouping has been challenged, too; several studies demonstrated a temporal difference between various grouping processes showing, for example, an earlier of impact of grouping by proximity than by similarity of shape (Ben-Av & Sagi, 1995; Han & Humphreys, 1999; Han, Humphreys, & Chen, 1999; Kurylo, 1997).

Consistent with this last idea that there may be multiple processes involved in perceptual organization, two forms of grouping have been identified: the process of unit formation that determines which elements belong together or what goes with what and the process of shape formation or configuring that determines the shape of the grouped elements based on the interrelationships of the elements (Koffka, 1935; Rock, 1986). This distinction between grouping and configuring will turn out to be critical in understanding the neuropsychological data and the differential contribution of configuring in relation to object recognition. In particular, we show that the product of grouping (in the sense of element clustering) as reflected in grouping elements into rows and columns may be preserved following brain damage but that configuring the elements and apprehending the interrelationships of the grouped elements may be affected and have adverse consequences for the ability to recognize objects.

Along with presenting data to support the distinction between unit formation and configuring, we suggest that these processes are likely supported by different neural mechanisms. Although the lesions documented after brain damage in humans are notoriously poor for the purpose of establishing brain-behavior relationships and localizing very fine-grained processes, neuropsychological studies, in tandem with data from neuroimaging and neurophysiology, can provide important clues to the neural substrate involved in perceptual organization. We discuss these issues after the behavioral data are presented.

VISUAL AGNOSIA

To explore the psychological and neural mechanisms underlying perceptual organization, we conducted a series of studies with two individuals whose unfortunate impairment provides us with an ideal testing ground for investigating processes involved in perceptual organization and their relationship to object perception. The patients, SM and RN, suffer from a neuropsychological impairment, referred to as visual object agnosia, in which they are unable to recognize even familiar common objects presented to them in the visual modality (see Fig. 10.1 for examples of their error responses). This object recognition deficit cannot be attributed to a problem in labeling the stimulus per se (anomia) nor to a loss of semantics; presented with the same object in a different sensory modality, either haptically or auditorily, they have no problem in naming it or providing detailed and rich descriptions of it. The deficit in visual agnosia, then, is a specific failure to access the meaning of objects from the visual modality (Farah, 1990; Humphreys & Riddoch, 2001; Ratcliff & Newcombe, 1982).

The patients we chose to study have a specific form of agnosia, in which the deficit apparently affects intermediate vision. The impairment has been referred to as integrative agnosia because the patients appear to have available to them the basic features or elements in a display but are then unable to integrate all aspects into a meaningful whole. For example, patient HJA performs well on a search task when identifying a target that does not require a combination of elements (for example, differentiating '/' from '|') but performs poorly when required to bind visual elements in a spatially parallel fashion across a field containing multiple stimuli, such as searching for an upright T among misoriented Ts (Humphreys, 1999; Humphreys & Riddoch, 1987; Humphreys, Riddoch, Quinlan, Price, & Donnelly, 1992).

The failure of these patients to integrate elements occurs equally with displays of two- and three-dimensional stimuli and with black-and-white and chromatic displays, although, in some cases, the presence of depth, color and surface cues may be of some assistance to the patients in segmenting the display (Chainay & Humphreys, 2001; Farah, 1990; Humphreys et al., 1994; Jankowiak, Kinsbourne, Shalev, & Bachman, 1992). These patients are also more impaired at identifying items that overlap one another compared with the same items presented in isolation. Interestingly and counterintuitively, in some patients, the presence of

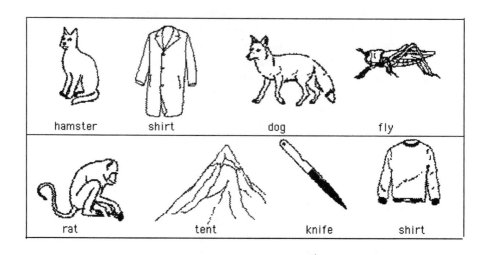

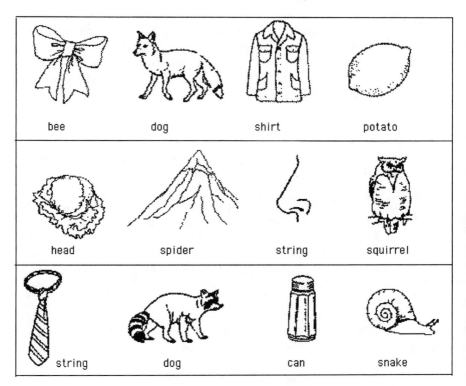

FIG. 10.1. Examples of black-and-white line drawings (from the Boston Naming test) and the responses of the patients to these pictures.

local information may even reduce the efficiency of visual recognition; in contrast with normal perceivers, some integrative agnosic patients (Butter & Trobe, 1994; Humphreys et al., 1992; Lawson & Humphreys, 1999; Riddoch & Humphreys, 1987) identified silhouettes better than line drawings whose internal details apparently led to incorrect segmentation. The silhouette advantage is thought to arise from the reduced need to segment and integrate elemental features relative to the line drawings. Another key feature of the disorder is the failure to carry out figure-ground segregation; patient FGP, for example, cannot even determine the presence of a X when it is superimposed on a noisy background (Kartsounis & Warrington, 1991). Finally, and critically for our purposes, these agnosic patients seem to be impaired at grouping; for example, patient NM was impaired at detecting the presence of a target letter when it was defined by multiple oriented line segments in a display with distractors of different orientations (Ricci, Vaishnavi, & Chatterjee, 1999). The same was true when the target was defined by color, luminance, or motion features relative to the distractors (Marstrand, Gerlach, Udesen, & Gade, 2000). Note that when the demands for element integration are low, as in making same/different judgments about two stimuli that share area and brightness but not shape (aspect ratio is manipulated from square to rectangle; Efron, 1968), the patients performed well.

Case Histories

Our two patients, SM and RN, are male, right-handed and English speaking. Both have been diagnosed as having visual agnosia and participated in several previous studies (Behrmann, 2003; Behrmann & Kimchi, 2003; Gauthier, Behrmann, & Tarr, 1999; Marotta, Behrmann, & Genovese, 2001; Williams & Behrmann, 2002). Neither patient has a field defect. SM has visual acuity corrected to 20/20, and RN has normal acuity.

SM sustained a closed head injury in a motor vehicle accident in 1994 at the age of 18. Despite extensive injuries, he recovered extremely well, and the only residual deficit is the visual agnosia. Fig. 10.2 presents MRI images for SM demonstrating the site and extent of his inferior temporal lobe lesion (Marotta et al., 2001). Note that, although SM is right-handed, he has some weakness on the right side because his arm was badly damaged in the accident, so he uses his left hand intermittently. RN suffered a myocardial infarction during bypass surgery in 1998 at the age of 39. He does not have a focal lesion on his MRI scan; the absence of a circumscribed lesion from a patient who has sustained brain damage following a myocardial infarction is not uncommon.[1] Because the neuropil is generally preserved after such an incident, even if the neurons themselves are affected, a circumscribed lesion may not be detectable even with high-resolution imaging.[2]

---

[1] We thank Dr H. B. Coslett for discussing RN's neurological status with us.

[2] We attempted a functional imaging scan on RN, but he is too large to remain in the scanner for any length of time, so these data could not be obtained.

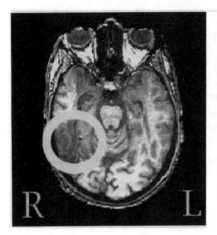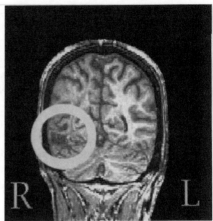

FIG. 10.2.   Structural scan from SM showing the localization of the
lesion to the right inferior temporal lobe. From "What Does Visual
Agnosia Tell Us About Perceptual Organization and Its Relationship to
Object Perception?" by M. Behrmann and R. Kimchi, 2003, *Journal
of Experimental Psychology: Human Perception and Performance,
29*(1), pp. 19–42. Copyright 2003 by APA. Reprinted with permission.

Both patients performed normally on those subtests of the Birmingham Object
Recognition Battery (BORB; Riddoch & Humphreys, 1993) that tap low-level or
early visual processes, including judging line length, orientation, size, and gap
position. That both patients can derive considerable visual information is further
supported by their copying performance; both patients produce reasonably good
copies of a target object or a scene (see Fig. 10.3 and 10.4), although they do so
slowly relative to normal subjects and in a labored and segmental fashion. Both
patients also performed within normal limits on more complex visual tasks, such as
matching objects based on minimal features or when one object was foreshortened.
Importantly, however, both patients were impaired on the BORB subtests, which
evaluate discrimination of overlapping shapes, and both performed in the impaired
range on the object decision subtests (task: "is this a real object or not?"), as is
usually the case with patients with integrative agnosia. In contrast with some
integrative agnosic subjects, neither SM nor RN performed better with silhouettes
than with line drawings. Examples of stimuli from these various perception tests
are shown in Fig. 10.5.

Both patients performed normally in naming objects presented to them in the
haptic modality, while blindfolded, or in the auditory modality, including naming
the very objects they failed to recognize when presented visually. The preserved
naming performance and ability to define the objects rule out both an anomia and
a semantic deficit as the underlying cause of the agnosia. The patients also did
not have available to them information about the display that they could indicate

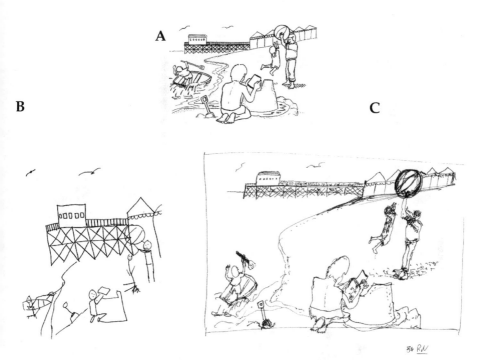

FIG. 10.3. Display of a beach scene with the (A) original and copies by (B) SM and (C) RN, who both took an extraordinary amount of time to complete this. From "What Does Visual Agnosia Tell Us About Perceptual Organization and Its Relationship to Object Perception?" by M. Behrmann and R. Kimchi, 2003, *Journal of Experimental Psychology: Human Perception and Performance, 29*(1), pp. 19–42. Copyright 2003 by APA. Reprinted with permission.

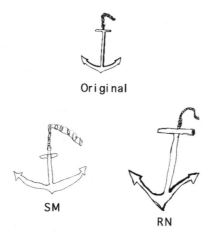

FIG. 10.4. Display of individual object (anchor) with the original and copies by SM and RN.

A   B

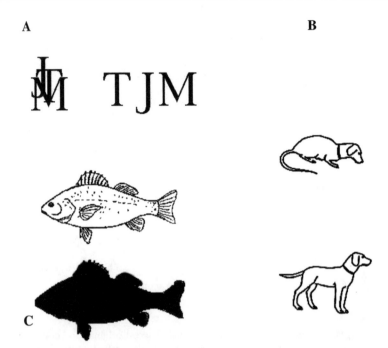

C

FIG. 10.5.   Examples of (A) overlapping and individual letters, (B) line drawings for object decision and (C) silhouettes for object identification. From "What Does Visual Agnosia Tell Us About Perceptual Organization and Its Relationship to Object Perception?" by M. Behrmann and R. Kimchi, 2003, *Journal of Experimental Psychology: Human Perception and Performance, 29*(1), pp. 19–42. Copyright 2003 by APA. Reprinted with permission.

through another output modality, such as gesture, as is the case in subjects with optic aphasia. The deficit for SM and RN is clearly in the inability to recognize images presented in the visual modality.

Both patients read accurately but slowly as tested in a naming latency task with words of different lengths presented individually on the computer screen. Whereas normal readers show minimal, if any, effect of the number of letters on word recognition within this range (three to eight letters in length), the subjects both showed raised intercepts as well as slopes, relative to control subjects. Whereas SM read 117/120 words correctly, with a slope of 104 ms for each additional letter, RN read 95/120 words correctly with a slope of 241 ms for each additional letter. In addition to the object and word agnosia, both patients are impaired at recognizing faces (i.e., suffer from prosopagnosia), and their face recognition deficit has also been explored in some of the previous publications (Gauthier et al., 1999; Marotta, McKeeff, & Behrmann, 2002).

Object Recognition Abilities

To document the object recognition deficits of the patients and compare this problem across the patients, we had them identify objects presented on a computer screen as black-and-white line drawings from the Snodgrass and Vanderwart (1980) set. Each object appeared individually for an unlimited exposure duration and the reaction time (RT) and accuracy were recorded. The patients differed in their ability: SM identified a total of 66% (171/260) of the objects, whereas RN identified only 51% (132/160). The errors made by the patients are mostly visual confusions (see Fig. 10.1). Neither subject appeared to be exhibiting a speed-accuracy trade-off because SM required an average of 2.14 s per image, whereas RN averaged 8.52 ms per image, confirming the greater impairment in RN than SM. We previously obtained naming data on the same stimulus set from a group of normal control subjects with no history of neurological illness whose mean accuracy was 96.4% and mean reaction time was 884.67 ms (Behrmann, Nelson, & Sekuler, 1998). Both patients showed accuracy and RTs more than 3 SD from the mean of these normal subjects.

As expected given their diagnosis of visual agnosia, both patients are impaired at object recognition as reflected in their accuracy and response times. Their long reaction times for correct identifications suggest that they build up their object representations slowly and in a segmental fashion. We also note that RN is significantly impaired relative to SM in both accuracy and RT, a finding that becomes important later.

DERIVATION OF GLOBAL SHAPE

Global/Local Processing in Hierarchical Stimuli

One obvious reason why integrative agnosic patients might fail to recognize objects is that they cannot derive the global form or shape because they fail to group or integrate the elements. We explored this possibility using the now-standard stimulus, the Navon-type hierarchical display, in which a global letter is made up of local letters having either the same or different identity as the global letter (see Fig. 10.6A). Half the trials consist of consistent letters, in which the global and the local letters shared identity (a large H made of smaller Hs and a large S made of small Ss), and the other half consist of inconsistent letters, in which the letters at the two levels had different identities (a large H made of small Ss and a large S made of small Hs). This type of paradigm has been used to tap grouping and element integration (Enns & Kingstone, 1995; Han & Humphreys, 1999; Han et al., 1999). In the version of the task we used, a stimulus appears on the computer screen, and, in different blocks of trials, subjects identify the letter at either the global or local level. All else being equal, in normal individuals, the global letter is identified

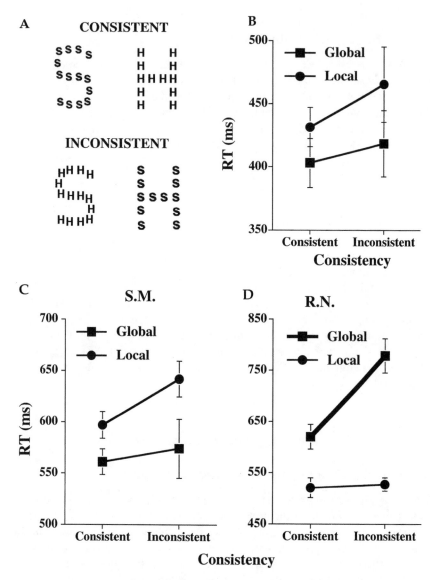

FIG. 10.6. (A) Hierarchical stimuli, made of two letters, *H* and *S*, which are composed of *H*s or *S*s. Mean millisecond responses times for (B) control subjects, (C) SM and (D) RN to indicate letter identify as a function of consistency between the local and global levels. Note the difference in the *y*-axis across the three graphs. From "What Does Visual Agnosia Tell Us About Perceptual Organization and Its Relationship to Object Perception?" by M. Behrmann and R. Kimchi, 2003, *Journal of Experimental Psychology: Human Perception and Performance, 29*(1), pp. 19–42. Copyright 2003 by APA. Reprinted with permission.

faster than the local letter, and conflicting information between the global and the local levels exerts asymmetrical global-to-local interference (Navon, 1977). Although the mechanisms underlying this global advantage are still disputed, the phenomenon is robust and is observed under various exposure durations, including short ones (Navon, 1977; Paquet & Merikle, 1984; Yovel, Yovel, & Levy, 2001; see Kimchi, 1992, for a review), suggesting that normal subjects can easily and quickly perceive the global configuration of hierarchical patterns. If the patients are impaired at grouping the local letters, they would have problems deriving the global configuration and would therefore be slowed in detecting the global letter. Additionally, if their processing is driven mostly by the local elements, then we might observe interference from the local identity when subjects identify the global, inconsistent letter.

Along with the patients, we tested a group of nonneurological control subjects, all of whom had corrected-to-normal visual acuity by self-report and, with the exception of one, were right-handed. The normal participants completed 192 experimental trials, whereas the patients completed 384 experimental trials across two sessions. Before each block, participants were verbally instructed to respond to the global or local letters. Each trial was initiated with a central fixation cross of 500 ms duration. This was immediately replaced by one of the four possible stimuli, which remained on the screen until a response was made. Participants were instructed to press the right key on the button box to indicate a response of S or the left key for it H. The order of the blocks and response designation was counterbalanced across subjects. Mean correct RTs for the global and local identification are presented in Fig. 10.6 as a function of stimulus consistency, for the normal participants (Panel B) and for each of the patients (Panel C and D).

The normal subjects were extremely accurate in identifying the letters, reporting 96.3% correctly and showed a small but significant global advantage of 15 ms. There was no difference between consistent and inconsistent items and no significant interaction between globality and consistency, although numerically it looks like there is some interference from the global identity onto the local identification. The absence of strong interference effects is not unusual given the unlimited exposure duration (Paquet & Merikle, 1984), foveal presentation (Pomerantz, 1983), and spatial certainty (Lamb & Robertson, 1988).

Both patients were also highly accurate, with SM and RN achieving 98.9% and 99.1% accuracy, respectively, but they differed markedly in their pattern of performance as reflected in their RT data. SM's pattern of performance was not that different from that of the normal participants: He showed a significant global advantage of 58 ms, and no consistency effect nor an interaction between globality and consistency, although, as in the normal subjects, there was a numeric trend for global-to-local interference.

RN exhibited a dramatically different pattern, consistent with the predictions we made: There was a clear local advantage, with local letters identified 174 ms faster than global letters. He was also 149 ms faster for consistent over inconsistent stimuli, but this consistency effect was qualified by an interaction with globality.

Although there was only a 7-ms difference between consistent and inconsistent trials in the local condition, there was a 159-ms slowing for the inconsistent over consistent trials in the global condition, reflecting strong local-to-global interference. Thus, although RN was accurate, his performance was very different from that of normal observers. Instead of exhibiting a global advantage, he exhibited a clear local advantage. That RN's performance was nevertheless accurate may suggest that eventually he can derive the global configuration but it is a very laborious and time-consuming process for him. Alternatively, RN may be unable to derive a coherent global configuration but can perform global discrimination on the basis of some local cues or some partial global information. This may be a rather slow process, but, given enough time, it can lead to accurate performance.[3] As we discuss later, further investigations of RN's performance seem to support the latter rather than the former account.

The findings from the global/local task reveal a major discrepancy in the performance of the two patients. SM performed qualitatively similarly to normal participants: Responses were faster with global than local stimuli, and there was a trend toward global-to-local interference. RN, on the other hand, was faster with local than global letters and showed strong interference from the local letter onto global identification when there was inconsistency between the two.

A finer analysis of the data revealed another interesting difference between SM and RN. When making global identifications, both patients responded faster to *H* than to *S*. However, SM responded to the global *H* made of *H*s (537 ms) as fast as to the global *H* made of *S*s (544 ms). RN, on the other hand, was 133 ms faster in responding to the global *H* made of *H*s (605 ms) than to the global *H* made of *S*s (738 ms), and, furthermore, the former was the only case in which his global identification was nearly as fast as his local identification of *H* (565 ms).

Presumably, the discrepancy between the patients in their ability to apprehend normally the global configuration of patterns composed of elements reflects different types of deficits in perceptual organization or perhaps different levels of deficits. Assuming that the local elements of the hierarchical letters are grouped by proximity, or similarity, or both (the elements are identical and close to one another), RN seems unable to use these grouping principles to derive the global configuration; he can derive some global structure only when collinearity between elements is present (as in the case of *H* made of *H*s). SM, on the other hand appears able to derive a global configuration even when simple collinearity is not present in the image. We pursue this issue further in later experiments.

A similar discrepancy between global/local performance exists between two other patients in the literature. HJA, perhaps the most extensively studied patient with integrative agnosia, showed an advantage for global over local identification and showed no interference of any kind (Humphreys, 1999; Humphreys & Riddoch,

---

[3]This is why accuracy measures alone are coarse and do not reveal the whole story: There are many different ways in which one can achieve high accuracy.

2001). In contrast, NM, who is also a very good example of an integrative agnosic patient, was almost unable to identify the global letter even at unlimited exposure duration (Ricci et al., 1999) and favored reporting the local components.

The variability observed across patients on this task suggests that a problem in deriving the global structure of hierarchical stimulus might not be a core element of integrative agnosia. This conclusion might be premature, however. It is now well-known that a variety of stimulus and task factors affect the balance between global and local processing, including the type of hierarchical stimuli used, the attentional task (divided or focused), and the mode of response (forced choice, go-no-go; Kimchi, 1992; Yovel et al., 2001). Thus, the variability in the pattern of results obtained across patients might be a function of the different testing conditions used with different patients. Alternatively, because perceptual organization refers to a multiplicity of processes, it is possible that patients do vary and that integrative agnosia might manifest in different ways across different individuals. Here, the testing conditions were the same for the two patients, and the stimuli used were favorable for perceiving the global configuration because they were made of many small elements, which increase the salience of the global over the local letters (e.g., Yovel et al., 2001). Under these conditions and with unlimited exposure duration, SM was able to derive the global configuration, but RN was not. As we show later, under more stringent testing conditions, even SM exhibits an impairment in global processing. These findings further support the claim that differences in testing conditions may lead to variability in outcome, but they also suggest that integrative agnosia might manifest in different ways across different individuals. Because such individuals are rare, the opportunity to systematically analyze all their perceptual skills in depth is not that easy, so the source of this cross-patient variability remains to be definitively determined.

Hierarchical Processing and Spatial Frequency Analysis

Before we describe the patients' abilities to derive global form in further detail, we need to explore an alternative interpretation for the findings we obtained, and this concerns the relationship between spatial frequency analysis and global/local processing. Several researchers suggested an involvement of spatial filters, based on spatial frequency channels, operating at early visual processing (Ginsburg, 1986) in the perception of global and local structures. For example, in a number of these studies, no latency advantage for global over local processing was found when low spatial frequencies were removed from hierarchical stimuli (Badcock, Whitworth, Badcock, & Lovegrove, 1990; Hughes, Fendrich, & Reuter-Lorenz, 1990; Lamb & Yund, 1993; Shulman, Sullivan, Gish, & Sakoda, 1986; Shulman & Wilson, 1987), suggesting that the global advantage effect is mediated by low spatial frequency channels. Thus, one possible explanation for the patients' differential inability to perceive the global form of a hierarchical stimulus might concern a fundamental

limitation in processing low spatial frequency information. The obvious prediction from this in relation to the patients is that RN, who appears to process stimuli
almost entirely at the local level, should be impaired at processing low-frequency
displays, resulting in an increased low spatial frequency threshold, relative to control subjects, whereas SM, who shows some global form processing, should not
show as much of an increase in this threshold.

To document the spatial frequency thresholds for the patients and controls, we
established, for each individual, the log contrast thresholds at 1, 3, 5, 10, and 30
cycles per image (cpi) using Matlab. In each trial, a fixation point appeared on the
screen for 1 s. After 200 ms, an image appeared for 200 ms, and this was replaced
by a blank screen for an additional 200 ms (see Fig. 10.7A for example of images).
A second image then appeared for 200 ms, and it, in turn, was replaced by a blank
screen for 200 ms. At this point, the subject was required to decide whether the
first or second image contained the grating. If the response was correct, a more
difficult discrimination (decreased contrast by 0.2) was presented on the next trial.
If the response was incorrect, the contrast was increased by 0.2. Feedback was
provided after each trial, and subjects received practice trials at the beginning. A
log contrast threshold was determined for each cpi using method of limits. In this
particular Matlab function, threshold is defined as the value of contrast that makes
the subject respond at 82% correct, and this is the value plotted for each subject
in Fig. 10.7B for each cpi.

As is evident from Fig. 10.7B, neither patient showed any difficulty in detecting
either low-or-high frequency gratings, performing well within the normal boundaries. There is also no obvious correlation between the patients' performance on
the spatial frequency measure and the ability to perceive the local or global form
of the stimulus. Both patients performed close to the control mean for the higher
frequency displays. SM, who was able to perceive the global configuration and
showed a global advantage with the Navon-type figures, showed the slightly poorer
low-frequency threshold than the controls and than RN, whereas this should be the
other way around to account for the hierarchical data. Also, RN, who processed
the hierarchical stimuli locally, has thresholds for the low spatial frequency that
are as good as the best control subject, and, therefore, this cannot account for his
failure to perceive the global configuration.

Having ruled out the possibility that the discrepancy between the two patients
in their perception of the hierarchical stimuli is due to differential limitations
in analyzing spatial frequency information, we now examine more closely their
performance on other tasks of perceptual organization.

Microgenetic Analysis of the Perceptual
Organization of Hierarchical Stimuli

To explore in further detail the patients' abilities to group local elements, we
focused more specifically on grouping processes and examined the time course of

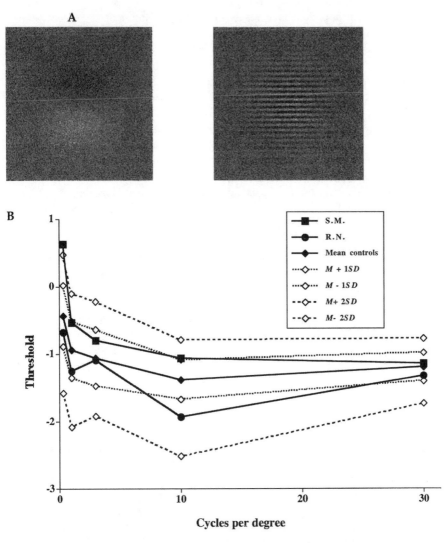

FIG. 10.7.   (A) Examples of displays of 1 and 30 cycles per inch used for establishing spatial frequency thresholds. (B) Log contrast thresholds as a function of cycles per image, including the mean for normal participants (and 1 and 2 *SD*) and for SM and RN. From "What Does Visual Agnosia Tell Us About Perceptual Organization and Its Relationship to Object Perception?" by M. Behrmann and R. Kimchi, 2003, *Journal of Experimental Psychology: Human Perception and Performance, 29*(1), pp. 19–42. Copyright 2003 by APA. Reprinted with permission.

the perceptual organization of hierarchical stimuli. This approach, often referred to as a microgenetic approach, involves examining the evolution of the percept rather than just the final outcome of the organizational processes. To conduct this analysis, we adopted the primed matching paradigm, which has been used successfully for this purpose (Kimchi, 1998, 2000, this volume). The basic procedure (Beller, 1971) is as follows: Participants view a priming stimulus followed immediately by a pair of test figures, and they must judge, as rapidly and accurately as possible, whether the two test figures are the same or different. The speed of same responses to the test figures depends on the representational similarity between the prime and the test figures: Responses are faster when the test figures are similar to the prime than when they are dissimilar to it. By constructing test figures that are similar to different hypothesized representations of the prime and varying the prime duration, we can tap earlier and later internal representations (Kimchi, 1998, 2000; Sekuler & Palmer, 1992). Thus we can assess implicitly the participants' perceptual representations and the time course of their organization.

The priming stimuli were hierarchical patterns (global diamonds made up of circles) of two types: a few-element pattern and a many-element pattern. The few-element prime was a diamond made of four relatively large circles, and the many-element prime was a diamond made of 16 relatively small circles. Each test stimulus consisted of two hierarchical patterns. There were two types of test pairs defined by the similarity relations between the test figures and the prime (see Fig. 10.8): the element-similarity (ES) test pairs, in which the test figures were similar to the prime in their local elements but differed in global configuration, and the configuration-similarity (CS) test pairs, in which the figures were similar to the prime in global configuration but differed in local elements. Priming effects of the configuration would manifest in faster correct same RTs for the CS than for the ES test pairs, whereas priming effects of the elements would manifest in faster same RTs for the ES than for the CS test pairs.

Each trial was initiated with a central fixation dot of 250-ms duration, followed by a priming stimulus. The presentation time for the prime was equally and randomly distributed among 40, 90, 190, 390, and 690 ms. Immediately after the presentation of the prime, the test display appeared and stayed on until the participant responded. The test display contained two figures presented on either side of the location previously occupied by the prime. At this point, participants had to decide whether the two figures were the same or different and to respond as accurately and quickly as possible using the response keys. All the combinations of the factors of prime duration, test type, and response were randomized within block with each combination occurring on an equal number of trials. Two sessions were administered, each on a separate day a few weeks apart, with two blocks (one of few-element and one of many-element patterns) in each session. Altogether each patient completed 640 trials. Sixteen practice trials were completed for each of the few- and many-element patterns before the experimental trials.

Mean correct same RTs for prime-test similarity (ES, CS) are plotted in Fig. 10.9 as a function of prime duration for each prime type (few-element and

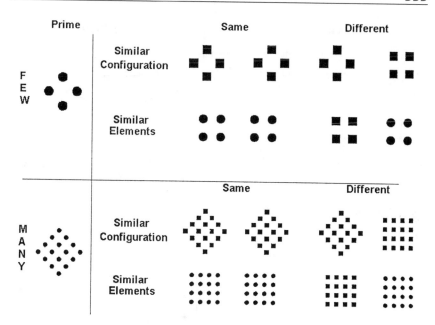

FIG. 10.8. Primed match paradigm: primes, consisting of few and many elements, are followed after varying stimulus onset asynchrony (SOAs) by test pairs which require same or different responses and which are similar to the prime in elements or configuration. From "What Does Visual Agnosia Tell Us About Perceptual Organization and Its Relationship to Object Perception?" by M. Behrmann and R. Kimchi, 2003, *Journal of Experimental Psychology: Human Perception and Performance, 29*(1), pp. 19–42. Copyright 2003 by APA. Reprinted with permission.

many-element patterns) for SM and RN (Panels B and C, respectively), and the normal data (from Kimchi, 1998) are in Panel A. Like the control subjects, both SM and RN performed well on this task, making very few errors (normal participants: 4.1%; SM 4%; RN 1%), and we do not examine the error data further.

As can be seen in Fig. 10.9A, few- and many-element patterns produced different patterns of results for normal participants. For the few-element patterns, responses to ES test pairs were faster than responses to the CS test pairs at 40-, 90-, and 190-ms prime duration, and the difference diminished at the longer prime durations of 390 and 690 ms. For the many-element patterns, responses to CS test pairs were faster than responses to ES at the early durations of 40 and 90 ms. The pattern of RTs reversed at the intermediate durations of 190 and 390 ms: ES produced faster responses than CS test pairs, and at 690 ms both element and configuration were available for priming with a tendency for faster RTs to CS test pairs. These results have been interpreted as suggesting that, for normal participants, the elements of the few-element patterns are represented initially, and the global configuration is then consolidated with time. In contrast, in the

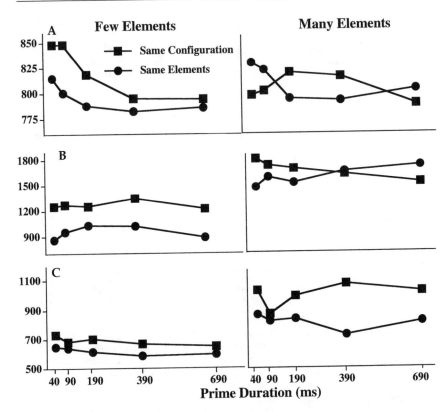

FIG. 10.9. (A) Mean of median correct same RTs for (A) the normal participants for few and many elements displays as a function of prime duration for the two prime-similarity conditions (element similarity, ES, and configuration similarity, CS) and mean responses for (B) SM and (C) RN under the same conditions. From "What Does Visual Agnosia Tell Us About Perceptual Organization and Its Relationship to Object Perception?" by M. Behrmann and R. Kimchi, 2003, *Journal of Experimental Psychology: Human Perception and Performance*, 29(1), pp. 19–42. Copyright 2003 by APA. Reprinted with permission.

many-element patterns, there is early representation of the configuration (as in the forest before the trees; Navon, 1977), the elements then become individuated, and finally both the configuration and elements are represented and accessible (Kimchi, 1998, this volume).

For the few-element patterns, in contrast with the normal participants who seemed to derive the global configuration over time, neither SM nor RN appeared to be able to derive a global configuration, even at the longest exposure duration of 690 ms. Both patients showed faster RTs to the ES test pairs, and there was no effect of prime duration on this element advantage. Previous research suggested that for patterns composed of few, relatively large elements, the local elements are perceived by normal individuals as figural parts of the overall form (Goldmeier, 1936/1972; Kimchi & Palmer, 1982), and the local elements and the global form are perceptually integral (Kimchi, 1988; Kimchi & Palmer, 1985). The two patients, however, seem unable to integrate the local elements into a global entity, so they fail to perceive the local elements as figural parts of an overall form and, rather, perceive them as discrete, unrelated entities.

For the many-element patterns, again in contrast with the normal participants, neither patient exhibited an early advantage for the configuration. Rather, RN showed an advantage for the ES test pairs as early as 40 ms, and this element advantage remained fairly unchanged over the entire time course so that the global configuration was not available to him even at the longest duration of 690 ms. SM also did not show any early advantage for the CS test pairs either, although he eventually showed a tendency for faster RT for CS than ES test pairs at the longest duration of 690 ms.

In addition to the differences between the patients and the normal participants, there are also some differences between RN and SM. First, the difference in RTs for many- and few-element patterns was larger for RN (510 ms) than for SM (256 ms), reflecting the greater difficulty in processing the many-element patterns for RN than for SM.[4] Second, for RN, the ES advantage for the many-element patterns was larger than for few-element patterns, whereas the opposite was true for SM. Third, whereas no effect whatsoever of prime duration on prime-test similarity was observed for RN, a tendency for a reversal in the relative advantage of ES and CS was observed for SM at the longest duration for the many-element patterns.

Taken together, these differences between the patients suggest that in the case of SM, although there is no evidence for the early rapid grouping of many elements that characterizes normal perception, grouping processes do operate with many elements. Eventually these grouping processes can lead to the perception of the global configuration. This finding is consistent with his performance on the Navon-type figures, in which, with unlimited exposure duration, SM showed a global advantage, similar to normal participants. RN, on the other hand, seems unable to group the elements into a global configuration even when conditions and time favor grouping, and this, too, is consistent with his performance on the Navon-type figures.

Microgenetic Analysis of Line Configurations

Thus far, both patients are clearly impaired at grouping multiple elements (presumably by proximity and by similarity) into a global configuration, and RN seems to be more impaired at this than SM. Interestingly, the only instance in which RN

---

[4]We have to be somewhat cautious about this statement in light of the fact that RN's RTs to the few-element patterns were rather short (almost shorter than those of the normal participants).

showed some indication of forming a global configuration was with the *H* made of *H*s in the Navon-type figures, in which collinearity between the local elements can be exploited. We examined further the patients' ability to group line segments into a configuration by collinearity and also by closure. Previous research demonstrated the perceptual dominance of configuration even for disconnected line segments (Kimchi, 1994; Pomerantz & Pristach, 1989; Rensink & Enns, 1995), suggesting that disconnected line segments are grouped into a configuration and that this grouping occurs early and rapidly (Kimchi, 2000; Rensink & Enns, 1995) and possibly even independently of the number of elements (Donnelly, Humphreys, & Riddoch, 1991). We again adopted a microgenetic approach using line segments and compared the performance of the patients to that of normal individuals (Kimchi, 2000, Experiment 1).

The priming stimuli used in this experiment (see Fig. 10.10) were line configurations (a diamond and a cross)[5] that varied in the connectedness of the line components (no gap, small gap, and large gap) and were presented at various exposure durations. We assumed that the line segments of the cross were likely to be grouped by collinearity, whereas the line segments of the diamond were more likely to be grouped by closure. The relatability theory (Kellman & Shipley, 1991; Shipley & Kellman, 1992), which formalizes the Gestalt principle of good continuation, suggests that the visual system connects two noncontiguous edges that are relatable so that the likelihood of seeing a completed figure increases systematically with the size of the angle that must be interpolated, with the 50% threshold occurring at around 90°. According to this criterion, the cross-configuration is characterized by high relatability (an angle of 180°—collinearity) and the diamond configuration by low relatability (an angle of 90°). The diamond configuration, however, possesses closure, whereas the cross does not.

In the experiment, there were two types of same-response test pairs defined by the similarity relation between the test figures and the prime. The figures in the configuration-similarity test pair were similar to the prime in both configuration and line components, whereas the figures in the component-similarity test pair were similar to the prime in lines but dissimilar in configuration. For this set of stimuli, we assumed priming effects of the configuration would manifest in faster correct same RTs for the configuration-similarity than for the component-similarity test pairs. No difference in RT between the two types of test pairs was expected due to component priming because both types of test pairs are similar to the prime in line components.

The sequence of events in each trial was the same as in the experiment (described previously), except that the prime was presented for one of only four durations: 40,

---

[5]In addition to the diamond and cross prime, Kimchi (2000, Experiment 1) used a random array of dots for which prime-test similarity was considered neutral and served as a baseline condition. To simplify the experiment for the patients, we omitted the neutral prime because the performance of the normal participants serves as the control for the patients.

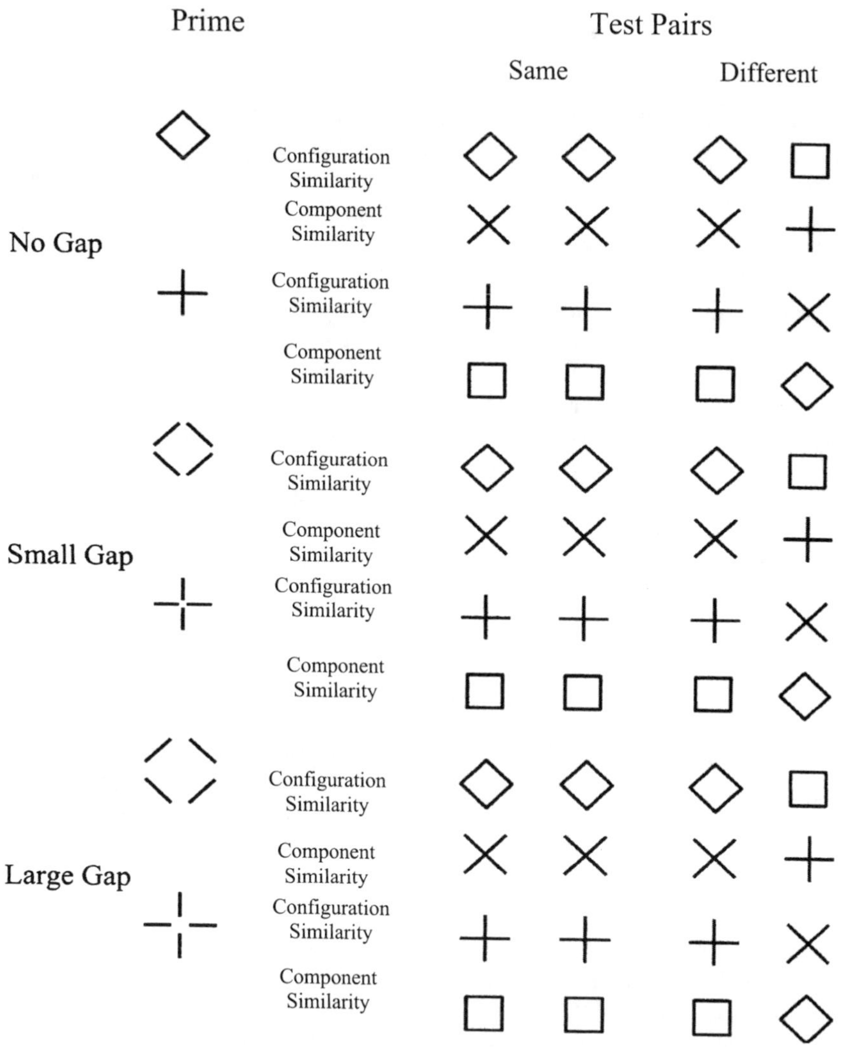

FIG. 10.10. The priming stimuli and the same- and different-response pairs used in the (a) no-gap condition, (b) small-gap condition, and (c) large-gap condition. When the prime is a diamond made of four oblique lines and the test pair is two outline diamonds, prime-test similarity is configuration similarity; when the test pair is two Xs, prime-test similarity is component similarity. When the prime is a cross, made of two vertical and two horizontal lines, and the test pair is two outline crosses, prime-test similarity is configuration similarity and when the test pair is two outline squares, prime-test similarity is component similarity. From "What Does Visual Agnosia Tell Us About Perceptual Organization and Its Relationship to Object Perception?" by M. Behrmann and R. Kimchi, 2003, *Journal of Experimental Psychology: Human Perception and Performance, 29*(1), pp. 19–42. Copyright 2003 by APA. Reprinted with permission.

90, 190, or 390 ms. The three different gap conditions were manipulated between blocks (between subjects for the normal subjects). All combinations of the factors of prime type, prime duration, test type, and response were randomized within block, with each combination occurring on an equal number of trials. For each gap condition, there were six blocks of 160 experimental trials each, preceded by a block of 15 practice trials.

Like the normal participants, SN and RN made very few errors on this task (errors: normal participants 1.4%; SM 0.2%; RN 0.7%). In light of the small number of errors, no further analysis is undertaken, and we turn to the RT data. Mean correct same RTs for each prime-test similarity relation (component similarity, configuration similarity) are plotted in Fig. 10.11 as a function of prime duration for each gap condition for the two prime types (diamond and cross) for SM and RN (Panels B and C, respectively). The results for the normal subjects are used as the benchmark against which to evaluate the patient data and are plotted in Fig. 10.11 (Panel A). Analyses of the correct same RTs for the normal partici-pants (Kimchi, 2000, Experiment 1) showed that prime type (diamond or cross) did not interact significantly with priming effects, prime duration, and gap condi-tion, and, therefore, the data for the normal participants are collapsed across prime type.

For the normal participants, configuration similarity produced faster RTs than component similarity as early as 40 ms for the no gap and the small gap conditions, and there was no effect of prime duration on this configuration advantage. No sig-nificant difference between configuration similarity and component similarity was observed for the large gap condition, but no relative dominance of the component was observed either (for details see Kimchi, 2000, Experiment 1; this volume).[6] These results have been interpreted as suggesting that for normal individuals, disconnected line segments are rapidly organized into configurations, provided collinearity (the cross prime) or closure (the diamond prime) is present. Strong proximity between the line segments (as in the no-gap and small-gap conditions) facilitates grouping by closure or collinearity more than does weak proximity (as in the large-gap condition), but connectedness does not seem to be necessary for rapid grouping.

The results for SM (Fig. 10.11B) showed a significant effect of prime type with faster RTs for crosses than diamonds and a significant effect of duration with faster RTs as duration increases. There was also a significant effect of prime-test similarity that interacted with prime type. As can be seen in Fig. 10.11B, RTs for configuration similarity were significantly faster (by an average of 117 ms) than RTs for component similarity for the diamond prime, but no difference between

---

[6]It is important to note that when RT for the component-similarity test pairs was compared with baseline performance, no facilitation for the component-similarity test pair was observed even for the large-gap condition, suggesting that even under relatively weak proximity between the lines, there was no relative dominance of the component lines.

the two test types was observed for the cross prime. The configuration advantage decreased with an increase in gap size, as indicated by the significant interaction between prime-test similarity and gap condition, and it increased with prime duration, as indicated by the significant interaction between prime-test similarity and prime duration.

The results for RN showed a significant effect of prime-test similarity that varied with gap condition. There was a significant advantage for configuration similarity over line similarity for the no gap condition (averaged 51 ms) and the small gap condition (averaged 33 ms), roughly equal across the two prime types, but no significant difference between configuration similarity and component similarity was observed for the large-gap condition. Like SM, RN's RTs were faster when the prime was a cross than a diamond, but prime type did not interact significantly with prime-test similarity, prime duration, and gap condition.

RN showed a priming effect of the configuration both for the diamond and for the cross primes that decreased with gap size. As long as the gaps between the line components were relatively small (i.e., relatively strong proximity), he was able to integrate them either by collinearity or by closure. SM, on the other hand, showed a priming effect of the configuration for the diamond prime but no priming effect for the cross prime. Because SM's responses, like RN's, were faster for the cross than for the diamond prime, it is unlikely that the absence of configuration advantage for the cross indicates that SM cannot use collinearity for grouping. Rather, this finding may result from SM's high sensitivity to closure. Given that the component-similarity test pair for the cross includes two squares and the configuration-similarity test pair includes two crosses (see Fig. 10.10), it is possible that although responses to the configuration-similarity test pairs were facilitated due to prime-test similarity, responses to the component similarity test pairs were facilitated due to closure, and, as a result, no difference between the two was obtained. It is not the case, then, that SM is impaired at grouping by collinearity, whereas RN is not, but rather that SM is more sensitive than RN to closure. Further support for this claim comes from the finding that the configuration advantage for the diamond is larger for SM (180, 125, and 48 ms, for the no-gap, small-gap, and large-gap, respectively) than for RN (54, 38, and –17 ms, for the no-gap, small-gap, and large-gap, respectively, see Fig. 10.11), and furthermore, RN, contrary to SM, does not show any configuration advantage but rather an element advantage for the large-gap condition. That is, strong proximity facilitated grouping by closure for RN, whereas, for SM, closure was strong enough to override weak proximity. Interestingly, the performance of the normal participants in the neutral prime condition also showed faster responses to the pair of squares than to the pairs of crosses (Kimchi, 2000, Experiment 1), suggesting a sensitivity of the normal participants to the property of closure.

To rule out the possibility that the difference between RN and SM in their responses to the cross prime is due to a difference in their ability to exploit collinearity, we compared their performance in an elementary contour interpolation task.

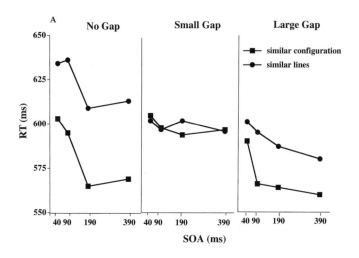

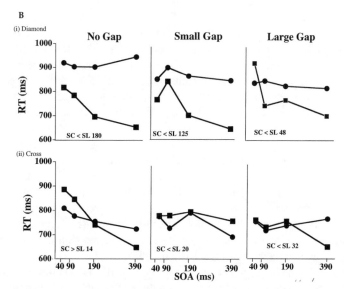

FIG. 10.11.   (A) Mean of median correct same RTs for the component similarity and configuration similarity as a function of prime duration for each gap condition for control subjects and mean responses for diamond and cross primes for (B) SM and (C) RN. For SM and RN, the differences in ms between the component similarity (SC) and line similarity (SL) conditions are also provided. From "What Does Visual Agnosia Tell Us About Perceptual Organization and Its Relationship to Object Perception?" by M. Behrmann and R. Kimchi, 2003, *Journal of Experimental Psychology: Human Perception and Performance, 29*(1), pp. 19–42. Copyright 2003 by APA. Reprinted with permission.

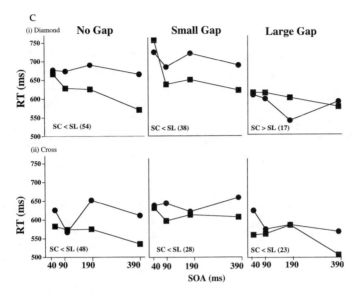

FIG. 10.11. (*Continued*)

CONTOUR INTERPOLATION

To test contour detection thresholds, we used a set of cards containing displays of a smoothly aligned, closed path of Gabor elements embedded in a random array of Gabor elements of the same spatial frequency and contrast, devised by Pennefather, Chandna, Kovács, Polat, and Norcia, (1999). In this test, cards containing the displays are presented individually to the subject, who is required to indicate the location of the contour formed by the Gabor patches. The critical manipulation or parameter, Δ, is the spacing between the adjacent elements in the background relative to the spacing between neighboring elements along the contour. The Δ ranges between 1.2 (card 2_1) to 0.5 (card 2_15) in steps of 0.05 (examples of these displays are presented in Fig. 10.12). This parameter expresses relative noise density and reflects, in a way, signal-to-noise ratio so that the smaller the Δ value, the easier detection. It has also been suggested that as Δ decreases, long range spatial interactions of oriented features, presumably mediated by low-level areas of visual cortex, are more involved. Given that early visual areas are preserved in both patients, we expect them both to perform normally. If they do so and there is no difference between them, this would further indicate that they both can exploit collinearity as a grouping heuristic. Establishing contour detection thresholds using this method has been successfully achieved previously with various pathological populations (Kovács, Polat, Pennefather, Chandna, & Norcia, 2000).

A   B

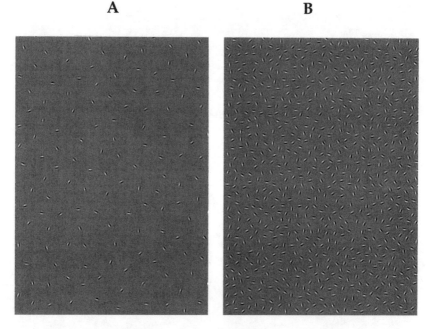

FIG. 10.12.   Examples of displays from Kovács et al. (2000) of contours made of local Gabor units. (A) easy, (B) difficult. From "What
Does Visual Agnosia Tell Us About Perceptual Organization and Its
Relationship to Object Perception?" by M. Behrmann and R. Kimchi,
2003, *Journal of Experimental Psychology: Human Perception and
Performance, 29*(1), pp. 19–42. Copyright 2003 by APA. Reprinted
with permission.

Both SM and RN completed this task easily and effortlessly. Importantly, both
attained thresholds within normal limits, with Δs of 0.6 and 0.65, respectively.
The norm is around 0.7 (Kovács et al., 2000). It is interesting to note, at this point,
that patient HJA also performed well on the present task, obtaining a threshold
of 0.65 (Giersch, Humphreys, Boucart, & Kovács, 2000). These findings indicate
that both our patients have a normal ability to integrate collinear elements into
contours and that there is no obvious difference between them in this ability. These
data can explain the finding of faster responses for the cross prime (presumably
grouping by collinearity) than for the diamond prime (presumably grouping by
closure) that was observed in the previous experiment for both patients. Further
support for their ability to integrate collinear elements comes from the results of
the Navon-type figures, in which even RN, who was generally unable to derive
the global configuration of the many-element patterns, was able to do so in the
case of *H* made of *H*s. Furthermore, the present findings support the claim that the
difference between RN and SM for the cross (see previous section) is unlikely

to arise from a differential sensitivity to collinearity but rather to a difference in their sensitivity to closure: SM is more sensitive to closure than is RN. The consistency in performance across the patients (SM, RN, and HJA) in the contour interpolation task endorses the notion that the integration of contours in a task such as this likely relies on visual processes mediated by earlier or lower level regions of visual cortex and that these areas are preserved in integrative agnosic patients.

GROUPING BY SIMILARITY IN LUMINANCE AND PROXIMITY

We assumed that in the hierarchical stimuli we used, the local elements are grouped into a global configuration by proximity, or by similarity, or both, and the inability of the patients to apprehend the global configuration reflects an impairment in grouping. However, as mentioned previously, perceptual organization is thought to involve two operations: element clustering, which determines which elements belong together, and shape formation or configuring, which determines the shape of the grouped elements (Rock, 1986; Trick & Enns, 1997). It is possible, then, that our patients are not impaired in clustering but rather in shape formation or configuring. That is, it is possible that they are able to group the elements of the hierarchical stimuli into a unit, but are unable to apprehend the relationships among the grouped elements so that the unit is not organized for them into a whole that has unique qualities such as shape. To explore this possibility we examined the performance of the two patients in simple grouping tasks: grouping into columns or rows by proximity and by similarity in luminance.

A display consisting of small circles, each 4 mm in diameter, appeared centered on a computer screen (see Fig. 10.13 for examples). In the proximity condition, the display contained 32 solid black circles, and the distance between them horizontally or vertically was manipulated to yield an organization of either rows or columns, respectively. The distance was either 4 or 8 mm from the center of one circle to the next, and, depending on the distance, the arrangement obeyed a rows or column organization. In the similarity condition, the elements were solid black or white circles, equally distant (4 mm), and the organization was determined by the alternation of the two colors, either in rows or columns. The subjects were instructed to indicate, for each display, whether an arrangement of rows or columns is present. There were 50 trials in each of the two organization conditions, rows or columns, and we measured both accuracy and RT.

Both patients performed well on this task as was true of the normal control subjects (controls: 93.3% in both cases). SM was correct 90% and 94% of the time in the proximity and similarity conditions, respectively, and RN was correct 100% of the time in both cases. That is, when proximity favored an organization of rows, the patients perceived rows, and when it favored an organization of columns, they

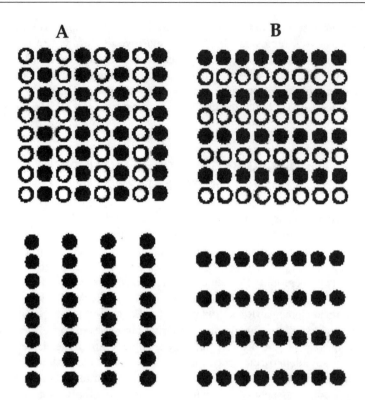

FIG. 10.13.   Arrangement of dots into (A) columns and (B) rows for grouping by similarity and by proximity. From "What Does Visual Agnosia Tell Us About Perceptual Organization and Its Relationship to Object Perception?" by M. Behrmann and R. Kimchi, 2003, *Journal of Experimental Psychology: Human Perception and Performance, 29*(1), pp. 19–42. Copyright 2003 by APA. Reprinted with permission.

perceived columns. The same was true when organization was based on similarity in luminance. These findings indicate that both patients are sensitive to grouping by proximity and by similarity in luminance and are able to determine the orientation of the grouped elements. If anything, whereas RN scored perfectly, SM made a few errors, possibly due to a speed accuracy trade-off because SM was much faster (proximity: 603 ms; similarity: 659 ms) than RN (proximity: 917 ms; similarity: 862 ms).

However, grouping by proximity and by similarity may not suffice for deriving the shape of the grouped elements. Interestingly, Kimchi and Razpurker-Apfeld (2001) found that grouping by similarity of luminance and color into columns or rows occurred earlier than grouping into arrows or triangles and that the former, but not the latter, occurred under conditions of inattention. This finding suggests that grouping is not a single process even when it is based on the same heuristic, but, rather, it involves operations that differ in their time course and attentional demands.

The findings of the present experiment suggest that the difficulty of our patients, and in particular RN, to apprehend the global configuration of hierarchical stimuli is not due to an impairment in simple grouping (i.e., in the sense of what goes with what) but presumably to an impairment in the ability to apprehend the interrelationships of the elements and to derive the emergent structure or shape.

SUMMARY OF FINDINGS

The goal of our research was to explore the psychological and neural processes involved in deriving structure and coherence from visual input. Many traditional theories of visual perception assume that perceptual organization processes operate early and preattentively to deliver candidate units for further processing, such as object identification. These theories make no attempt to distinguish in detail between the different perceptual organization processes nor to evaluate their relative contribution to object recognition. To address these issues, we investigated the behavior of two individuals with acquired integrative visual object agnosia, on tasks of object recognition and perceptual organization, with a specific emphasis on grouping elements into global forms. By understanding how the system breaks down, and how a perceptual organization deficit is related to impaired object recognition, we hoped to obtain insight into the normal processes of perceptual organization and object identification.

When required to integrate many small elements into a global configuration, SM, but not RN, was able to derive the global form, although he required more time to do this than did the normal participants. A microgenetic analysis of this integration process confirmed that, given enough time and sufficient data-driven support, he was eventually able to derive the global form. Importantly, normal perceivers unify a multielement stimulus early and quickly, reflecting their spontaneous bias to deal with such a stimulus as a unit rather than as disparate components, and only later do they individuate the elements. SM did not show this early and fast grouping of the many elements displays and only, with time, was he able to laboriously derive a global form. Even under optimal circumstances, RN failed to derive the global form from the image. When the stimulus was composed of only a few, relatively large elements, neither SM nor RN was able to extract a global structure. Under these conditions, normal subjects can apprehend the global structure despite the relative salience of the individual elements, and the global configuration becomes further consolidated with time. Note that the differences between the two patients and the difference between them and the normal participants in apprehending the global configuration of hierarchical stimuli cannot be attributed to a differential sensitivity to low spatial frequency information because both patients displayed spatial frequency threshold functions within normal limits.

In an investigation of the time course of the ability to group simple line segments into configurations by collinearity and by closure, we found that both patients were able to exploit these properties early on, as is also true of normal participants. However, SM was more sensitive to closure than was RN. Strong proximity facilitated grouping by closure for RN, but SM was able to group by closure even when proximity was weak. We should note that RN's performance here might even be mediated by collinearity at its limits (relatability at 90°), indicating that he might be even less sensitive to closure than we have suggested. Indeed, in a task that was designed specifically to evaluate the ability to integrate collinear elements into simple contours, both SM and RN performed like normal perceivers and did not differ from one another.

The final result was that, presented with the classic, simple Gestalt displays requiring grouping into rows or columns, both patients were able to group by proximity and by similarity of luminance and did not differ from one another or from the normal individuals.

In sum, both patients are able to group collinear elements into a contour, elements into simple rows or columns by proximity and by similarity in luminance or color, and simple line segments into simple configurations by closure. It is important to note, however, that although the basic grouping abilities of both patients seem intact under simple conditions, they nevertheless encounter difficulties under more difficult conditions as in segmenting overlapping shapes. In contrast with the seemingly intact basic grouping, there is a significant impairment in both patients in deriving global structure and apprehending a multielement stimulus as a whole with a specific shape, and the impairment is more marked in RN than in SM. RN fails to derive a global structure even under the most favorable conditions and unlimited time and is also less sensitive to closure than is SM. Critically, the patients differed from each other in the severity of their object recognition deficit, with SM performing significantly better than RN in both accuracy and latency.

DISCUSSION AND CONCLUSION

We now return to our original three questions, namely, the differences between various forms of perceptual organization, the relative contribution of these different processes to object recognition, and the neural systems subserving these mechanisms.

The first important conclusion is that not all organizational processes are created equal. Clearly, grouping by collinearity, proximity, and similarity by luminance and color was easily and equally well achieved by the patients, whereas this was not the case for grouping by closure. The relative preservation of grouping by collinearity is also evident in other agnosic patients, such as HJA (Giersch et al., 2000) and NM (Ricci et al., 1999), who are impaired at integrating low-level elements into a whole but are nevertheless able to extract contours from an image (see also patient FGP; Kartsounis & Warrington, 1991). The present data also clearly show that, although the patients are sensitive to basic grouping, they are not equally able to derive a global structure and shape, suggesting that they may be impaired (and to different degrees) in configuring shape formation (see also Humphreys, this volume).

The differential sensitivity to different forms of grouping is consistent with the idea that some perceptual organization processes may precede others; for example, some processes operate on fairly local components, such as edges, and map onto basic neurophysiological interactions quite early in the visual pathway (Kellman, 2000, this volume; Kovács, Kozma, Feher, & Benedek, 1999; Shipley & Kellman, 1992). This also fits well with recent neuroimaging and neurophysiological work (Lamme & Roelfsema, 2000; Lee, 2002; Sugita, 1999; Westheimer, 1999) suggesting that the ability to interpolate across discrete collinear elements arises from the lateral connections and long-range interactions in early (V1 and V2) visual cortex. Time constants associated with the V1 and V2 operations have been estimated at 45–50 ms and 70–90 ms in V1 and V2, respectively (Doniger et al., 2000; von der Heydt & Peterhans, 1989). Unfortunately, as is often the case in neuropsychological investigations and is true in our case, too, the lesion localization in our patients is not precise enough to yield definitive evidence for the neural structures that are involved, but our results are consistent with the neurophysiological and imaging findings. We know, for instance, that the early visual areas are preserved in SM and, although not definitely established, are likely intact in RN, too, given the absence of low-level deficits. It is these preserved visual regions that probably mediate the patients' ability to exploit collinearity and grouping by proximity and similarity in luminance.

In contrast with these rather simple forms of grouping, other forms of organization have more global influences, as in the case of closure and deriving a structured whole, and these more complex forms are probably mediated by more anterior regions of the visual system. Some evidence to support this claim, for example, comes from a recent high-density event-related potential study (Doniger et al., 2000) in which the amount of visual information in the image was incrementally increased with each subsequent presentation. The critical result was the existence of a bilateral occipito-temporal negative potential that tracked the amount of closure in the image; activation did not manifest in an all-or-none fashion at the point of closure but, rather, built incrementally over a number of preidentification levels. This finding suggests that this region is involved in the computation of closure rather than just registering its presence. Importantly, the peak of activation in this region occurred at approximately 290 ms, much later than the estimated onset of V1 or V2 activity. That perceptual closure is subserved by ventral occipito-temporal areas is also supported by recent hemodynamic and metabolic data (Gerlach et al., 2002) showing that the inferior occipital gyri (perhaps even including area V2) are involved in the integration of visual elements into perceptual wholes, irrespective of whether the wholes were familiar objects or not (see Georgopoulos et al., 2001, for similar evidence, and Gauthier & Tarr, 2002, for behavioral evidence on different forms of configuring and associated neural substrates).

The hypothesis we put forward entails that some organization processes precede others, and we linked these to brain structures on a continuum from more posterior to anterior regions. We do not, however, propose that the system operates in a purely serial and feedforward fashion. There is now ample evidence for bidirectional connectivity and mutual bottom-up and top-down reciprocity (Bullier & Nowak, 1995; Lee, 2002; von der Heydt, Zhou, & Friedman, this volume; Zhou, Friedman, & von der Heydt, 2000) and processing operating in a cascaded and interactive fashion in the visual system (see also Peterson, this volume). We do suggest, however, that there is a temporal advantage for some processes over others, and the order in which these processes takes place follows a posterior-anterior brain organization.

The finding that SM and RN are similar to one another in more basic, presumably low-level grouping operations, but show marked differences in their ability to derive a global form from a multielement display, strongly suggests that perceptual organization involves not only grouping in the sense of element clustering but also, presumably higher level, configuring and shape formation. It is in these more configural forms of grouping that the two patients differ from one another and in which RN is more impaired than SM. The distinction we made between grouping and shape formation/configuring may also help to clarify some confusion found in the literature on perceptual organization. For example, understanding the attentional demands of perceptual organization may depend on whether we refer to grouping (i.e., element clustering) or to configuring (i.e., shape formation). The former is more likely to occur under conditions of inattention than is the latter, and a failure to distinguish between the two organizational processes may lead to seemingly conflicting results. Also, when a task that is designed to assess grouping performance also requires shape formation, caution is necessary in interpretation. For example, Ricci et al. (1999) reported that patient NM is impaired in grouping (by luminance, color, and line orientation). However, the test that was administered to examine NM's grouping ability required her to identify a hierarchical letter embedded in a background of elements. Clearly, grouping alone (i.e., determining which elements belong together) is not sufficient for deriving the structure or the shape of the grouped elements in this case, and shape formation is also necessary. It is unclear, then, whether NM is impaired in grouping or in shape formation or in both.

The differences between the patients in their sensitivity to closure and their ability in configuring and shape formation parallels the difference between their object recognition performance in that RN is more impaired than SM in both accuracy and speed of object identification. Clearly both patients are able to group collinear elements into a contour, but there is more to an object than a contour, and it appears that it is the higher level processes that are critical for object recognition. This is supported by RN's object recognition errors, which reflect his inability to derive form with extent and surfaces and the reliance on simple contours to extract the outline of the shape. For example, shown a black-and-white line drawing of a tie, he identifies it as a string and, on another occasion, refers to a drawing of a nose as a string. In contrast to simple contours, objects are considered to be complex wholes: They have contours, but they also have extent, closure, and internal structure (Feldman, 1999, 2000; Sanocki & Sellers, 2001). Indeed, some studies have shown that, under some circumstances, the global shape outline (and perhaps some surface properties, as revealed for example when silhouettes are used as stimuli) may automatically induce activation of object representations (Boucart & Humphreys, 1992b; Boucart, Humphreys, & Lorenceau, 1995; Dell'Acqua, Job, & Grainger, 2001).

At the same time, it is conceivable that there are circumstances in which certain lower level grouping may suffice for object recognition; for example, when grouping by collinearity provides contours, and the object is easily recognizable from the contours. It may be also the case that object recognition may occur without a full apprehension of the whole (Davidoff & Warrington, 1999). For example, a real, familiar object may be recognized by a distinctive feature or part that is uniquely diagnostic of the object's identity. Thus, we do not claim that all forms of grouping and configuring (or shape formation) are always necessary for object recognition but rather that simple grouping is not sufficient for object recognition, whereas shape formation and configuring are critical for it.

Before concluding, we need to consider a final issue that emerges from the present findings and that concerns the relationship between spatial frequency analysis, performance on tasks evaluating global/local processing, and the relationship between these and the two cerebral hemispheres. With regard to spatial frequency and global/local processing, one view assumed a direct relationship between spatial frequency filters and global/local bias: High spatial frequency information supports the local analysis of the image, and low spatial frequency information supports the global analysis of the image (Hughes et al., 1990; Shulman et al., 1986; Shulman & Wilson, 1987). The data from our two patients challenge this assumption. Both patients exhibit normal spatial frequency thresholds in both the high- and low-frequency range, yet both are impaired (and differentially so) at deriving the global shape from multielement displays.

A rather different view on this matter focused on relative spatial frequency. According to Ivry and Robertson (1998; also Robertson & Ivry, 2000), there is a secondary stage of processing that is sensitive to the relative rather than absolute spatial frequencies in the image, and this stage is functionally asymmetric and associated with more cortical anterior regions than those that register the absolute frequencies. In this account, the difference between global and local information is a difference along a continuum of spatial frequency. With respect to the hemispheres, the claim is that the two hemispheres are biased toward different information along the same dimension of spatial frequency (Lamb, Robertson, & Knight, 1990; Robertson & Ivry, 2000), with the result that the right hemisphere is preferentially biased to process global information and the left hemisphere local information. Although our finding that the patients have normal spatial frequency thresholds is not incompatible with Ivry and Robertson's approach, within their perspective, there does not appear to be a clear way to accommodate the finding that the few- and many-element displays are processed differently by normal subjects and by one of our patients (SM) given that the spatial frequency of the elements is relatively higher than that of the configuration for both displays within their view. A potential further complication is that SM, who has a clearly defined right hemisphere lesion, is still able to derive the global form. In light of these findings, we suggest that the processing of global and local components is tied more to organizational processes than to differences along a continuum of spatial frequency and its relation to hemispheric biases.

This is not to say that the two hemispheres play equivalent roles in perceptual organization, because they apparently do not, but we suggest that the means whereby organization occurs is not primarily dependent on hemispheric-tuned spatial frequency filters. Although the neuroimaging studies obtain bilateral activation in posterior cortex in many integration tasks (Gerlach et al., 2002), this does not necessarily imply that there is an equal contribution of both hemispheres to this process. As revealed by patient HJA, a lesion to the right hemisphere alone can impair the ability to derive closure (Boucart & Humphreys, 1992a, 1992b). Moreover, the relatively greater contribution of the right hemisphere to perceptual organization is also observed in split-brain patients: Corballis, Fendrich, Shapley, and Gazzaniga (1999) showed that whereas both hemispheres seemed to be equally capable of perceiving illusory contours, amodal completion is more readily achieved by the right hemisphere.

In conclusion, we examined the perceptual organization and object recognition abilities of two visual agnosic patients to shed light on the nature of these psychological processes, how they relate to one another, and the possible underlying neural substrates. Our findings indicate that perceptual organization is not a unitary phenomenon but rather a multiplicity of processes, some of which are simpler, operate earlier, and are instantiated in lower level areas of visual cortex, such as grouping by collinearity. In contrast, other processes are more complex, operate later, and rely on higher order visual areas, such as grouping by closure and shape formation. It is these latter processes that are critical for object recognition. The failure to exploit these more complex, configural processes, despite the preserved ability to do basic grouping, gives rise to a deficit in object recognition. The implication of these findings is that the ability to organize elements into visual units is necessary but not sufficient for object identification and recognition. To appreciate the identity of an object, one must necessarily apprehend the internal structure and its emergent global form.

ACKNOWLEDGMENTS

Authorship on this chapter is assigned alphabetically and the work reflects an equal contribution by both authors. This research was supported by a grant from the National Institutes of Mental Health to M. Behrmann (MH57466) and a United States-Israel Binational Science Foundation grant to both authors. Some of the research was conducted while R. Kimchi was visiting Carnegie Mellon University and while M. Behrmann was visiting the Weizmann Institute.

This chapter was partly written while the first author was on sabbatical at the Weizmann Institute of Science, Israel. The sabbatical period was supported by grants from The Weston Visiting Professorship at the Weizmann Institute of Science, Israel; the James McKeen Cattell Sabbatical award; and NIMH grants MH54766 and MH54246. The authors thank Thomas McKeeff, who helped with the data collection and statistical analysis and Dr Ilona Kovács, who graciously provided the material for the contour interpolation experiment. The authors are also grateful to the patients for their good-hearted and continued involvement in these experiments.

REFERENCES

Badcock, C. J., Whitworth, F. A., Badcock, D. R., & Lovegrove, W. J. (1990). Low-frequency filtering and processing of local-global stimuli. *Perception, 19*, 617–629.

Behrmann, M. (2003). Neuropsychological approaches to perceptual organization: evidence from visual agnosia. In G. Rhodes & M. Peterson (Eds.), *Analytic and holistic processes in the perception of faces, objects and scenes*. New York: Oxford University Press.

Behrmann, M., & Kimchi, R. (2003). What does visual agnosia tell us about perceptual organization and its relationship to object perception? *Journal of Experimental Psychology: Human Perception and Performance, 29*(1), 19–42.

Behrmann, M., Nelson, J., & Sekuler, E. (1998). Visual complexity in letter-by-letter reading: "Pure" alexia is not so pure. *Neuropsychologia, 36*(11), 1115–1132.

Beller, H. K. (1971). Priming: Effects of advance information on matching. *Journal of Experimental Psychology, 87*, 176–182.

Ben-Av, M. B., & Sagi, D. (1995). Perceptual grouping by similarity and proximity: Experimental results can be predicted by intensity auto-correlations. *Vision Research, 35*, 853–866.

Boucart, M., & Humphreys, G. W. (1992a). The computation of perceptual structure from collinearity and closure: Normality and pathology. *Neuropsychologia, 30*(6), 527–546.

Boucart, M., & Humphreys, G. W. (1992b). Global shape cannot be attended without object identification. *Journal of Experimental Psychology: Human Perception and Performance, 18*(3), 785–806.

Boucart, M., Humphreys, G. W., & Lorenceau, J. (1995). Automatic access to object identity: Global information, not particular physical dimensions, is important. *Journal of Experimental Psychology: Human Perception and Performance, 21*, 584–601.

Bullier, J., & Nowak, L. G. (1995). Parallel versus serial processing: New vistas on the distributed organization of the visual system. *Current Opinion in Neurobiology, 5*, 497–503.

Butter, C. M., & Trobe, J. D. (1994). Integrative agnosia following progressive multifocal leukoen-cephalopathy. *Cortex, 30*, 145–158.

Chainay, H., & Humphreys, G. W. (2001). The real object advantage in agnosia: Evidence for a role of shading and depth in object recognition. *Cognitive Neuropsychology*, *12*(8), 175–191.

Corballis, P. M., Fendrich, R., Shapley, R. M., & Gazzaniga, M. S. (1999). Illusory contour perception and amodal boundary completion: Evidence of a dissociation following callosotomy. *Journal of Cognitive Neuroscience*, *11*(4), 459–466.

Davidoff, J., & Warrington, E. K. (1999). The bare bones of object recognition: Implications from a case of object recognition impairment. *Neuropsychologia*, *37*, 279–292.

Dell'Acqua, R., Job, R., & Grainger, J. (2001). Is global shape sufficient for automatic object identification? *Visual Cognition*, *8*(6), 801–822.

Doniger, G., Foxe, J. J., Murray, M. M., Higgins, B. A., Snodgrass, J. G., Schroeder, C. E., & Javitt, D. C. (2000). Activation timecourse of ventral visual stream object-recognition areas: High density electrical mapping of perceptual closure processes. *Journal of Cognitive Neuroscience*, *12*(4), 615–621.

Donnelly, N., Humphreys, G. W., & Riddoch, M. J. (1991). Parallel computations of primitive shape descriptions. *Journal of Experimental Psychology: Human Perception and Performance*, *17*(2), 561–570.

Driver, J., Davis, G., Russell, C., Turatto, M., & Freeman, E. (2001). Segmentation, attention and phenomenal visual objects. *Cognition*, *80*, 61–95.

Efron, R. (1968). What is perception? *Boston Studies in Philosophy of Science*, *4*, 137–173.

Enns, J. T., & Kingstone, A. (1995). Access to global and local properties in visual search for compound stimuli. *Psychological Science*, *6*(5), 283–291.

Farah, M. J. (1990). *Visual agnosia: Disorders of object recognition and what they tell us about normal vision*. Cambridge, MA: MIT Press.

Feldman, J. (1999). The role of objects in perceptual grouping. *Acta Psychologica*, *102*, 137–163.

Feldman, J. (2000). Bias toward regular form in mental shapes. *Journal of Experimental Psychology: Human Perception and Performance*, *26*(1), 152–165.

Gauthier, I., Behrmann, M., & Tarr, M. J. (1999). Can face recognition really be dissociated from object recognition? *Journal of Cognitive Neuroscience*, *11*(4), 349–370.

Gauthier, I., & Tarr, M. J. (2002). Unraveling mechanisms for expert object recognition: Bridging brain activity and behavior. *Journal of Experimental Psychology: Human Perception and Performance*. *28*(2), 431–440.

Georgopoulos, A. P., Wang, K., Georgopoulos, M. A., Tagaris, G. A., Amirikian, B., Richter, W., Kim, S. G., & Ugurbil, K. (2001). Functional magnetic resonance imaging of visual object construction and shape discrimination: Relations among task, hemispheric lateralization, and gender. *Journal of Cognitive Neuroscience*, *13*(1), 72–89.

Gerlach, C., Aaside, C. T., Humphreys, G. W., Gade, A., Paulson, O. B., & Law, I. (2002). Brain activity related to integrative processes in visual object recognition: Bottom-up integration and the modulatory influence of stored knowledge. *Neuropsychologia*, *40*, 1254–1267.

Giersch, A., Humphreys, G., Boucart, M., & Kovács, I. (2000). The computation of occluded contours in visual agnosia: Evidence for early computation prior to shape binding and figure-ground coding. *Cognitive Neuropsychology*, *17*(8), 731–759.

Ginsburg, A. P. (1986). Spatial filtering and visual form information. In K. R. Boff, L. Kaufman, & J. P. Thomas (Eds.), *Handbook of human perception and performance* (pp. 1–41). New York: Wiley.

Goldmeier, E. (1972). Similarity in visually perceived forms. *Psychological Issues*, *8*(Suppl. 1, Whole 29). (Original work published 1936).

Han, S., & Humphreys, G. W. (1999). Interactions between perceptual organization based on Gestalt laws and those based on hierarchical processing. *Perception and Psychophysics*, *61*(7), 1287–1298.

Han, S., Humphreys, G. W., & Chen, L. (1999). Parallel and competitive processes in hierarchical analysis: Perceptual grouping and encoding of closure. *Journal of Experimental Psychology: Human Perception and Performance*, *25*(5), 1411–1432.

Hughes, H. C., Fendrich, R., & Reuter-Lorenz, P. (1990). Global versus local processing in the absence of low spatial frequencies. *Journal of Cognitive Neuroscience, 2,* 272–282.

Humphreys, G. W. (1999). *Integrative agnosia.* In G. W. Humphreys (Ed.), *Case studies in vision* (pp. 41–58). London: Psychology Press.

Humphreys, G. W., & Riddoch, M. J. (1987). *To see but not to see: A case-study of visual agnosia.* Hillsdale, NJ: Lawrence Erlbaum Associates.

Humphreys, G. W., & Riddoch, M. J. (2001). Neuropsychological disorders of visual object recognition and naming. In F. Boller & J. Grafman (Eds.), *Handbook of neuropsychology* (Vol. 4, pp. 159–180). North-Holland: Elsevier Science.

Humphreys, G. W., Riddoch, M. J., Donnelly, N., Freeman, T., Boucart, M., & Muller, H. M. (1994). Intermediate visual processing and visual agnosia. In M. J. Farah & G. Ratcliff (Eds.), *The neuropsychology of high-level vision* (pp. 63–101). Hillsdale, NJ: Lawrence Erlbaum Associates.

Humphreys, G. W., Riddoch, M. J., Quinlan, P. T., Price, C. J., & Donnelly, N. (1992). Parallel pattern processing and visual agnosia. *Canadian Journal of Psychology, 46*(3), 377–416.

Ivry, R., & Robertson, L. C. (1998). *The two sides of perception.* Cambridge, MA: MIT Press.

Jankowiak, J., Kinsbourne, M., Shalev, R. S., & Bachman, D. L. (1992). Preserved visual imagery and categorization in a case of associative visual agnosia. *Journal of Cognitive Neuroscience, 4,* 119–131.

Kartsounis, L., & Warrington, E. K. (1991). Failure of object recognition due to a breakdown in figure-ground discrimination in a patient with normal acuity. *Neuropsychologia, 29,* 969–980.

Kellman, P. J. (2000). An update on Gestalt psychology. In B. Landau, J. Sabini, E. Newport, & J. Jonides (Eds.), *Essays in honor of Henry and Lila Gleitman.* Cambridge, MA: MIT Press.

Kellman, P. J., & Shipley, T. F. (1991). A theory of visual interpolation in object perception. *Cognitive Psychology, 23,* 141–221.

Kimchi, R. (1988). Selective attention to global and local levels in the comparison of hierarchical patterns, perception and psychophysics, *43,* 189–198.

Kimchi, R. (1992). Primacy of wholistic processing and global/local paradigm: A critical review. *Psychological Bulletin, 112*(1), 24–38.

Kimchi, R. (1994). The role of wholistic/configural properties versus global properties in visual form perception. *Perception, 23,* 489–504.

Kimchi, R. (1998). Uniform connectedness and grouping in the perceptual organization of hierarchical patterns. *Journal of Experimental Psychology: Human Perception and Performance, 24*(2), 1105–1118.

Kimchi, R. (2000). The perceptual organization of visual objects: A microgenetic analysis. *Vision Research, 40,* 1333–1347.

Kimchi, R., & Razpurker-Apfeld, I. (2001). Perceptual organization and attention. Paper presented at the 42nd meeting of the Psychonomics Society. Orlando, Florida, November.

Kimchi, R., & Palmer, S. (1982). Form and texture in hierarchically constructed patterns. *Journal of Experimental Psychology: Human Perception and Performance, 8*(4), 521–535.

Kimchi, R., & Palmer, S. E. (1985). Separability and integrality of global and local levels of hierarchical patterns. *Journal of Experimental Psychology: Human Perception and Performance, 11*(6), 673–688.

Koffka, K. (1935). *Principles of Gestalt psychology.* New York: Harcourt Brace Jovanovich.

Kovács, I., Kozma, P., Feher, A., & Benedek, G. (1999). Late maturation of visual spatial integration in humans. *Proceedings of the National Academy of Sciences, 96*(21), 12204–12209.

Kovács, I., Polat, U., Pennefather, P. M., Chandna, A., & Norcia, A. M. (2000). A new test of contour integration deficits in patients with a history of disrupted binocular experience during visual development. *Vision Research, 40,* 1775–1783.

Kurylo, D. D. (1997). Time course of perceptual grouping. *Perception and Psychophysics, 59*(1), 142–147.

Lamb, M., & Yund, E. W. (1993). The role of spatial frequency in the processing of hierarchically organized structure. *Perception and Psychophysics, 54*, 773–784.

Lamb, M. R., & Robertson, L. (1988). The processing of hierarchical stimuli: Effects of retinal locus, location uncertainty, and stimulus identity. *Perception and Psychophysics, 44*, 172–181.

Lamb, M. R., Robertson, L. C., & Knight, R. T. (1990). Component mechanisms underlying the processing of hierarchically organized patterns—Inferences from patients with unilateral cortical lesions. *Journal of Experimental Psychology: Learning, Memory and Cognition, 16*, 471–483.

Lamme, V. A. F., & Roelfsema, P. R. (2000). The distinct modes of vision offered by feedforward and recurrent processing. *Trends in Neurosciences, 23*(11), 571–579.

Lawson, R., & Humphreys, G. W. (1999). The effects of view in depth on the identification of line drawings and silhouettes of familiar objects. *Visual Cognition, 6*(2), 165–195.

Lee, T. S. (2003). Computational and neural processes of attentive perceptual organization. In R. Kimchi, M. Behrmann, & C. Olson (Eds.), *Psychological and neural mechanisms of perceptual organization*. Mahwah, NJ: Lawrence Erlbaum Associates.

Mack, A., Tang, B., Tuma, R., Kahn, S., & Rock, I. (1992). Perceptual organization and attention. *Cognitive Psychology, 24*, 475–501.

Marotta, J. J., Behrmann, M., & Genovese, C. (2001). A functional MRI study of face recognition in patients with prosopagnosia. *Neuroreport, 12*(8), 959–965.

Marotta, J. J., McKeeff, T. J., & Behrmann, M. (2002). The effects of inversion and rotation on face processing in prosopagnosia. *Cognitive Neuropsychology, 19*(1), 31–47.

Marr, D. (1982). *Vision*. San Francisco: W. H. Freeman.

Marstrand, L., Gerlach, C., Udesen, H., & Gade, A. (2000). Selective impairment of intermediate vision following stroke in the right occipital lobe. *Journal of the International Neuropsychological Society, 6*, 381.

Moore, C., & Egeth, H. (1997). Perception without attention: Evidence of grouping under conditions of inattention. *Journal of Experimental Psychology: Human Perception and Performance, 23*(2), 339–352.

Navon, D. (1977). Forest before trees: The precedence of global features in visual perception. *Cognitive Psychology, 9*, 353–383.

Neisser, U. (1967). *Cognitive psychology*. New York: Appleton Century Crofts.

Palmer, S., Neff, J., & Beck, D. (1996). Late influences on perceptual grouping: Amodal completion. *Psychonomic Bulletin and Review, 3*(1), 75–80.

Palmer, S. E. (2003). Perceptual organization and grouping. In R. Kimchi, M. Behrmann, & C. Olson (Eds.), *Perceptual organization in vision: Behavioral and neural processes* (pp. 3–43). Mahwah, NJ: Erlbaum.

Paquet, L., & Merikle, P. M. (1984). Global precedence: The effect of exposure duration. *Canadian Journal of Psychology, 38*, 45–53.

Pennefather, P. M., Chandna, A., Kovacs, I., Polat, U., & Norcia, A. M. (1999). Contour detection threshold: Repeatability and learning with "contour cards." *Spatial Vision, 2*(3), 257–266.

Pomerantz, J. R. (1983). Global and local precedence: Selective attention in form and motion perception. *Journal of Experimental Psychology: General, 112*(4), 516–540.

Pomerantz, J. R., & Pristach, E. A. (1989). Emergent features, attention, and perceptual glue in visual form perception. *Journal of Experimental Psychology: Human Perception and Performance, 15*, 635–649.

Ratcliff, G., & Newcombe, F. A. (1982). Object recognition: Some deductions from the clinical evidence. In A. W. Ellis (Ed.), *Normality and pathology in cognitive functions* (pp. 147–171). New York: Academic Press.

Rensink, R., & Enns, J. T. (1995). Preemption effects in visual search: Evidence for low-level grouping. *Psychological Review, 102*, 101–130.

Ricci, R., Vaishnavi, S., & Chatterjee, A. (1999). A deficit of intermediate vision: Experimental observations and theoretical implications. *Neurocase, 5*, 1–12.

Riddoch, M. J., & Humphreys, G. W. (1987). A case of integrative visual agnosia. *Brain, 110*, 1431–1462.

Riddoch, M. J., & Humphreys, G. W. (1993). *Birmingham Object Recognition Battery*. Hillsdale, NJ: Lawrence Erlbaum Associates.

Robertson, L. C., & Ivry, R. (2000). Hemispheric asymmetries: Attention to visual and auditory primitives. *Current Directions in Psychological Science, 9*(2), 59–64.

Rock, I. (1986). The description and analysis of object and event perception. In K. R. Boff, L. Kaufman, & J. P. Thomas (Eds.), *Handbook of perception and human performance* (Vol. 33, pp. 1–71). New York: Wiley.

Rock, I., & Brosgole, L. (1964). Grouping based on phenomenal proximity. *Journal of Experimental Psychology, 67*, 531–538.

Rock, I., Nijhawan, R., Plamer, S. E., & Tudor, L. (1992). Grouping based on phenomenal similarity of achromatic color. *Perception, 21*, 779–789.

Sanocki, T., & Sellers, E. (2001). Shifting resources to recognize a forming object: Dependencies involving object properties. *Visual Cognition, 8*(2), 197–235.

Sekuler, A. B., & Palmer, S. E. (1992). Perception of partly occluded objects: A microgenetic analysis. *Journal of Experimental Psychology: General, 121*(1), 95–111.

Shipley, T. F., & Kellman, P. (1992). Perception of occluded objects and illusory figures: Evidence for an identity hypothesis. *Journal of Experimental Psychology: Human Perception and Performance, 18*, 106–120.

Shulman, G. L., Sullivan, M. A., Gish, K., & Sakoda, W. J. (1986). The role of spatial-frequency channels in the perception of local and global structure. *Perception, 15*, 259–273.

Shulman, G. L., & Wilson, J. (1987). Spatial frequency and selective attention to local and global information. *Neuropsychologia, 18*, 89–101.

Snodgrass, S. G., & Vanderwart, M. A. (1980). A standardised set of 260 pictures: Norms for name agreement, image agreement, familiarity and visual complexity. *Journal of Experimental Psychology: Learning, Memory and Cognition, 6*, 174–215.

Sugita, Y. (1999). Grouping of image fragments in primary visual cortex. *Nature, 401*, 269–272.

Treisman, A. (1982). Perceptual grouping and attention in visual search for features and for objects. *Journal of Experimental Psychology: Human Perception and Performance, 8*, 194–214.

Treisman, A. (1983). The role of attention in object perception. In O. J. Braddick & A. C. Sleigh (Ed.), *Physical and biological processing of images* (pp. 316–325). New York: Springer Verlag.

Trick, L. M., & Enns, J. T. (1997). Clusters precede shapes in perceptual organization. *Psychological Science, 8*, 124–129.

von der Heydt, R., & Peterhans, E. (1989). Mechanisms of contour perception in monkey visual cortex. *Journal of Neuroscience, 9*(5), 1731–1748.

von der Heydt, R., Zhou, H., & Friedman, H. S. (2003). Neural coding of border ownership: Implications for the theory of figure-ground perception. In R. Kimchi, M. Behrmann, & C. Olson (Eds.), *Perceptual organization in vision: Behavioral and neural processes* (pp. 281–304). Mahwah, NJ: Erlbaum.

Westheimer, G. (1999). Gestalt theory reconfigured: Max Wertheimer's anticipation of recent developments in visual neuroscience. *Perception, 18*, 5–15.

Williams, P., & Behrmann, M. Object categorization and part integration: Experiments with normal perceivers and patients with visual agnosia. Manuscript submitted for publication.

Yovel, G., Yovel, I., & Levy, J. (2001). Hemispheric asymmetries for global and local visual perception: Effects of stimulus and task factors. *Journal of Experimental Psychology: Human Perception and Performance, 27*(6), 1369–1385.

Zhou, H., Friedman, H. S., & von der Heydt, R. (2000). Coding of border ownership in monkey visual cortex. *Journal of Neuroscience, 20*(17), 6594–6611.

11 Binding in Vision as a Multistage Process

Glyn W. Humphreys
University of Birmingham

Damage to areas of the brain concerned with visual processing can lead to selective disorders of visual perception. In many instances, these disorders affect the processing of some aspects of the visual world but not others. For example, patients can have selective loss of color vision without necessarily having an impairment of form perception or motion vision (Heywood & Cowey, 1999). In contrast, patients can have a gross impairment in motion vision without suffering loss of color perception (Heywood & Zihl, 1999). Likewise there can be marked damage to form perception along with maintenance of the ability to reach and grasp objects using properties of form, or, contrariwise, impaired reaching and grasping from vision along with spared object perception (e.g., see Jeannerod, 1997; Milner & Goodale, 1995, for reviews). This neuropsychological evidence suggests that there is a fractionation of visual processing within the brain, with different regions specialized for coding contrasting properties of the world—form, color, motion, location, and so forth. The argument is further supported by evidence from neurophysiology, where cells in different cortical areas show response preferences for particular visual properties (e.g., color specialization in area V4, motion in area MT; see Cowey, 1994; Desimone & Ungerleider, 1989; Zeki, 1993), and from functional imaging data in humans, where there is selective activation of different cortical sites depending on the visual property being manipulated (e.g., see Tootell et al.,

1995; Ungerleider & Haxby, 1994; Watson et al., 1993). Indeed, even within a single visual domain, such as form perception, there will be multiple cells at early stages of vision that code the image independently and in parallel. However, for coherent representations of whole objects to be derived, activity must be integrated across these cells, so that, for example, local image features become grouped into the shapes that support recognition and action. I refer to this process of integrating image features, both between and within visual dimensions, as visual binding. In this chapter I use neuropsychological evidence on the fractionation of visual processing to argue that binding is not a single operation but instead can be decomposed into multiple stages, each of which may offer a probabilistic interpretation of how image features are interrelated. I link this argument to converging evidence from experimental psychology and neurophysiology, which suggests that forms of binding can be achieved at early stages of vision to be verified by later stages perhaps using reentrant feedback.

SINGLE SOLUTION ACCOUNTS OF BINDING

There have been two major solutions offered for the binding problem in vision. One is that features are linked on the basis of time. The best-known account of this kind is that binding is contingent on temporal synchrony in the firing of neurons (e.g., see Eckhorn, 1999; Singer & Gray, 1995). A temporal code for binding can be derived if neurons responsive to the features of a single object fire at the same time, while those responsive to the features of other objects fire at a different time. As a consequence of this, features can be bound to each object based on the temporal difference in the firing of the contrasting cell assemblies. This account is supported most strongly by physiological evidence showing time-locked firing of cells when stimulus elements group (see Singer & Gray, 1995, for a review). There is also behavioral evidence from humans for temporal synchronization in the input being important for feature binding (e.g., Elliot & Muller, 1998; Fahle, 1993).

A second account is that binding is achieved only by visual processing going serial—for example, by attentional enhancement applied to the location of each object in the field (or attentional filtering of objects at all unattended regions of field or both; see later discussion). Cells at higher levels of the visual system can have large receptive fields (e.g., see Gross, Rocha-Miranda, & Bender, 1972)—a property useful for achieving viewpoint invariance in object recognition. However viewpoint invariance may only be achieved in this way at the risk of incorrect feature binding, which could occur if cells are activated by features belonging to different objects that happen to fall within the same receptive field. Attention to a location can increase the activation of features that fall there (see Brefczynski & de Yoe, 1999; Hillyard, Vogel, & Luck, 1998), and it can also reduce effects of stimuli at unattended regions (e.g., Moran & Desimone, 1985). This may allow features at an attended location to activate high-level cells without suffering competition from features falling at unattended locations. Hence, there can be binding only of the features belonging to the attended object. The idea that binding is modulated by attention to location is highlighted by the well-known feature integration theory (FIT) of visual attention (Treisman, 1998; Treisman & Gelade, 1980). To explain why the features of a whole object become bound, though, a more elaborated account may be needed. For example, if attention is only to one part of a stimulus, feedback from processes concerned with object coding may be needed so that features are integrated across the complete form (e.g., see Humphreys & Riddoch, 1993; Vecera & Farah, 1994, for this proposal).

These approaches are not mutually inconsistent, and one way that attention may generate a competitive advantage in processing is by improving the synchrony of firing for attended elements. Nevertheless, both the attentional and temporal synchrony accounts offer single solutions to the binding problem. In contrast to this, neuropsychological evidence suggests that the binding process can fractionate— there can be selective disorders affecting the binding of different properties of objects. A multistage account of binding may be needed.

FRACTIONATING THE BINDING PROCESS IN FORM PERCEPTION

In the view of I outlined, one type of visual binding operates when the form elements making up an object group together to yield a coherent description distinguishing a figure from the background of other features in the field. In the disorder of integrative agnosia (Humphreys, 1999; Riddoch & Humphreys, 1987), there can be a breakdown in this process of binding the form elements into a coherent object description to segment it from the ground. Interestingly, one but not other types of visual binding appear to be affected in such patients, consistent with the argument for multiple types of binding in vision.

Agnosic patients may be impaired at making simple perceptual judgments about objects. Nevertheless, the same patients can reach and grasp objects appropriately (e.g., Milner & Goodale, 1995). In integrative agnosia, patients can copy the objects they misidentify without there being gross mislocalization of object parts (from one side of space to another; Humphreys & Riddoch, 1987). Hence, despite severe misperceptions (documented later), patients can retain the ability to integrate visual stimuli into a stable spatial representation. Objects remain correctly bound to their spatial locations.

Despite there being binding of form and location, other types of binding seem to be damaged. For example, there may be poor discrimination of simple Gestalt grouping relations based on proximity and similarity (e.g., Milner et al., 1991). There may also be poor grouping of the parts of single objects. Thus, the integrative agnosic patient HJA, when given a black-and- white photograph of a paintbrush remarked, "It appears to be two things close together; a longish wooden stick and a shorter, darker object, though this can't be right or you would have told me [that there were two objects rather than one present]" (see Humphreys & Riddoch, 1987). Butter and Trobe (1994) similarly reported a patient who thought that there were several objects present when given single line drawings to identify. Indeed, integrative agnosic patients can find it even more difficult to identify line drawings than silhouettes of the same stimuli (Butter & Trobe, 1994; Lawson & Humphreys, 1999; Riddoch & Humphreys, 1987). This suggests that the internal details in line drawings are actually unhelpful for such patients, perhaps because such details provide cues to break up the coding of the whole objects into separate segments. This is consistent with some form of an impairment in the interplay between grouping and segmentation. If the grouping of parts to wholes is relatively weak when compared with segmentation operations between parts, then recognition of the whole can be impaired.

Further evidence for impaired grouping of parts to wholes in integrative agnosia comes from studies showing abnormal reductions in performance when fragmented forms are presented (Boucart & Humphreys, 1992) and when overlapping forms are given (Butter & Trobe, 1994; DeRenzi & Lucchelli, 1993; Riddoch & Humphreys, 1987). These stimuli stress the processes involved in grouping and organizing the spatial relations between edge contours within an object and in segmenting contours within objects from those in background forms, relative to when single objects are presented with full contours.

These deficits in integrative agnosia demonstrate that object recognition depends on processes that bind edge contours into their correct spatial relations and that support appropriate segmentation between elements in the figure and the ground. In these patients grouping and segmentation processes are impaired by the damage to their ventral visual system, even though stimuli can be localized.

Recently, Giersch, Boucart, Kovacs, and I examined these impairments in binding shape information in some detail with the integrative agnosic HJA (Giersch, Humphreys, Boucart, & Kovács, 2000). A first study evaluated what may be one of the earliest stages of the binding of shape—the ability to link contour elements into elongated contours. HJA was given stimuli, such as those shown in Fig. 11.1, composed of multiple Gabor patches. In one part of each image, a target formed by collinear Gabor patches grouped to create a circular shape. Distractor patches, at random orientations, could fall at random locations within the image. When the spacing between the contours in the target is kept constant, the ease of detecting the target decreases as more distractor elements are present. From this we can calculate a threshold for detecting the target as a function of the number of distractors in the image (see Kovács, 2000). Somewhat to our surprise, HJA had a normal threshold in this task. We conclude that the process of binding local edge fragments into a contour is intact.

The good performance on the contour detection task contrasts with HJA's performance on other tasks in which contours had to be integrated into more holistic shapes. One example is presented in Fig. 11.2. HJA was given the stimulus configuration shown at the top of each shape triplet (presented here within a single box),

FIG. 11.1. Display of Gabor patches with some local elements aligned to form a shape from grouping by collinearity.

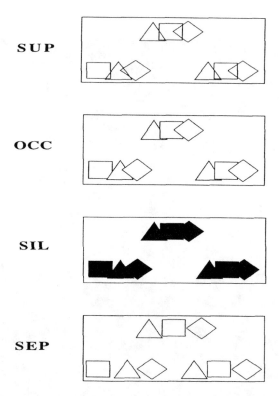

FIG. 11.2.   Example displays of the type used by Giersch et al. (2000). On each trial the top shapes in each box were presented first, followed by the lower shapes on the left and right of the screen. The task was to choose which of the bottom shapes matched the top one.

followed by the two other stimuli presented later (these were exposed on the screen latter where the original shape triplet had appeared). The task was to match the original configuration to one of the two following ones. The configurations were exposed as overlapping line drawings (SUP), occluded shapes (OCC), silhouettes (SIL), and spatially separated shapes (SEP). We found that HJA was abnormally impaired with occluded shapes, even relative to the more complex stimuli in which all contours were depicted (condition SUP). In addition, HJA was most impaired when there was just a small area of occlusion for the background shapes so that a narrow distance separated the broken parts of their edge contours. A difficulty under this circumstance suggests that HJA was computing the occluded edges of the background shapes, but these edges then disrupted performance. For example, occluded edges, once computed, may increase the difficulty of perceptual organization because these edges have to be suppressed when they are formed behind an occluder to prevent them from being part of the final conscious percept.

Another example of HJA's impaired ability to organize occluded figures appro-priately can be derived from his performance on simple copying tasks. Fig. 11.3 illustrates example copies of both nonoccluded (Fig. 11.3A) and occluded shapes (Fig. 11.3B). With nonoccluded shapes, HJA made no errors, and he never drew a connecting line within the shape. In contrast, with occluded shapes, HJA did some-times mistakenly draw in the occluded line as it were present in the front shape (see Fig. 11.3(B)(i) and (C)(ii)). This supports the argument that HJA did compute the occluded edge from the visible collinear edges in the background shape, but this virtual line was sometimes used as if it were really present. Other errors with occluded shapes are shown in Fig. 11.3(B)(ii) and (iii). These included segmen-tation of the background shape based on the T junctions between the foreground

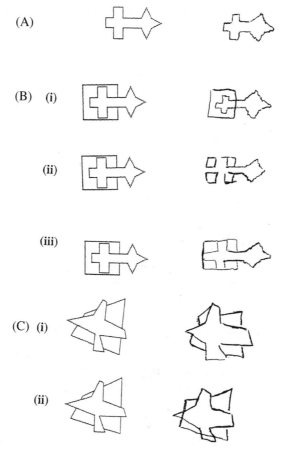

FIG. 11.3. Examples of the stimuli given to HJA for copying (on the left) along with some example copies (on the right).

and background shapes and inappropriate continuation of the foreground contours to join background contours. Also, with some complex background shapes (as in Fig. 11.3(C)(i)), there were some apparent failures to group collinear edges. These data from drawing tasks indicate an abnormal problem in computing the appropriate spatial relations between foreground and background shapes from two-dimensional edges. Although occluded edges can be completed, they may be labeled incorrectly as far as their depth relations are concerned. This then allows occluded lines to be represented as visible lines in the foreground. In addition, there can be grouping between edges in foreground and background shapes when edges are continued incorrectly along an occluded edge. It is also of interest to note that, although HJA had difficulty in depicting depth relations from line drawings, he had no general problems in depth perception. HJA has good perception of stereoscopic depth (Humphreys & Riddoch, 1987), and he uses the depth cues of stereopsis and motion parallax, from head movements, to help him identify real objects (Chainay & Humphreys, 2001).

The data have important implications for understanding visual binding. First, they indicate that the binding of edge elements into holistic shapes takes place after local-orientated elements are bound into edges (and indeed after edges are computed from occluding objects). HJA's ability to compute connected edges from collinear fragments is relatively intact, but binding of contours within shapes is disrupted. Second, contour completion with occluded stimuli operates before figure-ground relations are coded—if this were not the case, it would be difficult to understand how occluded contours could be represented in the foreground. From this last point, I further conclude that the binding of contours into holistic shapes operates in conjunction with the assignment of figure-ground relations within the image after elements have been bound into contours. HJA's deficits are caused by bilateral lesions affecting the lingual, fusiform and posterior, inferior temporal gyri (see Riddoch, Humphreys, Gannon, Blott, & Jones, 1999, for an MRI scan). From this we may conclude that the process of binding contours into more holistic shapes, impaired in HJA, involves these posterior, inferior regions of ventral cortex. HJA's ability to group orientated elements into contours, though, seems to be supported by earlier visual areas (including V1) spared by the lesions. There is consistent evidence for grouping by collinearity within such early cortical regions (e.g., Gilbert, Ito, Kapadia, & Westheimer, 2000).

SEPARATING THE BINDING OF FORM FROM THE BINDING OF FORM AND SURFACE DETAIL

Neuropsychological deficits after damage to the parietal lobes can contrast quite strikingly with those found after damage to ventral (occipito-temporal) regions of the brain. For example, although localization is generally preserved after ventral damage, patients with parietal lesions can show poor localization of visual stimuli (e.g., Stark, Coslett, & Saffran, 1996; see also DeRenzi, 1982; Ungerleider & Mishkin, 1982, for early reviews). Similarly, when copying stimuli, patients with unilateral parietal damage can mislocalize parts of objects and reproduce stimuli from the contralesional side of space on the ipsilesional side (Bisiach, Capitani, Luzzatti, & Perani, 1981), and, in tasks such as reading aloud the letters within a letter string, parietal patients can make numerous mislocalization errors, reporting the letters in the wrong spatial order (e.g., Baylis, Driver, Baylis, & Rafal, 1994; Hall, Humphreys, & Cooper, 2001; Shallice & Warrington, 1977). This suggests that visual forms may be computed correctly but are poorly bound to space.

Parietal damage can also lead to impaired binding between shape and surface information in objects. Friedman-Hill, Robertson, and Treisman (1995) reported that a patient (RM) with Balint's syndrome,[1] following bilateral parietal damage, made abnormally large numbers of illusory conjunction (IC) errors under prolonged viewing conditions when asked to identify multiple colored letters (see also Cohen & Rafal, 1991, for similar results in the contralesional field of patients with unilateral parietal damage). For example, given the presence of a red A and a blue B in the field, RM might report that there was a red B and a blue A. With normal subjects, IC errors can be induced but only when stimuli are presented relatively briefly and full attention is prevented (e.g., Treisman & Schmidt, 1982; though see Donk, 1999). The ICs found with RM under free viewing conditions demonstrate an impairment in binding. This could be accounted for in various ways. One possibility is that there is inaccurate localization of stimuli along each dimension (form and color), preventing accurate integration; an alternative is that there is a deficit in attending to the locations of stimuli, which allows features from both stimuli to be coded by cells at higher levels of the visual system (cf. Treisman, 1998).

These results suggest that the parietal lobe is important for linking visual stimuli to some stable representation of space and also for controlling attention to the locations of stimuli. Consequently, parietal damage produces both poor visual localization of shapes and poor integration of shape and surface detail when there are multiple, competing shapes and surfaces present. The cooccurrence of impaired visual localization and integration of shape and surface detail is consistent with the basic tenet of FIT—that attention to location generates feature binding in multielement displays (see Treisman, 1998). A further possibility, though, is that integration across stimulus dimensions is disrupted directly by the coarse spatial representation found in parietal patients. I consider these proposals further after presenting data on feature binding after parietal damage.

Although, as I have noted, parietal damage is associated with disruption to some types of visual binding, other types of binding seem to be relatively intact. For

---

[1]The term Balint's syndrome is applied to patients showing two primary behavioral symptoms: poor identification of multiple visual stimuli (simultanagnosia) and poor visual localization, following the first description of such a case by Balint (1909).

instance, whole-word reading can be relatively preserved in patients with bilateral parietal lesions, even when abnormally high numbers of mislocalization errors are made in letter report tasks (Baylis et al., 1994; Hall et al., 2001). Apparently, word forms can be derived even though explicit letter localization is poor. Similarly, mislocalization errors involve the migration of whole forms (letters), consistent with the letter features themselves being bound before mislocalization occurs. Also patients who make an abnormally high number of color-form IC errors can still be relatively intact at recognizing single objects (Robertson, Treisman, Friedman-Hill, & Grabowecky, 1997). Again, apparently, there remains some ability to bind parts within objects.

A particularly dramatic example of binding continuing to operate despite parietal damage comes from studies of visual extinction, where binding between elements can even dictate whether the elements are detected. Visual extinction occurs when patients are able to report the presence of single stimuli presented in their contralesional field but cannot report (or sometimes even detect) the same stimulus when it is presented simultaneously with an item on the ipsilesional side (e.g., Karnath, 1988). The phenomenon is consistent with a brain lesion producing a spatial bias in visual selection so that the ipsilesional stimulus is selected in preference to the contralesional one. Interestingly, several studies showed that extinction is reduced by grouping between the ipsi- and contralesional stimuli. This has been found when ipsi- and contralesional shapes have collinear edges (Gilchrist, Humphreys, & Riddoch, 1996) when they have common brightness, are connected, and when the ipsilesional item extends to surround the contralesional one, (see Humphreys, 1998). Effects can also be modulated by whether two elements fall in appropriate occlusion relations behind objects (Mattingly, Davis, & Driver, 1997) and by whether they together form a familiar shape (e.g., a – and > making up a →; see Ward, Goodrich, & Driver, 1994). Effects of grouping on extinction can even occur based on the activation of stored representations alone. Kumada and Humphreys (2001) showed that there was less extinction for two-letter words (be, go) relative to two-letter nonwords (bo, ge, created by exchanging the letters across the words), even though there are no bottom-up cues that favor the grouping of letters in words compared with nonwords. Similarly, there can be less extinction for parts of a compound word than for equivalent parts in a matched noncompound (e.g., for COW in COWBOY relative to SUN in SUNBOY; Behrmann, Moscovitch, Black, & Mozer, 1990). These data suggest that the letters became bound and were selected together because they activated a common stored representation (with a word but not a nonword, or with a compound word but not with a noncompound). In all of these examples, the grouping effects also take place despite the presence of parietal damage. This fits with the argument that some forms of binding take place in neural areas unaffected by parietal damage.

Extinction can also be biased by the goodness of objects. For example, Humphreys, Romani, Olson, Riddoch, and Duncan (1994) compared the selection of stimuli that differed in how well their parts grouped into a shape. Though single stimuli could be detected, there was impaired detection of the less-good stimulus when both were presented simultaneously. This occurred even though one patient (GK, see later discussion) was severely impaired at localizing the stimuli that were selected relative to a fixed reference point (a fixation cross). This suggests that there is binding of elements into a more global shape despite there being both parietal damage and poor spatial localization. Neither explicit localization nor the preservation of the parietal lobes are prerequisites for the binding of form elements.

BINDING FORM AND SURFACE DETAILS IN BALINT'S SYNDROME (SIMULTANAGNOSIA)

I noted that bilateral damage to the parietal lobes may lead to the occurrence of abnormally high numbers of IC responses when multiple stimuli are exposed, under conditions where normal subjects make few such errors (Friedman-Hill et al., 1995). Yet patients with parietal lesions can also be sensitive to the effects of grouping on extinction. What are the relations between these two apparently contrasting results?

Humphreys, Cinel, Wolfe, Olson, and Klempen (2000) examined this issue in a patient with Balint's syndrome, GK. GK suffered bilateral parietal lesions in 1986 and subsequently presented with a number of neuropsychological impairments, including simultanagnosia (see Cooper & Humphreys, 2000), attentional dyslexia (Hall et al., 2001), and a mild problem in word finding. He also showed visual extinction. With stimuli presented above and below fixation, extinction is influenced by the perceptual goodness of the stimuli—good stimuli tend to be reported, and poor stimuli are extinguished, irrespective of their spatial positions (Humphreys et al., 1994). Spatial extinction occurs with lateral presentations, with right-side items tending to be reported and left-side items extinguished. Interestingly, there is less spatial extinction when stimuli group relative to when they do not group (see Boutsen & Humphreys, 2000; Gilchrist et al., 1996; Humphreys, 1998). The effects of grouping on both spatial and nonspatial extinction indicate that some forms of binding continue to operate, despite GK's parietal lesions and neuropsychological deficits.

In contrast to the binding processes apparent when grouping leads to recovery from extinction, GK (like other Balint's patients) showed poor binding when asked to report the surface and shape properties of multiple items in the field. Given three colored letters and asked to report the color and identity of just the one at fixation, GK made about 32% IC responses, miscombining either the shape or color of the central letter with one of the other stimuli. There were few errors with single items (see also Friedman-Hill et al., 1995).

We assessed the relations between the apparently intact binding in recovery from extinction and the impaired binding that leads to ICs in color and form by

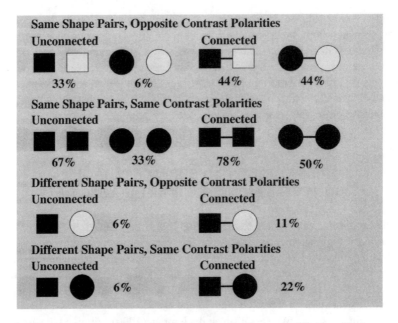

FIG. 11.4.   The shapes given to GK in a study comparing the effects of grouping on extinction and illusory conjunctions. On each trial, only one pair of shapes was presented, against the background of a complete grey screen. One shape fell to the left and one to the right of fixation.

presenting GK with shapes such as those presented in Fig. 11.4 (Humphreys et al., 2000). Shapes fell to the left or right of fixation, and two shapes, when present, could group in a variety of ways. Both could be squares (same shape and aligned collinear edges) or circles (same shape only), the shapes could have the same or opposite contrast polarities (both white, both black, or one white and one black, against a grey background), and the shapes could be connected or unconnected. All combinations of shapes appeared in the different shape and contrast polarity conditions (i.e., each shape appeared equally to the left or right of fixation, as did each contrast polarity). The stimuli were presented at the center of a computer monitor for 1 s, and GK was asked to report the shapes and letters present. The results were quite clear (see Fig. 11.4). Single shapes were reported at a high level (87% correct for single shapes in the left field and 90% correct for single shapes in the right), and, when two shapes were present, report of both was better when they grouped. Thus, when the two shapes were the same, performance improved relative to when they differed; performance also improved when the shapes had the same rather than opposite contrast polarities, and it improved when the shapes were connected relative to when they were unconnected. In the two shape conditions GK made many extinction-type errors, where he reported the presence of only one shape. The rate of extinction errors was affected by grouping. When the stimuli had different shapes and contrast polarities, extinction responses were made on 67% of the trials with unconnected shapes (GK then reported the shape and color of the stimulus in his right field). However, when the same stimuli were connected, extinction occurred on just 33% of the trials. These data confirm previous findings on the effects of grouping on extinction (Boutsen & Humphreys, 2000; Gilchrist et al., 1996; Humphreys, 1998).

As well as making extinction errors, GK also made errors by misreporting the properties of the stimuli (Humphreys et al., 2000). Sometimes, when the stimuli had different shapes and contrast polarities, some errors were made by pairing the shape in the right field with surface information from the item on the left and vice versa (e.g., black square, white cirlce → white square, black circle). We termed these feature exchange errors. These errors could be illusory conjunctions of shape and surface detail, or they could simply be feature misidentifications. We tested this by comparing the number of feature misidentifications made in other conditions where feature exchange errors could not occur because the two stimuli shared one of the critical attributes (e.g., the stimuli had the same color or the same shape). On these trials, unambiguous feature misidentifications could be made by reporting an attribute not present in the display (e.g., white square, black square → white square, black circle; here the response circle is labeled a feature misidentification because this shape was not present). Feature exchange errors could result from two concurrent feature misidentifications to the two stimuli present on a trial. The likelihood of feature exchange errors occurring by chance, then, can be estimated from the probability that two feature misidentifications errors would occur on the same trial (taking the data from the unambiguous feature misidentification trials). Fig. 11.5 gives the rates of observed feature exchanges, relative to those expected by chance combinations of feature misidentifications. Feature exchange errors occurred at a much higher rate than would be expected from chance feature misidentifications. We conclude that feature exchanges were indeed illusory conjunctions of shape and surface properties belonging to different stimuli. The data presented in Fig. 11.5 also illustrate that feature exchange errors tended to occur with more frequency when the shapes were connected than when they were unconnected. However, the opportunity for feature exchange errors was higher when the stimuli were connected because there were fewer extinction responses on those trials. When the probabilities for chance combinations of feature misidentifications were adjusted for this (with expected feature exchanges on 0.6% of the trials with connected stimuli, as opposed to 0.3% of the trials with unconnected items), then the rates of feature exchange errors did not differ for connected and unconnected shapes.

The finding of Humphreys et al. (2000), that ICs of shape and surface detail were not clearly affected by a grouping factor such as connectedness, contrasts with data from control subjects. For example, Prinzmetal, Treiman, and Rho (1986) used displays of colored letters and found that illusory reports of letter-color combinations

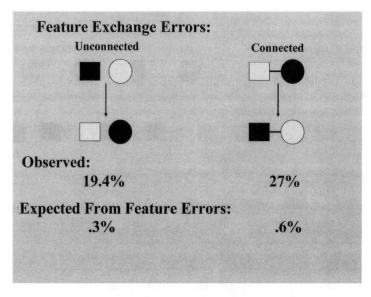

FIG. 11.5. Example of illusory conjunction and feature error responses that could be made to displays where the shapes differed and had opposite contrast polarities.

were more likely when the different colored letters occurred within a syllable boundary relative to when they occurred across syllable boundaries. Migrations of color were more frequent between letters within a syllabic group. Similarly, ICs of color and form are affected by common movement of the items (Baylis, Driver, & McLeod, 1992). Using the same displays as those employed with GK, Humphreys et al. also confirmed that control subjects made increased numbers of ICs with grouped than with ungrouped shapes (see Fig. 11.6). In contrast, for GK, grouping influences extinction, but it does not strongly constrain his report of how shape and surface details combine.

From these results, Humphreys et al. (2000) suggest that GK does have a deficit in linking the shape and surface details of objects together, but this problem occurs after shapes have been bound into perceptual groups. Because shape grouping has already taken place, surface properties tend to migrate between whole shapes. Such problems might arise for a variety of reasons. For example, it could be that GK has difficulty in attending to the common location occupied by shape and surface information so that shapes and surface details from different objects continue to compete for selection. Normal subjects may show effects of grouping on ICs of shape and surface detail (e.g., Baylis et al., 1992; Prinzmetal et al., 1986) because attention is biased to the area occupied by a dominant group (see Humphreys & Riddoch, 1993; Vecera & Farah, 1994, for accounts of how this might come about). This bias limits the likelihood that illusory conjunctions will incorporate

Effect of Grouping With Controls

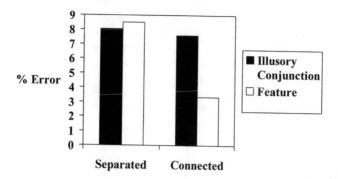

FIG. 11.6. Data from control subjects examining the effects of grouping on illusory conjunctions of form and surface detail (see Humphreys et al., 2000).

properties of stimuli outside the attended group. However, if the parietal damage sustained by GK reduces the impact of attention on a particular grouped object, then properties of separate stimuli may still be miscombined.

If the binding of shape and surface information depends on an interaction between ventral and dorsal visual streams, then we might also expect ICs of shape and surface detail to occur after ventral damage. To the best of my knowledge, such errors have not been reported in patients with ventral lesions, but it is also true that this has been little tested. It may also be the case that shape binding within the ventral system in such patients is sufficient to constrain the mapping of surface details to those shape representations that are formed. Errors in shape description, rather than shape-surface binding, are then apparent. Irrespective of whether this last speculation is correct, further study of such patients will be important for establishing detailed knowledge of how shape and surface details are linked by the brain.

BINDING TO WHAT LEVEL? THE ROLE OF FAMILIAR VISUAL REPRESENTATIONS AND STORED KNOWLEDGE

Although I discussed evidence that shape information can be bound successfully in the ventral visual system, even when patients have parietal damage, it remains the case that unilateral parietal damage can disrupt object and word recognition. For example, in the syndrome of neglect dyslexia, patients fail to report letters at one end of a word, and their comprehension can be based on their naming error rather than on the word as presented (e.g., TRACE → RACE, running; Ellis, Flude,

& Young, 1987). Such errors could arise if the parietal system helps a stimulus activate stored knowledge, even if its parts are initially bound. Then, if attention directed through the parietal lobe is biased to one side of the stimulus (due to a unilateral lesion), misidentifications could occur because features on the attended side are weighted more strongly in the recognition process.

It may also be that only some forms of visual binding are achieved without activation from the parietal system. As I noted, there is considerable evidence that image features such as collinearity, common contrast polarity, connectedness and closure can be computed in patients with parietal lesions (Gilchrist et al., 1996; Humphreys, 1998; Ward et al., 1994). However, computation of more complex visual representations may be dependent on stimuli activating stored knowledge. Thus, though patients with Balint's syndrome may read words relatively well despite their bilateral parietal damage (Baylis et al., 1994), they can be very sensitive to factors such as the visual familiarity of the word forms. For example, Hall et al. (2001) reported that the reading of mixed case stimuli (e.g., MiXeD) was extremely impaired. Furthermore, acronyms (e.g., BBC, IBM) could be identified if shown in their normal upper case format but not if presented in lower case (bbc, ibm), even though familiar words could be better identified in lower rather than upper case (table vs. TABLE). Hall et al. proposed that reading here was dependent on recognition of the familiar, whole visual pattern. Acronyms are familiar in their upper case form and thus were best identified when presented in that format. Words are more familiar in lower case format, and thus were advantaged when presented in that form. With each kind of stimulus, the individual letters in the strings were identified rather poorly. These results are consistent with the undamaged ventral system responding to a familiar visual word form. However, recognition based on letter processing was disrupted, presumably because that is mediated by the parietal system. The parietal system may be important for sustaining attention across the whole stimulus, improving the resolution of the letters across the strings. Where binding is dependent on fine-grained feature properties coded across complex stimuli, the parietal system may still play an important role.

FAST, PARALLEL BINDING IN NORMAL VISION

The neuropsychological data I summarized suggest that several forms of binding can operate in vision:

- There is an initial process of binding oriented elements into edge contours, and this can be distinguished from processes that bind contours into more holistic shapes and that segment them from background stimuli. The former process can remain intact when the latter is impaired (as in patient HJA; Giersch et al., 2000).

- The process of binding shape to surface detail can be separated from the processes involved in binding together shape elements. Shape binding can be relatively preserved, shown when shape grouping reduces visual extinction, even when there is a marked disturbance of the process that links shapes and surfaces (as in patient GK; Humphreys et al., 2000).
- Some forms of shape binding can operate within the ventral visual system, whereas the binding of shape to surface detail seems dependent on involvement of the dorsal as well as the ventral visual stream.

How do these conclusions relate to work on binding in normal (intact) vision?

Consider my argument that there is an early stage of processing in which oriented edge fragments are bound into contours, which is followed by a later process of binding contours into more holistic shapes. This two-stage account fits with proposals made by Kellman and Shipley (1991; Shipley & Kellman, 1992). These investigators argued that both visible and occluded contours are computed from local, oriented operators, and the outputs of these operators are then used to compute more global shape representations. For HJA, the local operators appear to still compute occluded contours, but he is then impaired at integrating the contour with the other contours present (Giersch et al., 2000). HJA has bilateral damage affecting the lingual and fusiform gyri and the inferior posterior temporal gyrus. His deficits in integrating contours into shapes suggest that this binding process normally operates in these now-damaged visual areas of cortex. In contrast to this, HJA's ability to group oriented fragments into edges is relatively preserved, consistent with this ability relying on preserved regions of early visual cortex (V1/V2). Both physiological studies on nonhuman primates and fMRI studies with humans show that these early regions of visual cortex are activated by illusory contours (Grosof, Shapley, & Hawken, 1993; Mendola, Dale, Fischl, Liu, & Toottell, 1999; Redies, Crook, & Creutzfelt, 1986; Sheth, Sharma, Rao, & Sur, 1996; von der Heydt & Peterhans, 1989) and that global perceptual structures can emerge from long-range interactions between the neurons in these regions (Gilbert et al., 2000; Gilbert & Wiesel, 1989). However, I suggest that the computation of more complex spatial relations, where multiple edges are integrated into holistic shapes, depends on later visual areas that competitively weight one emerging perceptual group against others (including parts within a single object; see my earlier example of segmentation of a paintbrush). These later, integrative processes are impaired in HJA (see also Riddoch & Humphreys, 1987).

The evidence from GK fits with the argument that (at least some types of) binding in the form system takes place within ventral cortex. GK, like other patients with parietal damage, shows relatively intact binding of known shapes; for example, object recognition is generally preserved, and grouping between form elements reduces extinction. Despite this, GK is grossly impaired at selecting multiple shapes and at localizing stimuli once selected (see Humphreys et al., 1994, for evidence on localization). Explicit localization of visual elements is not necessary for binding to operate.

The evidence that grouping reduces extinction is of theoretical interest because it suggests that grouping can operate prior to attention being brought to bear on the shapes present. Because patients may not even be able to detect a contralesional stimulus unless it groups with the ipsilesional item, it appears that the grouping relationship is formed pre-attentively. This runs contrary to an attentional account of binding, which stresses that binding is dependent on attention being applied to a spatial region to favor those features over others in the field (cf. Treisman, 1998). However, it should be noted that the effects of binding on extinction have typically been shown using relatively simple visual displays where, when the elements group, only a single object is present. It may be that attention is useful, if not also necessary, when multiple shapes are present and when there is increased competition for selection of the features between the different objects.

A stronger argument, that attention is not necessary for form binding even with multiple stimuli, comes from studies of normal visual search. Here there are data showing that search for targets defined by conjunctions of form elements can be efficient and apparently spatially parallel under some circumstances. For example, search is efficient when the distractor items are homogeneous and can be formed into a separate group from the conjunction target (Duncan & Humphreys, 1989; Humphreys, Quinlan, & Riddoch, 1989). Search is also efficient if all the form elements present group into a single two- or three-dimensional object (Donnelly, Humphreys, & Riddoch, 1991; Humphreys, & Donnelly, 2000), or, if, once grouped, the target has a unique three-dimensional orientation compared with the homogeneous distractors (Enns & Rensink, 1991). Highly efficient search, with slopes often less than 10 ms/item, is unlikely to stem from the serial application of visual attention (see Crick, 1984, for a discussion of biologically plausible mechanisms of serial search).

One interpretation of these data is that there is grouping of visual features into object descriptions at different levels—local elements into parts and local parts into more holistic objects, including representing the whole display as a single object if all the elements present form a coherent group (Duncan & Humphreys, 1989). If the display-level description supports the discrimination between targets and distractors—for example, by matching a template of the target—then search is highly efficient. However, if the grouped description is not useful for target discrimination (e.g., if grouping binds together targets and distractors, rather than helping targets and distractors segment; see Rensink & Enns, 1995), then attention may be required to help segment the stimuli in the display. This may be achieved by activating features within some regions of the display over others, which may bias grouping to take place over selective parts of the display. In this view, preattentive binding, which appears to operate within the ventral visual system, must normally be allied with attentional segmentation to enable individual objects to be segmented and identified in complex (multiobject) scenes.

My other neuropsychological finding, that ICs of shape and surface detail can be dissociated from the relatively intact binding of form information, can be linked to computational approaches to vision, such as the FAÇADE model of Grossberg and colleagues (e.g., Grossberg & Mingolla, 1985; Grossberg & Pessoa, 1998). These authors propose that visual coding depends on two distinct operations. First, a process of boundary formation is conducted within a boundary contour system (BCS). This system uses grouping processes such as collinearity and good continuation to form bounded contours of shapes. Second, a process of filling in is conducted within the bounded regions, an operation performed by a feature contour system (FCS). Activation within the FCS generates the surface properties of objects. For patients such as GK, processing within the BCS appears to be relatively intact, but there is a deficit within the FCS so that surface information is not always correctly bound to the appropriate shape.

We can also ask about the nature of the deficit in binding form and surface detail. On an attentional account, GK's impairment is caused by damage to his visual attentional system, which prevents activation of the common location shared by the color and form of an object. Due to this impairment in attention, colors from several objects are available to be combined with a given shape; illusory conjunctions result. An alternative view, though, is that the deficits are caused by poor co-registration of the locations of colors and shape within a master map of locations within the parietal lobe. Because there is overlapping coregistration of features, colors from one object may be misattributed to another.

This last view differs from an attentional account because accurate co-registration would make it possible for color and shape to be combined, even without attention to their common location. For patients such as GK, though, co-registration is disrupted by lesions to the master location map. Interestingly, there is evidence from search in normal subjects for superadditivity when multiple form-color conjunctions are present (Linnell & Humphreys, 2001; Mordkoff, Yantis, & Egeth, 1990), which is consistent with the conjunctions being coded in a spatially parallel manner. Similarly there can be superadditivity in segmentation tasks when form and color boundaries coincide (Kubovy, Cohen, & Hollier, 1999). These last results suggest that bindings of color and form do not necessarily depend on selective attention, though the parietal role may still play an important mediating role for co-registration.

In normal observers there is also evidence that ICs are sensitive to grouping between stimuli (Baylis et al., 1992; Prinzmetal et al., 1986; see also Fig. 11.6). This was not the case for GK, though there were clear effects of grouping on extinction (Humphreys et al., 2000). The data from normal subjects may be explained in terms of there being interactions between form grouping in the ventral visual system and activation within the parietal lobe. Grouping between elements in one location may lead to increased associated activation for neurons within the parietal lobe representing the same location, and this may reduce the likelihood of coregistration with surface information from other locations. GK's parietal damage may limit these interactions. As a consequence, surface details from multiple objects may compete to be registered with shape information, even when the objects do not group.

In sum, the results from detailed neuropsychological case studies with patients such as HJA and GK can provide important new insights into the nature of binding operations in vision, and they can be linked to a framework for binding processes in normal vision.

ACKNOWLEDGMENTS

This work was supported by grants from the European Union and from the Medical Research Council, United Kingdom. I am extremely grateful to HJA and GK for all their time and for their ability to make research fun as well as interesting. My thanks go also to all of my colleagues who contributed to the different parts of the work reported here: Muriel Boucart, Caterina Cinel, Anne Giersch, Nikki Klempen, Illona Kovacs, Andrew Olson, Jane Riddoch, and Jeremy Wolfe.

REFERENCES

Balint, R. (1909). Psychic paralysis of gaze: Optic ataxia, and spatial disorder of attention. *Manatschrift fur Psychiatrie und Neurologie, 25,* 51–81.

Baylis, G. C., Driver, J., Baylis, L. L., & Rafal, R. D. (1994). Reading of letters and words in a patient with Balint's syndrome. *Neuropsychologia, 32,* 1273–1286.

Baylis, G. C., Driver, J., & McLeod, P. (1992). Movement and proximity constrain miscombinations of colour and form. *Perception, 21,* 201–218.

Behrmann, M., Moscovitch, M., Black, S. E. E. E., & Mozer, M. C. (1990). Perceptual and conceptual mechanisms in neglect: Two contrasting case studies. *Brain, 113,* 1163–1183.

Bisiach, E., Capitani, E., Luzzatti, C., & Perani, D. (1981). Brain and conscious representation of outside reality. *Neuropsychologia, 24,* 739–767.

Boucart, M., & Humphreys, G. W. (1992). The computation of perceptual structure from collinearity and closure: Normality and pathology. *Neuropsychologia, 30,* 527–546.

Boutsen, L., & Humphreys, G. W. (2000). Axis-based grouping reduces visual extinction. *Neuropsychologia, 38,* 896–905.

Brefczynski, J. A., & de Yoe, E. A. (1999). A physiological correlate of the "spotlight" of visual attention. *Nature Neuroscience, 2,* 370–374.

Butter, C. M., & Trobe, J. D. (1994). Integrative agnosia following progressive multifocal leukoencaphalopathy. *Cortex, 30,* 145–158.

Chainay, H., & Humphreys, G. W. (2001). The real object advantage in agnosia: Evidence of a role for shading and depth in object recognition. *Cognitive Neuropsychology, 18,* 175–191.

Cohen, A., & Rafal, R. D. (1991) Attention and feature integration: Illusory conjunctions in a patient with a parietal lobe lesion. *Psychological Science, 2,* 106–110.

Cooper, A. C. G., & Humphreys, G. W. (2000). Coding space within but not between objects: Evidence from Balint's syndrome. *Neuropsychologia, 38,* 1607–1615.

Cowey, A. (1994). Cortical visual areas and the neurobiology of higher visual processes. In M. J. Farah

& G. Ratcliff (Eds.), *The neuropsychology of high-level vision.* pp. 3–31. Hillsdale, N.J.: Lawrence Erlbaum Associates.

Crick, F. (1984). The function of the thalamic reticular spotlight: The searchlight hypothesis. *Proceedings of the National Academy of Sciences, 81,* 4586–4590.

DeRenzi, E. (1982). *Disorders of space exploration and cognition.* New York: Wiley.

DeRenzi, E., & Lucchelli, F. (1993). The fuzzy boundaries of apperceptive agnosia. *Cortex, 29,* 187–215.

Desimone, R., & Ungerleider, L.G. (1989). Neural mechanisms of visual processing in monkeys. In E. Boller & J. Grafman (Eds.), *Handbook of neuropsychology. II.* Amsterdam: Elsevier Science.

Donk, M. (1999). Illusory conjunctions are an illusion: The effects of target-nontarget similarity on conjunction and feature errors. *Journal of Experimental Psychology: Human Perception and Performance, 25,* 1207–1233.

Donnelly, N., Humphreys, G. W. & Riddoch, M. J. (1991). Parallel computation of primitive shape descriptions. *Journal of Experimental Psychology: Human Perception and Performance, 17,* 561–570.

Duncan, J., & Humphreys, G. W. (1989). Visual search and stimulus similarity. *Psychological Review, 96,* 433–458.

Eckhorn, R. (1999). Neural mechanisms of visual feature binding investigated with microelectrodes and models. *Visual Cognition, 6,* 231–266.

Elliott, M. A., & Muller, H. M. (1998). Synchronous information presented in 40Hz flicker enhances visual feature binding. *Psychological Science, 9,* 277–283.

Ellis, A. W. W. W., Flude, B., & Young, A. W. (1987). Neglect dyslexia and the early visual processing of letters in words and nonwords. *Cognitive Neuropsychology, 4,* 439–464.

Enns, J., & Rensink, R. A. (1991). Preattentive recovery of three-dimensional orientation from line drawings. *Psychological Review, 98,* 335–351.

Fahle, M. (1993). Figure-ground discrimination from temporal information. *Proceedings of the Royal Society, B254,* 199–203.

Friedman-Hill, S., Robertson, L. C., & Treisman, A. (1995). Parietal contributions to visual feature binding: Evidence from a patient with bilateral lesions. *Science, 269,* 853–855.

Giersch, A., Humphreys, G. W., Boucart, M., & Kovács, I. (2000). The computation of occluded contours in visual agnosia: Evidence for early computation prior to shape binding and figure-ground coding. *Cognitive Neuropsychology, 17,* 731–759.

Gilbert, C., Ito, M., Kapadia, M., & Westheimer, G. (2000). Interactions between attention, context and learning in primary visual cortex. *Vision Research, 40,* 1217–1226.

Gilbert, C., & Wiesel, T. N. (1989). Columnar specificity of intronsic horizontal and corticocortical connections in cat visual cortex. *Journal of Neuroscience, 9,* 2432–2442.

Gilchrist, I., Humphreys, G. W., & Riddoch, M. J. (1996). Grouping and extinction: Evidence for low-level modulation of selection. *Cognitive Neuropsychology, 13,* 1223–1256.

Goodrich, S. J., & Ward, R. (1997). Anti-extinction following unilateral parietal damage. *Cognitive Neuropsychology, 14,* 595–612.

Grosof, D. H., Shapley, R. M., & Hawken, M. J. (1993). Macaque V1 neurons can signal "illusory" contours. *Nature, 257,* 219–220.

Gross, C. G., Rocha-Miranda, C. E., & Bender, D. B. (1972). Visual properties of neurons in inferotemporal cortex. *Journal of Neurophysiology, 35,* 96–111.

Grossberg, S., & Mingolla, E. (1985). Neural dynamics of form perception: Boundary completion, illusory figures, and neon color spreading. *Psychological Review, 92,* 173–221.

Grossberg, S., & Pessoa, L. (1998). Texture segregation, surface representation and figure-ground separation. *Vision Research, 38,* 2657–2684.

Hall, D., Humphreys, G. W., & Cooper, A. C. G. (2001). Neuropsychological evidence for case-specific reading: Multi-letter units in visual word recognition. *Quarterly Journal of Experimental Psychology, 54,* 439–467.

Heywood, C. A., & Cowey, A. (1999). Cerebral achromatopsia. In G. W. Humphreys (Ed.), *Case studies in the neuropsychology of vision.* pp. 17–40. London: Psychology Press.

Heywood, C. A. & Zihl, J. (1999). Motion blindness. In G. W. Humphreys (Ed.), *Case studies in the neuropsychology of vision.* pp. 1–16. London: Psychology Press.

Hillyard, S. A., Vogel, E. K., & Luck, S. J. (1998). Sensory gain control (amplification) as a mechanism of selective attention: Electrophysiological and neuroimaging evidence. *Philosophical Transactions of the Royal Society, B353,* 1257–1270.

Humphreys, G. W. (1998). Neural representation of objects in space: A dual coding account. *Philosophical Transactions of the Royal Society, B353,* 1341–1352.

Humphreys, G. W. (1999). Integrative agnosia. In G. W. Humphreys (Ed.), *Case studies in the neuropsychology of vision* (pp. 41–58). London: Psychology Press.

Humphreys, G. W., Cinel, C., Wolfe, J., Olson, A., & Klempen, N. (2000). Fractionating the binding process: Neuropsychological evidence distinguishing binding of form from binding of surface features. *Vision Research, 40,* 1569–1596.

Humphreys, G. W., & Donnelly, N. (2000). 3D constraints on spatially parallel shape processing. *Perception and Psychophysics, 62,* 1060–1085.

Humphreys, G. W., Quinlan, P. T., & Riddoch, M. J. (1989). Grouping processes in visual search: Effects with single- and combined-feature targets. *Journal of Experimental Psychology: General, 118,* 258–279.

Humphreys, G. W., & Riddoch, M. J. (1987). *To see or not to see: A case study of visual agnosia.* Hillsdale, NJ: Lawrence Erlbaum Associates.

Humphreys, G. W., & Riddoch, M. J. (1993). Interactions between object and space vision revealed through neuropsychology. In D. E. Meyer & S. Kornblum (Eds.), *Attention and performance XIV* (pp. 143–162). Cambridge, MA: MIT Press.

Humphreys, G. W., Romani, C., Olson, A., Riddoch, M. J., & Duncan, J. (1994). Non-spatial extinction following lesions of the parietal lobe in humans. *Nature, 372,* 357–359.

Jeannerod, M. (1997). *The cognitive neuroscience of action.* Oxford: Blackwells.

Karnath, H.-O. (1988). Deficits of attention in acute and recovered visual hemi-neglect. *Neuropsychologia, 26,* 27–43.

Kellman, P. J., & Shipley, T. F. (1991). A theory of visual interpolation in object perception. *Cognitive Psychology, 23,* 141–221.

Kovács, I. (2000). Human development of perceptual organization. *Vision Research, 40,* 1301–1310.

Kubovy, M., Cohen, D. J., & Hollier, J. (1999). Featured integration that routinely occurs without focal attention. *Psychonomic Bulletin & Review, 6,* 183–203.

Kumada, T., & Humphreys, G. W. (2001). Lexical recovery from extinction: Interactions between visual form and stored knowledge modulate visual selection. *Cognitive Neuropsychology, 18,* 465–478.

Lawson, R., & Humphreys, G. W. (1999). The effects of view in depth on the identification of line drawings and silhouettes of familiar objects. *Visual Cognition, 6,* 165–196.

Linnell, K., & Humphreys, G. W. (2001). Spatially parallel processing of within-dimension conjunctions. *Perception, 30,* 49–60.

Mattingly, J. B., Davis, G., & Driver, J. (1997). Pre-attentive filling in of visual surfaces in parietal extinction. *Science, 275,* 671–674.

Mendola, J. D., Dale, A. M., Fischl, B., Liu, A. K., & Tootell, R. B. H. (1999). The representation of illusory and real contours in human cortical visual areas revealed by functional magnetic resonance imaging. *Journal of Neuroscience, 19,* 8560–8572.

Milner, A. D., & Goodale, M. A. (1995). *The visual brain in action.* Oxford, UK: Oxford University Press.

Milner, A. D., Perrett, D. I., Johnston, R. S., Benson, P. J., Jordan, T. R., Heeley, D. W., Bettucci, D., Mortara, F., Mutani, R., Terazzi, E., & Davidson, D. L. W. (1991). Perception and action in "visual form agnosia." *Brain, 114,* 405–428.

Moran, J., & Desimone, R. (1985). Selective attention gates visual processing in the extra-striate cortex. *Science, 229,* 782–784.

Mordkoff, J. T., Yantis, S., & Egeth, H. E. (1990). Detecting conjuncitons of color and form in parallel. *Perception and Psychophysics, 48,* 157–168.

Prinzmetal, W., Treiman, R., & Rho, S. H. (1986). How to see a reading unit. *Journal of Memory and Language, 25,* 461–475.

Redies, C., Crook, J. M., & Creutzfelt, O. D. (1986). Neural response to borders with and without luminance gradients in cat visual cortex and dorsal lateral geniculate nucleus. *Experimental Brain Research, 61,* 49–81.

Rensink, R. A., & Enns, J. (1995). Pre-emption effects in visual search: Evidence for low-level grouping. *Psychological Review, 102,* 101–130.

Riddoch, M. J. & Humphreys, G. W. (1987). A case of integrative visual agnosia. *Brain, 110,* 1431–1462.

Riddoch, M. J., Humphreys, G. W., Gannon, T., Blott, W., & Jones, V. (1999). Memories are made of this: The effects of time on stored knowledge in a case of visual agnosia. *Brain, 122,* 537–559.

Robertson, L. C., Treisman, A., Friedman-Hill, S., & Grabowecky, M. (1997). A possible connection between spatial deficits and feature binding in a patient with parietal damage. *Journal of Cognitive Neuroscience, 9,* 295–317.

Shallice, T., & Warrington, E. K. (1977). The possible role of selective attention in acquired dyslexia. *Neuropsychologia, 15,* 31–41.

Sheth, B. R., Sharma, J., Rao, S. C., & Sur, M. (1996). Orientation maps of subjective contours in visual cortex. *Science, 274,* 2110–2115.

Shipley, T. F., & Kellman, P. J. (1992). Perception of partly occluded objects and illusory figures: Evidence for an identity hypothesis. *Journal of Experimental Psychology: Human Perception and Performance, 18,* 106–120.

Singer, W., & Gray, C. M. (1995). Visual feature integration and the temporal correlation hypothesis. *Annual Review of Neuroscience, 18,* 555–586.

Stark, M., Coslett, H. B., & Saffran, E. (1996). Impairment of an egocentric map of locations: Implications for perception and action. *Cognitive Neuropsychology, 13,* 481–524.

Tootell, R. B. H., Reppas, J. B., Kwong, K., Malach, R., Born, R. T., Brady, T. J., Rosen, B. R., & Belliveau, J. W. (1995). Functional analysis of human MT and related visual cortical areas using magnetic resonance imaging. *Journal of Neuroscience, 15,* 3215–3230.

Treisman, A. (1998). Feature binding, attention and object perception. *Philosophical Transactions of the Royal Society, 353,* 1295–1306.

Treisman, A., & Gelade, G. (1980). A feature-integration theory of attention. *Cognitive Psychology, 12,* 97–136.

Treisman, A., & Schmidt, H. (1982). Illusory conjunctions in the perception of objects. *Cognitive Psychology, 14,* 107–141.

Ungerleider, L. G., & Haxby, J. V. (1994). "What" and "where" in the human brain. *Current Opinions in Neurobiology, 4,* 157–165.

Ungerleider, L. G., & Mishkin, M. (1982). Two cortical visual systems. In D. I. Ingle, M. A. Goodale, & R. J. W. Manfield (Eds.), *Analysis of visual behavior.* pp. 549–586. Cambridge, MA: MIT Press.

Vecera, S. P., & Farah, M. J. (1994). Does visual attention select objects or locations? *Journal of Experimental Psychology: General, 123,* 146–160.

von der Heydt, R., & Peterhans, E. (1989). Mechanisms of contour perception in monkey visual cortex. I. Lines of pattern discontinuity. *Journal of Neuroscience, 9,* 1731–1748.

Ward, R., Goodrich, S., & Driver, J. (1994). Grouping reduces visual extinction: Neuropsychological evidence for weight-linkage in visual selection. *Visual Cognition, 1,* 101–130.

Watson, J. D. D., Myers, G. R., Frackowiak, R. S. J., Hajnal, V. J., Woods, R. P., Mazziota, J. C., Ship, S., & Zeki, S. (1993). Area V5 of the human brain: Evidence from a combined study using positron emission tomography and magnetic resonance imaging. *Cerebral Cortex, 3,* 79–84.

Zeki, S. (1993). *A vision of the brain.* Oxford, UK: Blackwell.

IV

Computational Approaches to Perceptual Organization

12 Perceptual Completion and Memory

David W. Jacobs
University of Maryland

This paper sketches an approach to the computational modeling of perceptual organization (PO). I see PO as an integral part of cognition. This means viewing PO as a process of object recognition, in which a generic model of the collective properties of objects is used, instead of a specific model of individual objects. That is, PO is part of the process of visual memory. I also take the view that processes analogous to PO can play a similar role in nonvisual memory. Memory is an interaction between some novel situation or memory cue and prior knowledge. I propose that memory proceeds by first using generic models to analyze the current situation. The results then trigger more specific items in memory. This process can be repeated until a good fit is found between specific memory items and the current cue. In this view, PO is the first step in the process of bringing our prior knowledge of the world into alignment with a current image of it.

To make this argument concrete I discuss specific models of illusory contour formation (Williams & Jacobs, 1997a, 1997b) and word memory (Jacobs, Rokers, Rudra, & Liu, 2002). These models address just one aspect of PO, that of the completion of a fragmented object. This occurs in vision when illusory contours fill in the gaps between the visible contours of a surface. It can occur in a word memory task when the presence of some letters in a word trigger the memory of the entire word. Although there is no percept in word memory that is analogous to the percept of an illusory contour, I present a model in which a similar filling-in acts as a precursor to word recall.

I also make use of one simple way of building a generic model of objects in memory, that of a one-dimensional Markov model (see, e.g., Geman & Geman, 1984, for important work on the use of Markov models in vision; Mumford, 1994 for a discussion of Markov models of contours; and Zhu, 1999, for a different approach to characterizing Gestalt laws using Markov models). This treats both a contour and a word as a one-dimensional string. A Markov model is a probabilistic model of contours or strings that assumes that the local properties of the object depend on their spatial neighborhood but are otherwise independent of the properties of more distant parts of the object. This is a simple approximation to the true complexities of the world. I do not argue that such Markov models can capture all phenomena in perceptual organization. However, they can capture a good deal and offer a concrete example of how a generic model can be used for perceptual completion and as part of a recognition process.

I treat PO, and memory in general, as the process of combining a model with current knowledge to reconcile the two. This is a computationally well-understood process when Markov models are used. In the case of word memory, one can solve this problem using belief propagation (Pearl, 1988). To handle contours more novel techniques that are still quite related to belief propagation must be developed. This will lead to a simple, neurally plausible architecture for the computation of illusory contours. In this model, Williams & Jacobs (1997a) interprets illusory contours as representing a probability distribution on the position and orientation of image contours. This distribution takes account of the immediate image and the generic model of object shape. In the case of word memory, Jacobs et al. (2002) also use a generic model to compute a probability distribution on the possible ways of completing a word fragment. This is then incorporated into a model in which this probability distribution triggers individual words in memory. This model is similar in spirit to previous models that combine top-down and bottom-up information (e.g., Kosko, 1987; Rumelhart & McClelland, 1982; Ullman, 1996). Our model differs from these primarily in our use of Markov models. This allows PO to be interpreted as the exact solution to a probabilistic inference problem. We also use a Markov model as an intermediate feature set to mediate matching between input and memory.

Parts of this chapter appear also in Jacobs (2001), which describes in greater detail our work on PO. Here, I more briefly survey that work and discuss its relation to our model of memory. My main goal is to argue that perceptual organization can be viewed as a part of memory in general. Hopefully, this may suggest new ways of examining memory processes and of understanding PO.

GENERIC OBJECT MODELS: MARKOV MODELS

In illusory contour displays parts of the boundary of an object are made explicit by significant gradients in intensity. In other parts, there is no intensity gradient, though an illusory gradient is perceived. One can say that the visual system perceives a surface boundary based on information present in the image and also based on the general properties of the surfaces of objects. Such general properties may be that contours tend to smoothly continue from one place to another, that an object's surface sometimes blends into the background, that corners are often signals for occlusions, and so forth. This view goes back at least to the Gestalt psychologists. We have built on this view by modeling illusory contour formation as probabilistic inference that combines prior information about shape with the image.

To make this approach to illusory contours explicit requires a representation of one's prior expectations about object shape. I show how to capture this knowledge using Markov models. I begin by explaining what I mean by a Markov model. I explain this for the case of words, which are simplest. I then describe Markov models of contours, pointing out that these can capture many properties known to be important in PO.

Consider first a string of letters. A Markov model of these strings is a probabilistic model. It assigns a probability to each string, stating how likely it is to occur. One can think of this probability as a coarse estimate of the probability that this string will occur in an English text, for example. The model is Markov if the probability is estimated by taking the product of probabilities based on local portions of the string.

For illustrative purposes, I consider models based only on bigrams, that is, on pairs of letters. However, everything generalizes to larger neighborhoods of letters. So with a bigram model, the probability of finding the string *the* is estimated as the probability of finding a string starting with *t*, times the probability that a *t* will be followed by an *h*, times the probability that an *h* will be followed by an *e*, times the probability that an *e* will end a word. With such a model, the probability of the third letter being an *e* depends on the identity of the second letter. But once this identity is known, the first letter in the word has no effect on the probability of the third. That is, nonadjacent letters are conditionally independent given the identity of any intervening letters.

Another way to look at this is as follows: Suppose, using a bigram model, one wishes to guess the identity of the fourth letter in a string. Knowing that the fifth letter is an *s* would help because one knows that some letters are more likely to be followed by an *s* than others. If one didn't know the identity of the third letter, then knowing the second letter would also help. The second letter tells which letters are most likely to come third, and this tells about the probability of different letters

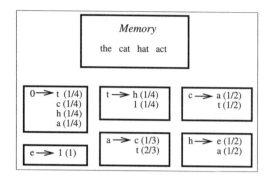

FIG. 12.1.   A Markov model for a small dictionary. The probability of each letter occurring is shown, given the preceeding letter.

coming fourth. But, if one does know the third letter, then also knowing the second letter doesn't help at all; it provides no additional information about the fourth letter.

As a quick example of a bigram model, suppose the entire dictionary consisted of the words: *the, cat, hat, act.* Denote the beginning of a word as *0,* and the end as *1,* so that the string *0t* means that a word begins with *t.* Fig. 12.1 describes bigram probabilities for a possible Markov model of this small dictionary. If one assumes that each of the four words really appears with a 1 in 4 probability, the Markov model produces strings that only approximate these probabilities. Each of these four words will have a nonzero probability of occurring, according to this Markov model. For example, *cat* will occur with probability $\frac{1}{4} \times \frac{1}{2} \times \frac{2}{3} \times \frac{3}{4} = \frac{1}{16}$. On the other hand, nonwords, such as *cthact,* will also occur.

This kind of Markov model is very compact compared with a full model of English. A full model might list the spelling of about 100,000 words. The bigram model described requires one to know 728 probabilities (the probability of each pair of letters occurring, plus the probability of each letter beginning or ending a word). In this sense they are a tremendously simplified model of the set of all words that one knows. As I show later, they provide computational advantages as well.

Markov models are widely studied in math. My description has been extremely informal, but a full, rigorous discussion can be found in Taylor and Karlin (1998), for example. Markov models have also been applied to language, most famously by Shannon (1951), and they form the basis for common compression algorithms. They have also been widely used in the computational study of vision (see, e.g., Chellappa and Jain, 1993).

Similarly, one can produce a compact, Markov model of contours. In this case, one evaluates the likelihood that a shape is an object boundary by looking separately at only small portions of the shape (see Fig. 12.2). At any one time, one only considers the portion of the shape that is visible through a small

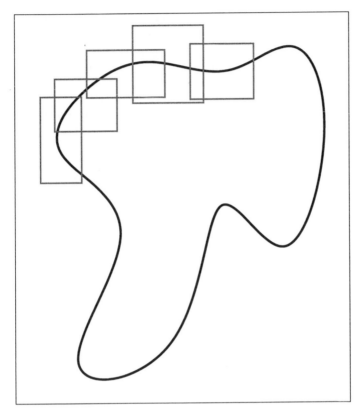

FIG. 12.2. In a local model of contour shape, the likelihood of a contour is found by sliding a small window around the contour, accumulating evidence.

window and forms a judgment about how likely this piece of the shape is to belong to an object boundary. One then combines information over the entire shape. The next section makes the computational advantages of such a simple shape model more explicit. The question I consider in this section is the extent to which such a local model of shape can be powerful enough to encode the properties of shape that seem to be used by the visual system in perceptual grouping.

The main difference between a Markov model of text and of contours is that contours are one-dimensional strings embedded in a two-dimensional world, whereas text is purely a one-dimensional string. Also, contours are continuous objects, but one can approximate them as being composed of a finite number of points that are strung together, such as a list of adjacent pixels along the contour. Then if one has a Markov model of shape, it just means that the probability of each point appearing with certain properties depends only on the properties of a specified set of neighbors, which can be inside a local window on the contour. If one says this model is low order, it means that this window isn't too big.

I describe shape models in which the probability that a point is on a boundary depends only on very local information. At times it is useful to think of the boundary as a discrete set of points, and at times it is useful to think of it as a continuous curve. In the first case, given two adjacent points on a contour, the direction between them approximates the tangent to the curve. Given three adjacent points, one can make a discrete approximation to the curvature of the curve based on the magnitude of the change in the tangent direction. With four points, one can determine the change in curvature to, for example, detect inflection points in the curve. If, on the other hand, one thinks of the boundary as a continuous curve, then rather than basing the measure of likelihood on a small number of points, one can base it on the first few derivatives of the curve. That is, one can base it directly on the tangent, curvature, or change in curvature. These are simply the limit of the properties that one can approximate using a small number of points, as these points get closer together.

One can see that the Gestalt property of good continuation can be encoded as a low-order Markov property of curves (Mumford, 1994). It has been noted that a curve that exhibits good continuation can be described as a curve with minimal amounts of curvature (e.g., Horn, 1981; Ullman, 1976). This can be measured as the energy of the curve, given by the equation

$$\int_{t \in \Gamma} \kappa^2(t)\, dt, \qquad (1)$$

where $\kappa(t)$ represents the curvature at a point t on the curve, Γ. In the discrete case, one can think of this measure as expressing a model of contours in which the probability of a point on the curve having a particular tangent direction depends only on the tangent at the previous point. The curvature is the normalized change in the tangent. Mumford (1994) suggests a stochastic model of contours in which the curvature is drawn from a normal distribution with 0 mean. In this case, the probability of a contour decreases as its energy increases; in fact, the negative log of the probability of a curve is its energy. This implies that models of illusory contour formation that consider the curve of least energy connecting two inducing elements can also be thought of as computing the likeliest shape drawn from a Markov model. This Markov model is just a generic model of shape that says shapes tend to be smooth. Fig. 12.3 provides an illustration of contours drawn from this and from other random processes.

This contour model has one parameter, the variance of the normal distribution on curvature. This controls how rapidly the orientation of a curve changes. Intuitively, if the variance is close to 0, the model will generate contours that are almost straight lines and that change direction very slowly. When variance is large, contours will become much more wiggly and reverse directions quickly.

Closure is another Gestalt property that can be encoded as a local property of a contour. A curve is closed if and only if every point on the curve has neighbors on

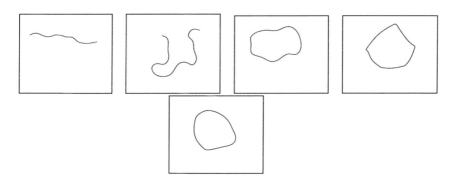

FIG. 12.3. These are schematic renderings of contours that might be generated by different random processes. On the left, is a contour whose probability is inversely related to its energy and where large curvatures are unlikely. Next, a contour from a similar process but with large curvatures less unlikely. In the bottom middle, a contour like this but restricted to be closed. Next, a closed contour in which large curvatures are unlikely but discontinuities in curvature, though rare, are not impossible. Finally, a closed contour in which inflection points have 0 probability.

both sides. An endpoint of the curve can be found locally. If one wants to enforce the property that object boundaries must be closed, one can say that such endpoints have 0 probability of occurring.

For a generic model of shape to be useful, it must assign a reasonable probability to the boundaries of objects that really occur. The model based on the energy of the curve has the disadvantage of not producing boundaries with corners. This is because the curvature of a contour is not defined at a discontinuity. When one discretely samples a boundary with a corner, one will assign a very high curvature at the location of the corner. This curvature will diverge to infinity as the sampling rate increases. This leads to the undesirable property that shapes with corners have 0 probability of occurring. If one wishes to use a shape model, for example, to produce illusory contours with corners, as seen in Koffka cross stimuli (e.g., Fig. 12.4; Sambin, 1974), the model must produce shapes with corners.

Thornber and Williams (1997) show that one can handle this by allowing a discontinuity to occur at any point on a contour, with some fixed, small probability. They use this to model the formation of illusory contours having corners. This is similar to the line process that is used in Markov random fields (e.g., Blake & Zisserman, 1987; Geman & Geman, 1984).

Such a shape model now has two parameters that indicate how curvy the contours are that it generates and how often they generate discontinuities. By adjusting these parameters, one can generate different sorts of shapes. For example, one can set curvature variance to 0 but allow for occasional discontinuities so that the contour never changes direction except at discontinuities. In this case, the shape

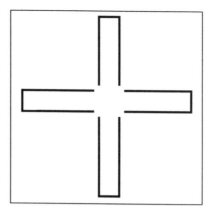

FIG. 12.4. A figure of the Koffka cross, in which subjects tend to see illusory contours with corners.

model produces polygons. Or one can set variance high and make discontinuities rare so that one gets rather wiggly shapes. In the world, the surface properties of a shape may change from one part of a shape to another. For example, much of a person's body may have a very smooth shape, whereas one's hair may have a much more wiggly shape. The models described until now will assign low probabilities to such shapes because if the parameters are chosen to make a smooth shape likely, they will make a wiggly shape unlikely, and vice versa. Shapes that have varying characteristics may be produced by a nonstationary Markov process. In such a process, the parameters of the model are also allowed to change stochastically. So as one moves along the contour, just as there is some small chance that a discontinuity will occur, there is also a small chance that the smoothness parameter will change so that a wiggly or smooth shape becomes more likely from that point on, until the parameters change again.

As a final shape property, I note that some aspects of convexity can also be captured by local shape models. This is because the transition on a contour from convex to concave, called an inflection point, is a local property of a shape. If one makes inflection points unlikely, then when part of a contour is convex, the ensuing parts of the contour will also be likely to be convex. This produces contours with long stretches that are either all convex or all concave. If inflection points are assigned 0 probability, then all contours generated will either be completely convex or completely concave (e.g., holes). In Liu, Jacobs, and Basri (1999) we consider at much greater length whether this kind of local model of convexity is adequate to model human sensitivity to convexity in contours.

In completion problems, fragments of contours are connected together into the boundaries of surfaces in spite of the presence of gaps. To determine the likelihood that a particular set of fragments come from a real object boundary, one therefore needs not only a model of object shape but also a model that can tell how likely a particular gap is to separate two contour fragments that come from the same object. For example, in amodal completion, a gap in the visible boundary of an object is caused by occlusion by another object. Grouping across gaps by proximity can also be captured using a low-order Markov model of shape. This too was done by Mumford (1994). To do this, when one looks at a local window of a shape that is being completed across a gap, one assigns some probability to the gap continuing across that small length. These local probabilities accumulate multiplicatively so that in crossing a long gap one pays a penalty that is the product of many local penalties. This represents the idea that it is increasingly unlikely for a contour to continue to remain hidden from view over an increasingly longer stretch of the image.

One can therefore build a model of contour shape and contour gaps that captures a number of Gestalt properties, such as good continuation, closure, convexity, and proximity. A visual system can use such a model to solve completion problems. In a contour completion problem, an image contains a number of contour fragments. The problem is to choose some of these fragments to join together so that they are perceived as the boundary of a surface. Using shape and gap models one can, for example, for any hypothesized grouping of fragments, determine whether the possible shape of the object fitting these fragments, and the associated gaps in it, are likely. This gives one a basis for choosing a preferred completion as the one that is most likely to be the boundary of an object. In spirit, this is much like many models of perceptual completion. My view emphasizes that an explicit probabilistic inference can explain perceptual completion. In Jacobs (1997) I present a more comprehensive discussion of the relationship between a much larger set of Gestalt grouping cues and local image properties. I now turn to the question of how to perform computations using Markov models.

COMPUTATION WITH MARKOV MODELS

A Markov model of contours or text is generic in the sense that it combines together in a simple form the properties of a large number of objects. The specifics of individual words or objects are lost, and only average local properties remain. Why use a generic model instead of, for example, just directly using a detailed model that includes every word or contour ever seen? The main reason is that a generic model, especially in the form of a Markov model, leads to tremendous computational simplicity.[1] I try to illustrate that now.

This chapter is limited to completion problems, in which part of a word or contour is given, and the remainder must be inferred using prior knowledge. I first show how Markov models can be used to compute contour completions.

---

[1]It may also be true that a generic model is useful in coping with novel objects, but this is aside from my main point.

Specifically, one computes the probability that contour is present in every position and orientation in an image. These probabilities can be directly related to the percept of an illusory contour. Then I show how a Markov model and text fragments can be used to compute the probability of each bigram (or n-gram) being present in a completed word. This has no direct perceptual correlate, but I show how it can play a role in a complete memory system. By analogy, I argue that in a similar way, perceptual grouping can play a role in a complete memory system.

The problem of completion in Markov models of strings has been solved using belief propagation. The problem is somewhat different for contours, and I describe an algorithm that is specific to computing with Markov models of contours. This algorithm can be mapped into a simple neural net. I then describe how belief propagation can be used directly on text fragments and discuss the close relationship between belief propagation and our method of contour completion.

Contour Completion

I now show concretely how a parallel, neurally plausible system can use Markov shape and occlusion models to compute the shape and salience of illusory contours. This section primarily summarizes the work in Williams and Jacobs (1997a, 1997b).

I describe the process of illusory contour formation using Kanizsa's famous example (Fig. 12.5) as an illustration (Kanizsa, 1979). In this case, a square is perceived as lying on top of and partially occluding four disks, although in fact only four black partial circles are physically present in the image. The visual system explains the missing edges of the square as due to the square's intensity nearly matching that of the background.

The image consists of 12 smooth curves in the form of 4 circular arcs, 1 for each partial circle, and 8 line segments. The junctions between the line segments

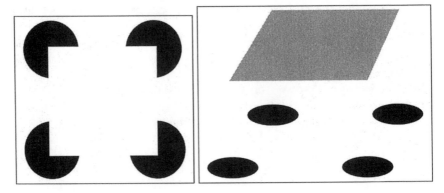

FIG. 12.5.   An example of an illusory contour figure (left) and its possible interpretation (right).

and circular arcs are sharp corners, which serve as a clue of the possible occlusion of one shape by another. This indicates that it is possible that the images of the partial circles are each formed by an object with a straight edge lying on top of an object with a circular arc. Creating an interpretation of the entire image can be viewed as the process of joining edge fragments into smooth surfaces that are most consistent with the image and the prior models of surface shape and occlusion and determining which of these surfaces lie on top of which. Such an approach is developed in, for example, Williams and Hanson (1996) or Nitzburg and Mumford (1990).

In this section I describe a solution to only one piece of this problem. Given two edge fragments, one determines some measure of the likelihood that they should be joined together in a single contour and the shape and salience of the possible completion between them. To do this, one computes a stochastic completion field. This tells, for every position and orientation in the image, the likelihood that there is an edge there, given both the priors and information about the position and orientation where illusory contours begin and end. Given the starting and ending points of an illusory contour, the stochastic completion field resembles, both in shape and salience, the percept of the illusory contour. Given different possible ways of connecting edge fragments into surfaces, the stochastic completion field tells the relative likelihood of these different completions. Therefore, one can see it as a precursor to illusory contour formation.

So one is faced with the following problem: Given the position, and orientation where a contour is supposed to begin and end, which we call source and sink positions, respectively, one wishes to compute, for every other position and orientation, $p = (x, y, \theta)$, in the image, the likelihood that the contour passes through there. One does this using a simple parallel network. First, one breaks the problem of whether a contour passes through p into two subproblems, illustrated in Fig. 12.6. These are finding the likelihood that a contour leaving the source point would pass through p, and the likelihood that the contour would continue on to a sink point. That is, one wants to consider all possible contours from the source to the sink, weighted by their likelihood according to a low-order Markov model, and measure the proportion that passes through each (x, y, θ). This can be expressed as the product of the likelihood that the contour will reach (x, y, θ) and the likelihood that it will go on to a sink because the model of likelihood is local; the likelihood of one part of the contour does not depend on the shape of the previous part of the contour.

One therefore computes a source field, giving for each (x, y, θ) the likelihood that a contour reaches that position from a source and a similar sink field and takes the product of these two. I now describe how to compute the source field, noting that the sink field is computed in exactly the same way because the model of contour probability is the same for both. I describe this computation in intuitive, nonrigorous language and refer the interested reader to Williams and Jacobs (1997a, 1997b) for a precise and rigorous description of the algorithm.

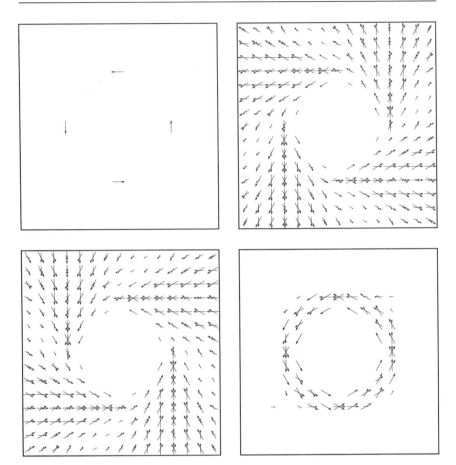

FIG. 12.6. This figure shows an example of source and sink fields when a contour is supposed to pass through four points equally spaced on a circle (top left). The top right shows the computed source field. The length of each vector indicates the probability that a contour passing through an initial position will reach the position and orientation of the vector. The bottom left shows the sink field. The bottom right is the product of the two, the stochastic completion field.

First, consider a somewhat idealized setting in which one ignores issues of discrete sampling. The algorithm proceeds iteratively, at the k'th iteration, finding for each position and orientation **p** the probability that a contour of length k will leave the source and end at **p**. This can be determined by looking at the probability that a contour reached each neighboring point of **p** on the $k - 1$'th iteration, and combining this with the probability that the contour would proceed to **p**. This can be done because the measure of probability is Markov. Consequently, the probability of a contour can be determined by taking the product of local probabilities. Each step from one point to the next on the contour is another local neighborhood, with another probability independent of previous ones. Finally, these probabilities are summed for all values of k, which implicitly assumes that the same contour is unlikely to pass twice through the same point.

In our experiments, the local measure of the likelihood contains a term to represent the smoothness, or good continuation of the contour, and a term to measure the likelihood of gaps. The good continuation term is based on a normal distribution of curvature, as previously described. Given a prior position and orientation for a curve, the orientation indicates the direction the curve is moving in; that is, it tells the position of the next point on the curve. So a point will precede **p** only if it is at an adjacent location, with an orientation pointing towards **p**. Furthermore, the difference between the orientation of the preceding point and the orientation of **p** tells how much the orientation of the curve has changed. The good continuation prior tells how likely any particular change in orientation is, penalizing large changes more than small. In sum, to determine the likelihood that a contour leaving a source winds up at **p** at its k'th point, one needs to look at the neighbors of **p** that point to it and multiply the probability that the contour is at those points at the $k - 1$'st step by the probability that they go on to **p** at the next step.

This description of the algorithm is radically oversimplified because I have ignored the issue of how one can perform these computations with a discrete set of computational units. In this case, only a discrete set of (x, y, θ) positions can be directly represented. Moreover, if one represents one particular (x, y, θ) position, the place that this position points to may not be directly represented. For example, if one unit represents the position $(17, 23, \pi/8)$, this points to contour locations with $(x, y) = (17 + \cos(\pi/8), 23 + \sin(\pi/8))$. But this location may lie in between points that are directly represented by units. To handle this problem, we use a continuous formulation of how the probability distribution representing the location of contours diffuses in position/orientation space given by a set of partial differential equations in Mumford (1994). These equations describe the likelihood of the contour position being at any particular place after any particular arc length as diffusing through the space of positions and orientations and is exact for the continuous case. One then uses numerical techniques designed to solve partial differential equations on a discrete grid. This allows one to accurately and stably approximate the computation of these probabilities using computational units that represent a discrete set of positions and orientations. The basic structure of this algorithm is as previously described, with each computational unit updating its probability based on its neighbor's values. However, when one unit does not point exactly to another, a contour through it must be considered to have some probability of reaching each of its neighbors on the next step, depending on how closely it points to each of them. Moreover, if some units are more than one step away, the contour must be given some probability of reaching these units and some probability of staying in the same position at the next step for its path to be accurately represented on average. This provides a stochastic representation of the contour's path through the network. Williams and Jacobs (1997b) contains details of this method. More recently, Zweck and Williams (2000) described a more accurate way of solving this partial differential equation with a related method but using a wavelet basis to represent positions and orientations.

In addition to judging likelihood based on good continuation, the algorithm also takes account of the likelihood of gaps. In modeling illusory contour formation, the entire contour from the source to the sink is a gap, in the sense that a contour is hypothesized even though no intensity edge is present in the image. Mumford (1994) suggested a model in which the probability of a gap of some length is set to a constant, and the probability of a longer gap is just the product of the probability of shorter gaps (i.e., the probability falls off exponentially with length). Williams and Jacobs (1997b) add to this the idea that the likelihood of an illusory contour crossing a gap in the image can be modulated by local brightness information. This means, for example, that one can make it unlikely for an illusory contour to cross an edge in the image. Edges are known to interfere with illusory contour information (e.g., Ramachandran, Ruskin, Cobb, Rogers-Ramachandran, & Tyler, 1994; Rock and Anson, 1979). On the other hand, if an illusory contour at some point actually follows a faint edge, one can reduce the penalty for gaps to the extent that this local information indicates that an edge may be present.

It is easy to integrate this gap penalty into the previous computational scheme. The local penalty for moving from one contour position to another is now modulated by the local intensity pattern, penalizing movement across a gap, penalizing even more movement across an edge, and penalizing less movement along an edge.

Some experimental results are shown with this system in Fig. 12.7, 12.8, and 12.9. The first two figures show results for simple illusory contour stimuli, whereas Fig. 12.9 shows how the stochastic completion field can be modulated by local intensity patterns. Williams and Jacobs (1997a, 1997b) contain many more experimental results.

I want to stress that although I have described this algorithm very informally, it computes illusory contour strength directly as the probability that positions and orientations lie on the boundary of an object, given the generic model of object shape and of the formation of gaps in object boundaries and subject to initial information about the position where the illusory contour may begin and end. In this sense, one has a precise, generic model of objects, and one interprets illusory contour formation as the recognition of the most likely position of generic objects.

I consider this to be a neurally plausible model because its computational requirements are modest and roughly matched to those of visual cortex. The method requires computational units for a discrete sampling of every position and orientation in the image. Such an array of neurons is known to be present in the visual cortex. These units only need to compute weighted sums of their neighbors' values. Fixed weight links between each unit and its neighbors can encode the probability

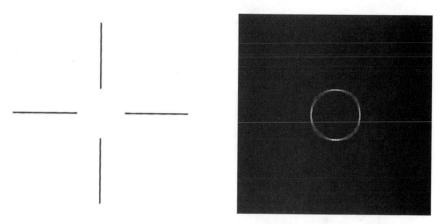

FIG. 12.7. On the left, an Ehrenstein figure. On the right, the stochastic completion field computed from it. Intensity at a pixel is proportional, on a log scale, to the probability at that position, summed over all orientations, for ease of visualization.

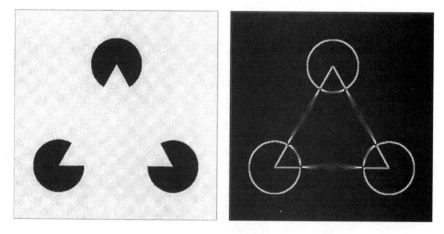

FIG. 12.8. The stochastic completion field for a Kanizsa figure.

of a contour passing from one unit to its neighbor. This requires a minimal amount of computation and connectivity in the network, probably much less than is actually present. This means that there are many simple ways of mapping the system into regions of the brain.

The model is distinguished by using both an explicit model of shape and occlusion and simple computational mechanisms. For example, Sha'ashua and Ullman (1988) proposed a method of computing the salience of contour fragments to which this model is quite related, in that both use a simple network of elements that each represents position and orientation. They pose their computation as a

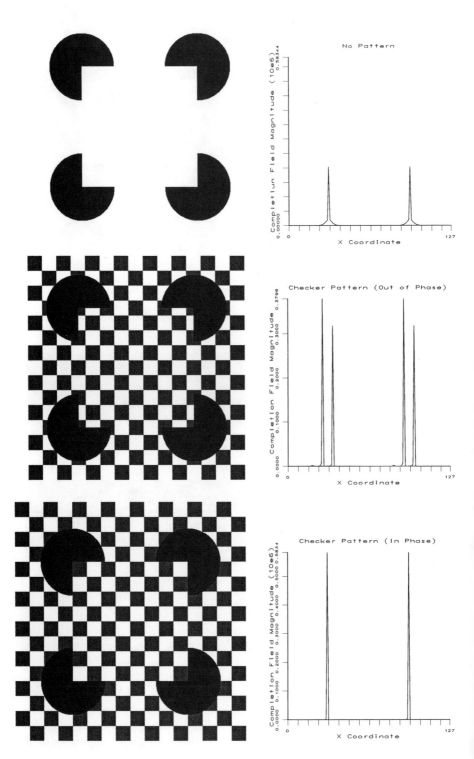

dynamic program, in which each element can update its value based only on its neighbors. The method I describe is different, however, in several key ways. First, one explicitly computes a likelihood measure based on a contour model, whereas Sha'ashua and Ullman proposed a more ad hoc cost function. Second, by posing likelihood propagation as a partial differential equation and solving it in this way, one is able to avoid many discretization artifacts. Alter and Basri (1997) discuss in detail a number of limitations of Sha'ashua and Ullman's scheme that arise from their ad hoc cost function and discretization problems. Third, by computing the product of a source and sink field, one ensures that only contours are considered that close a gap between the hypothesized starting and ending of an occlusion. Sha'ashua and Ullman rely on a more ad hoc approach to finding closed contours, which they recognize to be important for salience.

Heitger and von der Heydt (1993) propose a model that uses convolutions with large support and can be interpreted as something closer to the combination of a source and sink field. Guy and Medioni (1996) present a related model in which evidence for cocircularity is gathered over a large region, although this is not divided into evidence coming from two separate directions. Kumaran, Geiger, and Gurvits (1996) describe another related model, in which evidence about the presence of surfaces are diffused in two dimensions. Grossberg and Mingolla (1985) present a very comprehensive model based on convolution that attempts to account for a great many perceptual phenomena. The models of Heitger and von der Heydt (1993) and Grossberg and Mingolla (1985) are more directly inspired by neurophysiological data. The model I describe is closely related to these but shows how such a model can be derived as explicitly performing generic object recognition using probabilistic inference.

Belief Propagation

I now shift from contours to text. I consider the problem of recalling a known word from memory when only a fragment of that word is presented. This is not just a fragment completion problem; it is a memory problem. However, I show how fragment completion using a generic model can serve as the first step of a memory system. In this section I introduce the fragment completion problem and describe its

---

FIG. 12.9. (facing page) (a) Kanizsa square. (b) Stochastic completion field magnitude along the line $y = 64$. (c) Kanizsa square with out-of-phase checkered background (see Ramachandran, Ruskin, Cobb, Rogers-Ramachandran, & Tyler, 1994). (d) The enhancement of the nearest contrast edge is not noticeable unless the magnitudes are multiplied by a very large factor (i.e., approximately 1.0×10^6). (e) Kanizsa square with in-phase checkered background. (f) The peak completion field magnitude is increased almost threefold, and the distribution has been significantly sharpened.

solution using methods related to those used previously to model illusory contour formation. This also allows me to point out the connections between the illusory contour model I describe and belief propagation. Afterward, I show how this can be integrated into a complete memory system.

I consider memory cues based on the game Superghost. A Superghost cue consists of a sequence of letters, and a matching word contains all of these letters in this order but with possibly intervening letters. One writes a cue as *l*s*r*, where * indicates that the word may contain any number of letters here, including possibly none: *plaster* or *laser* match this cue.

As with illusory contours, portions of an object are present as cues, separated by gaps of unknown length, which must be filled in. Previously, I described how to use a generic Markov model and contour fragments to compute the probability that the true contour passed through each position and orientation of the image. In this section I describe how to use a generic model and text fragments to compute the probability that each bigram (set of two contiguous letters) is present in the true word. The algorithm can be extended to use Markov models of longer n-grams, but it is especially simple for bigrams.

I use the symbols 0 and 1 to indicate the beginning and end of a word, respectively. Then the superghost query *l*s*r can be thought of as implicitly 0*l*s*r*1. Suppose one wants to know how likely it is that the bigram *le* appears in the completion of this query. Then the Markov assumption means one can break this into a simple combination of the probability that it occurs in the completions of 0*l, l*s, s*r, and r*1. This is because the completion of one of these fragments is independent of the likelihood of various completions of the others.

So the problem reduces to one of answering questions such as the following: What is the probability that the completion of l*s contains the bigram *le*? To answer this, one derives a bigram model from the dictionary of words. One also needs a distribution describing gap lengths, that is, of the probability that a * stands for different numbers of missing letters. For this one can use essentially the same distribution that was used to model illusory contours. One assumes that the probability of a gap decreases exponentially with the length of the gap (but limit the maximum gap length to be five, to simplify computation).

For each possible gap length, one has a fixed number of bigrams, and one can represent the probabilistic relationship between them with a belief net (see Fig. 12.10). The probability distribution for each bigram depends on that of its neighbors and on any letters of the bigram that are given in the cue. One can solve this probabilistic inference problem exactly using belief propagation (Pearl, 1988).

In this method evidence about a bigram coming from the bigrams to the right is computed separately from the evidence coming from the left, and finally these two are combined. As a simple example of this process, consider the case where there is one missing letter between *l* and *s*. Going left to right, one computes the probability distribution for the first bigram, given that its first letter must be an *l*, and given also the Markov model of bigrams. Then, one can determine the

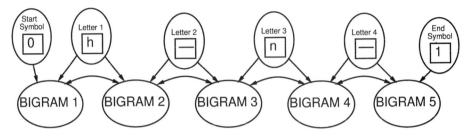

FIG. 12.10. This represents the conditional dependencies between the five bigrams that make up a four-letter word in our representation. The value of each bigram depends on its neighbors, and on the value of the letters in the query that are a part of that bigram. I use 0 and 1 as special symbols to denote the beginning and end of the word.

distribution for the second bigram, combining the distribution of the first with the knowledge that the second letter of the second bigram is s. One repeats this process going right to left. This gives two distributions for each bigram. One takes account of information to the left of the bigram, the other represents information to the right. These can be combined just by taking their product and normalizing. Details of this algorithm and an explanation as to why it is both correct and necessary (a more straightforward use of evidence can lead to an incorrect algorithm) can be found in Pearl (1988).

I have briefly described belief propagation here for two reasons. First, I wish to make the point that when one uses a generic Markov model, one can use it to precisely and efficiently calculate probability distributions on all possible completions of a text query. Secondly, I wish to point out the close connection between belief propagation and the model of illusory contour formation. With text, I have also described the compution of a stochastic completion field, giving the probability that each possible value for each bigram is in the completed word. In computing the stochastic completion field, one separately computes a source field and a sink field and then combines them. This separates evidence indicating a contour at a position into that coming from two different directions. Similarly, in belief propagation, evidence about a bigram must be computed separately for either side of the bigram. Finally, the source and sink fields are computed by locally propagating evidence, using the Markov model to indicate how the evidence at one position supports that at a neighboring one. These similarities are not accidental, of course. In both cases, one is solving the problem of propagating fragmentary evidence using a Markov model.

In general, I view perceptual organization as the process of using a generic model of objects to understand an image, determining which pieces belong together, which parts of the image are relevant or irrelevant, and how to fill in information that cannot be picked up directly in the image. The same processes will be important in any memory process. In any situation, one must parse information into subsets that each might match some item in memory. One wants to use relevant information to trigger appropriate items in memory while ignoring irrelevant information. And only some properties of a relevant memory will be present in the current situation. All this can be done with the aid of general properties of the items in memory. In this section, I discussed specifically how general knowledge about English words can be used to tell us how fragments of words might be completed into full words. This generic knowledge isn't powerful enough to tell exactly how to complete the fragments. But it can provide a starting point for the process of retrieving words from memory, as I now explain.

MEMORY

This section addresses the problem of retrieving items in memory from partial information. In particular, I focus on associative (or content-addressable) memory tasks. Although these tasks are very challenging computationally, people perform them quite well but not perfectly. I present a framework for performing memory tasks in which features are used to mediate the matching process between items in memory and an input query. Features therefore allow approximate matching while requiring much less processing and much less communication between potentially complex inputs and potentially huge memories. At the same time, the choice of features allows one to build a simple generic model of words that interacts with the input query.

Specifically, the memory, M, consists of all words in memory, with a weight associated with each, indicating how likely it is to match the current query. This is initialized with the prior probability of each word appearing in English (in our experiments, we initialize with a uniform weight). The intermediate feature space, F, represents every bigram, each with a weight. And I represents the input query.

The algorithm then proceeds according to the following iteration:

1. One builds a Markov model from the weighted memory, representing the frequency with which each bigram occurs.
2. One combines this Markov model with the input query to determine the probability that each bigram occurs in the completed word. This step was described in the previous section.
3. The previous step provides a probability distribution for each different bigram in the completed word. These are combined to determine the expected number of times each bigram occurs in the word. This assigns a single weight to each bigram.
4. Finally, one updates the weights of each item in memory. Given an estimated probability that each bigram appears in the word, one computes the probability of each word being correct by assuming independence and taking the product of the probability that each bigram of the word is in the input.

These four steps are repeated. Finally, the word with the highest weight is selected as the answer.[2]

This algorithm can be seen as an approximation to a standard iterative approach to finding the nearest neighbors between two sets. In a standard approach, one projects from one set to the other repeatedly, where each projection maps a point to its nearest neighbor in the other set. For convex sets, this iteration produces the points in each set that are closest. In our algorithm, a similar projection occurs but with an intermediate feature space standing between the memory and input. The success of this approach depends on the feature space, F. For efficiency it must be much simpler to compare F to I and M than it is to compare I and M directly. For accuracy, the feature space must be able to approximate M and I reasonably well. One can show analytically that, at least in simple cases, a good feature space guarantees effective performance. Another important point is that by treating M as a probability distribution over all words in memory one can make the memory space convex rather than just a discrete set of remembered items. This reduces problems of local minima in the search. We have applied this approach to two different problems, playing Superghost and recognizing partially occluded images. I discuss only the first here (for the second, see Jacobs and Rudra, 2000).

There has been a great deal of prior work on associative memory, which generally addresses the hangman problem, in which some of the letters of a word, and their exact position in the word, are given as a query. An example of a hangman query is l _ s _ r. Here, one is told, for example, that s is the third letter of the word. These queries are easier to handle computationally but seem less natural to human subjects.

Many recurrent neural networks have been proposed as models of hangman (Anderson, 1995, contains a review). Our model is similar in spirit to the interactive activation model Rumelhart & McClelland, 1982) of reading partly occluded words. In this model, letters that were present in the query activate words they are associated with, which in turn activate representations of possible missing or ambiguous letters. Our model differs in using a Markov model as an intermediate layer between the input query and the words in the dictionary. This allows one to handle Superghost queries naturally; it is not obvious how to extend models of hangman to handle Superghost. It also allows one to exactly compute the probability of each bigram occurring in the completed word, using belief propagation. The cost of this intermediate representation is that the input query is not brought directly in contact with the words in the dictionary. So there is no guarantee that the model will retrieve words that exactly match the query. I discuss the types of mistakes that the model makes and their relationship to human errors momentarily.

---

[2]Probably, this model should be augmented with a step that compares selected memory items to the input to see if they can match. If not, the weight of the selected word can be set to 0, and the iteration can repeat. However, in the experiments below I keep things simple by simply selecting a single answer and measuring how often this is correct.

Also similar in spirit to our approach is the bidirectional model of Kosko (1987s for more recent work see, e.g., Sommer and Palm, 1997). Our approach differs quite a bit from these, though, in that we maintain a complete memory of items and use features as an efficient intermediate step in matching. In maintaining a complete memory of words, our model is also related to the adaptive resonance models of Grossberg and collaborators (e.g., Carpenter & Grossberg, 1987; Grossberg, 1987). Again, our model differs from these in the use of Markov models as an intermediate representation for matching.

Our use of features is perhaps more related to feedforward neural nets and especially the information bottleneck approach of Tishby, Pereira, and Bialek 1999. Our work differs from feedforward methods in many ways, especially in that it is iterative and uses features symmetrically to relate the memory to input in both directions. Many other models iteratively combine top-down and bottom-up information (e.g., Hinton, Dayan, Frey, & Neal, 1995; Rao & Ballard, 1997). The structure of our algorithm is particularly related to methods like the wake-sleep algorithm of Hinton et al., although ours differs from these in many ways, especially our use of this for associative memory with complete memory of stored items. In spirit our approach is also similar to that of sequence-seeking counter streams (Ullman, 1996), although the way in which we relate top-down and bottom-up information is quite different.

Our use of a bigram representation of words is inspired by much previous work, especially that of Shannon (1951). Especially relevant to our work is that of Grimes and Mozer, (2001). Simultaneous with our work (Jacobs & Rudra, 2000), they use a bigram model to solve anagram problems, in which letters are unscrambled to match words in a dictionary. They also use a Markov model to find letter orderings that conform with the statistics of English spelling. Their model is quite different in how this is done, due to the different nature of the anagram problem. They view anagram solving as a mix of low-level processing and higher level cognitive processes, whereas it is our goal to focus just on lower level memory.

I consider three properties of human memory, discussing experiments that address the first property. First, human errors show consistent patterns. An obvious example of this is that it is easy to answer a Superghost problem with one letter given (e.g., *c*) or with most of the letters in a word given (e.g., *a*t*i*c*u*l*t*e*); it is generally much more difficult to answer cues with an intermediate number of letters given (e.g., *e*n*e*c*). Second, people are very flexible in the kinds of cues they can handle. For example, Superghost seems to require more difficult string matching than hangman, but people actually find Superghost easier. People can also handle mixed queries, such as *r*gm*c*, where the cue indicates that g and m appear contiguously in the answer. It is not always clear how existing memory models can handle such queries. Third, human memory can be primed by recent experience. For example, if one has studied a list of words and is then given a Superghost cue that matches a word on the list and a word not on the list, study will increase the chances of choosing the word on the list. Priming can be viewed as just another example of handling flexible cues. For example, one can be asked to think of a fruit that fits the cue *n*p*l*; being told to look for a fruit is a flexible cue that acts a bit as a prime to fruit names. It is not clear how to incorporate priming into some models of associative memory that do not maintain distinct representations of individual items in memory.

Previous work helps to elucidate the relative difficulty to people of different word memory problems. These have focused on hangman queries. Srinivas, Roediger, and Rajaram 1992, show it is easier to answer queries in which the letters present in a hangman question are contiguous rather than spread out (queries like arti_ _ _ _ _ rather than _ r _ i _ h _ k _). Olofsson and Nyberg (1992a, 1992b) and Srinivas et al. (1992) also show both that better recall on hangman queries occurs when letters presented occur contiguously at the beginning of a word rather than in the middle. When letters occur at the end of the word, queries are harder than when they occur at the beginning of the word but easier than queries with letters in the middle of the word. That is, queries like artic _ _ _ _ are easiest, then queries like _ _ _ _ choke, then _ _ ticho _ _.

We have compared our model to these results. To do so we modified our model to apply to hangman (by using the information provided in the query about the number of letters missing between two given letters). We ran the model using random queries and a dictionary of 6,040 eight-letter words. Our system produced results that show the same qualitative pattern as experiments on human subjects. That is, the model performed better on queries with contiguous letters and performed best when the beginning of the word is given, next best when letters at the end of the word are given, and worst with letters in the middle of the word. The model performs better with contiguous queries and queries at the beinning and end of the word because these provide more exact information about the bigrams present in the word. This is in part because we represent the first and last letters of the word as a separate bigram. It is interesting that our model, like humans, finds queries easier when the beginning of a word is given than when the end is given. This is in spite of our model treating the beginning and end of the word symmetrically and therefore results from the asymmetry of the statistics of spelling in English.

We have also experimented on human subjects to determine how performance on Superghost queries depends on the nature of the cue. We look at the ability of subjects to recall a valid English word that matches a query, within 10 seconds. All queries match at least one word in a standard dictionary. We categorize queries according to three variables. First is the length of the query. This is just the number of letters presented. Second is the overall frequency of all valid matches to the query in a standard English corpus. The third is the redundancy of a cue. Intuitively, this measures the extent to which each letter in the cue is needed to answer it correctly. More specifically, redundancy measures the probability that a word matching the query after removing one random letter would also match the full query. For example, the query *a*r*t*i*c*h*o*k* is highly redundant. The full query matches *artichoke* and *artichokes*. And if one removes any letter from the query the resulting, smaller query still only matches *artichoke* and *artichokes*. This means that not all letters in the query are really needed to find a correct answer. On the other hand, the query *a*r* is highly nonredundant because the query *a* matches many words that do not contain an *r*, and *r* matches many words without an *a*.

Our experiments demonstrate several effects. First, if one varies the length of otherwise randomly chosen queries, one finds a U-shaped performance curve. That is, subjects find very short (two- or three-letter), or very long (seven- or eight-letter) queries easier than queries of intermediate length. Second, when one controls for the frequency of the answers, the curve flattens, but the general effect persists. One explains these curves by looking at the redundancy of the queries. One finds that for a fixed length, queries of increasing redundancy are easier to answer. For a fixed redundancy, shorter queries are easier to answer. When one doesn't control for redundancy, longer queries are easier because they tend to be more redundant. But the data can be explained as the interaction of three performance characteristics of humans: queries that match more words, and more frequent words are easier; redundant queries are easier, and shorter queries are easier. Other effects arise from the nature of randomly chosen queries. For example, when one doesn't control for redundancy, longer queries tend to be easy because they tend to be highly redundant. But one can explain other patterns as side effects of the three main trends.

We compared these effects to simulations run with our model. In these simulations we generated Superghost queries. We again used a dictionary of 6,040 eight-letter words. Our simulations produced all the same qualitative trends as our experiments. In particular, our model found redundant cues significantly easier and found shorter cues easier when we controlled for redundancy. We also found a U-shaped performance curve when we did not control for redundancy. One discrepancy arose when we gave the model very low frequency cues that were not controlled for redundancy. These did not produce a U-shaped curve. This seems to be due to the fact that cues that matched very few words have a different pattern of redundancy, with short cues that match few words being especially nonredundant.

Perhaps the most unexpected result of these experiments is that when we control for frequency and redundancy, performance decreases with query length, both for human subjects and for our model. For nonredundant queries, all the information in the query is needed to get a correct answer. As query length increases, more information must be faithfully matched against items in memory. This seems to make these longer queries more difficult for people. Because the model uses intermediate features to mediate matching, some information present in the query is only approximately passed to memory, so performance also degrades. It is not clear which, if any, previous models of memory would show similar behavior; examining this question is a subject for future work.

It is also interesting that increasing the redundancy of queries makes them easier for people, although in retrospect this does not seem too surprising. I would expect that many computational models would show similar behavior. Certainly, this is an important criteria for any reasonable model to meet. It is also interesting that our model matches previous experiments that show how hangman queries with contiguous letters are easier than queries with fragmented letters. This seems to follow from our use of a Markov model of words and supports the psychological validity of such models. It is also interesting that by just using a Markov model, one finds that contiguous letters at the beginning of a word produce an easier cue than do letters at the end of the cue. One does not need to bias the representation to the beginnings of words to get this effect.

CONCLUSIONS

I have described a model of illusory contour formation in which a model that captures the general properties of contours is combined with image information to produce a stochastic completion field. This can be related to the percept of illusory contours but also serves as a representation of the probability distribution of contours consistent with the image. This casts illusory contour formation as a kind of object recognition process, in which a generic model of objects is recognized instead of a specific object.

I have also presented a model of memory in which processing an input query using a generic model is the first step of recall. In this model, a probability distribution describing the possible ways of completing a word fragment is computed using the general properties of words. The features of these completions are then compared with items in memory and used to sharpen the at first diffuse sense about what words might match the current query. This process is then repeated. This approach offers the potential to handle a wide range of possible queries (e.g., Superghost or mixed queries) because a complicated question doesn't need to be compared directly with every item in memory but only to a simplified model that combines all items. If this view is correct, then PO is the first step in visual memory and has analogs in all memory processes.

REFERENCES

Alter, T., & Basri, R. (1997). Extracting salient curves from images: An analysis of the saliency network. *International Journal of Computer Vision, 27*(1), 51–69.
Anderson, J. (1995). *An introduction to neural networks.* Cambridge, MA: MIT Press.
Blake, A., & Zisserman, A. (1987). *Visual reconstruction.* Cambridge, MA: MIT Press.
Carpenter, G., & Grossberg, S. (1987). Art 2: Self-organization of stable category recognition codes for analog input patterns. *Applied Optics, 26*, 4919–4930.

Chellappa, R., & Jain, A. (Eds.). (1993). *Markov random fields theory and application.* San Diego, CA: Academic Press.

Geman, S., & Geman, D. (1984). Stochastic relaxation, gibbs distributions, and the Bayesian restoration of images. *IEEE Transactions on Pattern Analysis and Machine Intelligence, 6,* 721–741.

Grimes, D., & Mozer, M. (2001). The interplay of symbolic and subsymbolic processes in anagram problem solving. In T. Leen, T. Dietterich, & V. Tresp (Eds.), *Advances in neural information processing systems 13.* pp 17–23. Cambridge, MA: MIT Press.

Grossberg, S. (1987). Competitive learning: From interactive activation to adaptive resonance. *Cognitive Science, 11,* 23–63.

Grossberg, S., & Mingolla, E. (1985). Neural dynamics of form perception: Boundary completion, illusory figures, and neon color spreading. *Psychological Review, 92*(2), 173–211.

Guy, G., & Medioni, G. (1996). Inferring global perceptual contours from local features. *International Journal of Computer Vision, 20*(1/2), 113–133.

Heitger, R., & von der Heydt, R. (1993). A computational model of neural contour processing, figure-ground segregation and illusory contours. In *International conference on computer vision.* pp. 32–40. Los Alamitos, CA: IEEE Computer Society Press.

Hinton, G., Dayan, P., Frey, B., & Neal, R. (1995). The "wake-sleep" algorithm for unsupervised neural networks. *Science, 268,* 1158–1161.

Horn, B. (1981). *The curve of least energy* [Memo]. Cambridge, MA: MIT AI Lab.

Jacobs, D. (2001). Perceptual organization as generic object recognition. In T. Shipley & P. Kellman (Eds.), *From fragments to objects: Segmentation and grouping in vision.* pp 295–329. Amsterdam, The Netherlands: Elsevier.

Jacobs, D. (1997). *What makes viewpoint invariant properties perceptually salient?* NEC TR #97–045.

Jacobs, D., Rokers, B., Rudra, A., & Liu, Z. (2002). Fragment completion in humans and machines. In T. Dietterich, S. Becker, & Z. Ghahramani (Eds) *Advances in neural information processing systems 14.* Cambridge, MA: MIT Press.

Jacobs, D., & Rudra, A. (2000). *An iterative projection model of memory* [Technical Report]. Washington, DC: NEC Research Institute.

Kanizsa, G. (1979). *Organization in Vision.* New York: Praeger.

Kosko, B. (1987). Adaptive bidirectional associative memory. *Applied Optics, 26*(23), 4947–4960.

Kumaran, K., Geiger, D., & Gurvits, L. (1996). Illusory surfaces. *Network: Computation in Neural Systems, 7,* pp. 33–60.

Liu, Z., Jacobs, D., & Basri, R. (1999). The role of convexity in perceptual completion. *Vision Research, 39,* 4244–4257.

Mumford, D. (1994). Elastica and computer vision. In C. Bajaj (Ed.), *Algebraic geometry and its applications.* New York: Springer-Verlag.

Nitzburg, M., & Mumford, D. (1990). The 2.1-D sketch. In *International conference on computer vision.* pp 138–144. Los Alamitos, CA: IEEE Computer Society Press.

Olofsson, U., & Nyberg, L. (1992a). Determinants of word fragment completion. *Scandanavian Journal of Psychology, 36*(1), 59–64.

Olofsson, U., & Nyberg, L. (1992b). Swedish norms for completion of word stems and unique word fragments. *Scandanavian Journal of Psychology, 33*(2), 108–116.

Pearl, J. (1988). *Probabilistic reasoning in intelligent systems.* San Francisco, CA: Morgan Kaufman.

Ramachandran, V., Ruskin, D., Cobb, S., Rogers-Ramachandran, D., & Tyler, C. (1994). On the perception of illusory contours. *Vision Research, 34*(23), 3145–3152.

Rao, R., & Ballard, D. (1997). Dynamic model of visual recognition predicts neural response properties in the visual cortex. *Neural Computation, 9*(4), 721–763.

Rock, I., & Anson, R. (1979). Illusory contours as the solution to a problem. *Perception, 8,* 665–681.

Rumelhart, D., & McClelland, J. (1982). An interactive activation model of context effects in letter perception: Part 2. The contextual enhancement effect and some tests and extensions of the model. *Psychological Review, 89,* 60–94.

Sambin, M. (1974). Angular margins without gradients. *Italian Journal of Psychology, 1,* 355–361.

Sha'ashua, A., & Ullman, S. (1988). Structural saliency: The detection of globally salient structures using a locally connected network. In *International conference on computer vision.* pp 321–327. Los Alamitos, CA: IEEE Computer Society Press.

Shannon, C. (1951). Prediction and entropy of printed English. *Bell Systems Technical Journal, 30,* 50–64.

Sommer, F., & Palm, G. (1998). "Bidirectional retrieval from associative memory" M. Jordan, M. Kearns, and S. Solla (Eds) In *Advances in neural information processing systems 10* pp. 675–681). Cambridge, MA: MIT Press.

Srinivas, K., Roediger, H., & Rajaram, S. (1992). The role of syllabic and orthographic properties of letter cues in solving word fragments. *Memory and Cognition, 20*(3), 219–230.

Taylor, H., & Karlin, S. (1998). *An introduction to stochastic modeling* (3rd ed.). San Diego, CA: Academic Press.

Thornber, K., & Williams, L. (2000). Characterizing the distribution of completion shapes with corners using a mixture of random processes. Pattern Recognition *33,* 543–553.

Tishby, N., Pereira, F., & Bialek, W. (1999). The information bottleneck method. In B. Hajek & R. Srinivas (Eds) *37th Allerton conference on communication, control, and computing.* pp 368–377. Urbana, IL: UIUC Press.

Ullman, S. (1976). Filling-in the gaps: The shape of subjective contours and a model for their generation. *Biological Cybernetics, 25,* 1–6.

Ullman, S. (1996). High-level vision. Cambridge, MA: MIT Press

Williams, L., & Hanson, A. (1996). Perceptual completion of occluded surfaces. *Computer Vision and Image Understanding, 64,* 1–20.

Williams, L., & Jacobs, D. (1997a). Stochastic completion fields: A neural model of illusory contour shape and salience. *Neural Computation, 9,* 837–858.

Williams, L., & Jacobs, D. (1997b). Local parallel computation of stochastic completion fields. *Neural Computation, 9,* 859–881.

Zhu, S. (1999). Embedding Gestalt laws in the Markov random fields. *IEEE Transactions on Pattern Analysis and Machine Intelligence, 21*(11), 1170–1187.

Zweck, J., & Williams, L. (2000). Euclidean group invariant computations of stochastic completion fields using shiftable-twistable functions. In *6th European conference on computer vision.* pp 100–116. Berlin: Springer-Verlag.

13 Neural Basis of Attentive Perceptual Organization

Tai Sing Lee
Carnegie Mellon University

Perceptual organization, broadly defined, is a set of visual processes that parses retinal images into their constituent components, organizing them into coherent, condensed, and simplified forms so that they can be readily interpreted and recognized. It generally includes many computational processes before object recognition, such as filtering, edge detection, grouping, segmentation, and figure-ground segregation. These processes are considered to be preattentive, parallel, and automatic (Treisman & Gelade, 1980) and mediated by feedforward and intra-areal mechanisms (Palmer, 1999). Attention, on the other hand, is thought to be driven by figure-ground organization, but not vice versa, even though some psychological evidence does suggest that later processes such as recognition and experience could influence earlier perceptual organization (Palmer, Neff, & Beck, 1996; Peterson & Gibson, 1991). The nature and the extent of top-down influence on perceptual organization thus remains murky and controversial. In this article, I first sketch a theoretical framework to reason about the computational and neural processes underlying perceptual organization. This framework attempts to unify the bottom-up organizational processes and the top-down attentional processes into an integrated inference system. I then discuss some neurophysiological experimental findings that lend strong support to these ideas.

THEORIES OF FEEDBACK

Marr's (1982) proposal that visual processing could be decomposed into a feedforward chain of relatively independent modules has had a strong influence on the vision community over the last 20 years. Neurophysiologists have focused on the detailed elucidation of single cells' properties and tuning in each cortical area, and computer scientists have attempted to formulate each computational module mathematically in isolation. Some psychological evidence seems to suggest feedforward computations may be sufficient in normal scene analysis. Thorpe, Fize, and Marlot (1996) demonstrated that people and monkeys could perform categorization tasks very rapidly and that event-related potentials (ERP) relevant to decision making can be observed in the prefrontal areas within 150 ms, apparently leaving little time for computations to iterate up and down the visual hierarchy. Much of visual processing, they argued, must be based on only feedforward mechanisms. In fact, many successful object detection and recognition algorithms are based on only feedforward algorithms (Lades et al., 1993; Rowley, Baluja, & Kanade, 1998; Schneiderman & Kanade, 1998). These algorithms typically use clustering or likelihood tests to classify patterns based on the configuration of responses of low-level features detectors, effectively bypassing the difficult perceptual organization problems. Hence, the dominant conceptual framework today on perceptual processing is still based on feedforward computations along a chain of computational modules (Palmer, 1999).

In recent years, it has become increasingly clear to computer scientists that many problems in perceptual organization are difficult to solve without introducing the contextual information of a visual scene (see Lee, Mumford, Romero, & Lamme, 1998). Psychologists and neural modelers have in fact long emphasized the importance of contextual feedback in perceptual processing (Dayan, Hinton, Neal, & Zemel, 1995; Grossberg, 1987; McClelland & Rumelhart, 1981; Mumford, 1992; Rao & Ballard, 1999; Ullman, 1994). Their arguments were inspired partly by psychological findings and partly by theoretical considerations and the knowledge that there is an enormous amount of recurrent anatomical connections among the cortical areas (Felleman & Van Essen, 1991).

The exact nature of information being fed back to the earlier areas, however, is far from being clear. There are three main proposals. The first suggests that feedback carries explicit hypotheses or predictions similar to model-based image rendering in computer graphics (Mumford, 1992, 1996a). The higher order hypothesis could feed back to suppress (or explain away) the earlier level descriptions that it can explain, as suggested in the predictive coding framework (Mumford, 1996a; Rao & Ballard, 1999). Alternatively, it could feed back to enhance (resonate with) the earlier representation that it is consistent with, facilitating perceptual completion, as suggested in the adaptive resonance/interactive activation framework (Grossberg, 1987; McClelland & Rumelhart, 1981).

In the second proposal, the information being fed back is more general and may be best understood in terms of top-down probabilistic priors in an inference framework (Dayan et al., 1995; Grenander, 1976, 1978, 1981; Lee & Mumford, in press; Tu & Zhu, 2002). Each area is endowed with its unique computational machinery and carries out its own special computation. The priors could be specific in the object domain but unspecific in the spatial domain or vice versa. They provide general guidance to influence, rather than to micromanage, the lower level inference.

A third proposal has recently become popular in the neuroscience community. In this proposal, feedback is primarily a mechanism for implementing selective attention (for a review, see Desimone & Duncan, 1995) and gain control (Prezybyszewski, Gaska, Foote, & Pollen, 2000). The mechanistic framework for attentional selection favored by neural modelers is called biased competition. Feedback in this framework serves to provide a positive bias to influence the competition at the earlier levels (Deco & Lee, 2002; Reynolds, Chelazzi, & Desimone, 1999; Usher & Niebur, 1996).

Despite some superficial contradictions, these three proposals are in fact quite similar at a certain level. They reflect the concerns of three different communities: the psychological/neural modeling, the statistical/artificial intelligence modeling, and the biological communities. I attempt to use a probabilistic inference framework rooted in the second proposal to reconcile and unify all these perspectives.

BAYESIAN INFERENCE IN THE VISUAL HIERARCHY

Visual processing may be conceptualized as what Helmholtz (von Helmholtz, 1867; Palmer, 1999) called the unconscious inference or what has been recently referred to as Bayesian inference (Knill & Richards, 1996). That is, we rely on contextual information and our prior knowledge of the world to make inferences about the world based on retinal data. Consider the image patch depicted in Fig. 13.1A. Seen alone it is merely a collection of spots and dots. However, when placed in a larger scene context (Fig. 13.1B), the same image patch assumes a more specific and richer meaning. The image in Fig. 13.1B is still quite ambiguous. It will take unfamiliar viewers a few minutes before they perceive the object in the scene. However, once they are told that the picture depicts a dalmatian dog sniffing the ground near a tree, the perception will start to crystallize in their minds. The spots and dots are transformed into the surface markings of the dog's body. Furthermore, if the same viewers were to see this image again in the future, their memory would help them see the dog instantly. This terrific example by R. C. James illustrates the important roles of both the global context and prior knowledge in perceptual inference.

From the Bayesian perspective, perceptual inference can be formulated as the computation to obtain the most probable causes of the visual scene by finding the a posteriori estimate S of the scene that maximizes $P(S|I, K)$, the conditional

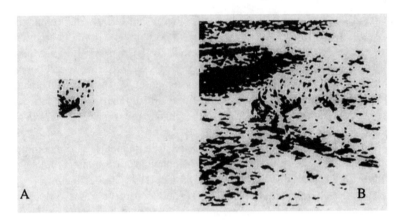

FIG. 13.1.   (A) An image patch of spots and dots. (B) The image patch
situated in a particular scene, as originally designed by R. C. James.

probability of a scene S given a particular image I and our knowledge of the world
K. By Bayes's theorem, this is given by,

$$P(S|I, K) = \frac{P(I|S, K)P(S|K)}{P(I|K)},$$

where $P(I|S, K)$ is the conditional probability of the image given the scene hy-
pothesis S and the prior knowledge K. S has a hierarchical description (e.g., edges,
eyes, face, person)—that is, it is in fact a collection of hypotheses at different
levels S_i with i indicating the level in the hierarchy. At a particular level i, one
can think of prior knowledge K as captured by the possible hypotheses at the other
levels (i.e., $P(S_{i-1})$, $P(S_{i+1})$, $P(S_{i+2})$, etc.). If we assume that a cortical area talks
primarily to an adjacent area, but not to more distant areas, then the hierarchy
can be considered to be roughly Markovian, and the probability distribution of
hypotheses at level i can be factorized as

$$P(S_i|I, K) = P(S_{i-1}|S_i)P(S_i|S_{i+1})/Z,$$

where Z is a normalization constant.

Let I be the information output by the retina, then

$$P(S_{lgn}|I, K) = P(I|S_{lgn})P(S_{lgn}|S_{v1})/Z_1,$$
$$P(S_{v1}|I, K) = P(S_{lgn}|S_{v1})P(S_{v1}|S_{v2})/Z_2,$$
$$P(S_{v2}|I, K) = P(S_{v1}|S_{v2})P(S_{v2}|S_{v4})/Z_3,$$

and so on, where Z's are normalization constants for each of the distributions, and

$S_{i=lgn,v1,v2,v4,it}$ describes the hypotheses generated at the respective area along the visual hierarchy.

For example, V1 receives input from the LGN and generates a set of hypotheses that might explain the LGN data. The generation is constrained by feedforward and intracortical connections specified by $P(S_{lgn}|S_{v1})$ (i.e., how well each V1 hypothesis S_{v1} can explain S_{lgn}). S_{v2} are the hypotheses generated by V2 based on its input from V1 and feedback from higher areas. V2 communicates directly to V1 but not to LGN. The feedback from V2 to V1 is given by the estimate that maximizes $S_{v2|I,K}$ weighted by feedback connections $P(S_{v1}|S_{v2})$ (i.e., how well S_{v2} can explain away S_{v1}). V1 is to find the S_{v1} (at its level of interpretation) that maximizes $P(S_{v1}|I, K) = P(S_{lgn}|S_{v1})P(S_{v1}|S_{v2})/Z$.

This scheme can then be applied again to V2, V4, and IT recursively to generate the whole visual hierarchy. Perception corresponds to each of the cortical areas finding its best hypothesis S_i, constrained by the bottom-up and the top-down information. Each cortical area is an expert at inferring some aspects of the visual scene. Unless the image is simple and clear, each area normally cannot be completely sure of its conclusion and has to harbor a number of candidate proposals simultaneously, waiting for the feedback guidance and possibly a change in the input interpretation to select the best hypothesis. The feedforward input drives the generation of the hypotheses, and the feedback from higher inference areas provides the priors to help select the most probable hypothesis. Information does not need to flow forward and backward from V1 to IT in big loops, which would take too much time per iteration. Rather, successive cortical areas in the visual hierarchy can constrain each other's inference in small loops instantaneously and continuously in a Markov chain. The system, as a whole, could converge rapidly and almost simultaneously to an interpretation of the visual scene.

EFFICIENT CODING IN THE HIERARCHY

Hierarchical Bayesian inference can tie together rather nicely the three plausible proposals on the nature of feedback and its role on perceptual organization. In fact, it helps to reconcile some apparent contradictory predictions from the pattern theory (Grenander, 1978; Mumford, 1996a; Rao & Ballard, 1999) and the resonance theory (Grossberg, 1987; McClelland & Rumelhart, 1981). In the hierarchical Bayes framework, many levels of descriptions (organizations) can coexist in the visual hierarchy, with the highest level of explanations most salient to visual awareness, or the cognitive and decision processes. The high-level description feeds back to attenuate the saliency of the lower level descriptions but should not annihilate them. This is an important but subtle distinction between this theory and Mumford's earlier interpretation of the pattern theory (Mumford, 1992, 1996a; Rao & Ballard, 1999). Most importantly, this top-down hypothesis also serves to eliminate the alternative hypotheses in the earlier

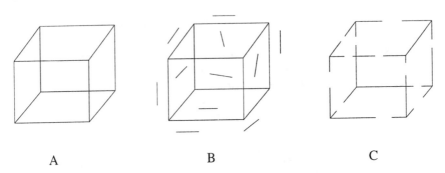

A   B   C

FIG. 13.2. (A) A Necker cube. (B) A cube with background noises.
(C) A cube with missing information.

level, suppressing more severely the responses of the neural ensembles that are representing the alternative hypotheses. Thus, the early-level hypothesis consistent with the higher level description is actually enhanced relative to the alternative hypotheses, as predicted by the resonance theory. In this way, this hierarchical Bayes engine contains both the explaining away element as well as the resonance element.

Let us use the Necker cube in Fig. 13.2A as an example. This line drawing can be immediately perceived as a cube, rather than a bunch of lines and junctions. The black dots, the most elementary-level description, are organized into lines. The lines, their positions, and the junctions are then organized into a three-dimensional interpretation at the higher level. The three-dimensional percept is the simplest description that explains all the evidences and is perhaps what first penetrates into our consciousness. The cube interpretation is then fed back to early visual areas to attenuate the saliency of the representations of line and edge elements because they have been explained. For this simple picture, all one can observe is the explaining away (i.e., attenuation of early visual neurons' responses). Fig. 13.2B shows the same picture that is corrupted with spurious noises. In this case, the theory predicts that the higher order hypothesis of a cube will suppress all the noise elements more severely than the edge elements that are consistent with the cube hypothesis, enhancing (resonating) the consistent earlier representation in a relative sense. This scheme is in fact a generalized form of efficient and sparse coding (Barlow, 1961; Field, 1994; Lewicki & Olshausen, 1999; Olshausen & Field, 1996; Rao & Ballard, 1999). On the other hand, the consequence of resonance is that the higher level hypothesis can help to complete missing information at the earlier levels. One can imagine that the V1 neurons at the location of the gap (location A) in Fig. 13.2C will be activated in the appropriate order to be consistent with the cube interpretation higher up. These theoretical predictions are precisely what my colleagues and I observed in the following neurophysiological experiments involving V1.

EVIDENCE IN THE EARLY VISUAL CORTEX

In the first experiment (Lee et al., 1998), my colleagues and I studied how V1 neurons responded to different parts of a texture stimulus (Fig. 13.3A). While a monkey was fixating on a red dot on the computer monitor, an image was flashed on the monitor for 330 ms. The image in this case was a texture strip subtending 4° of visual angle on a background of contrasting texture. The texture in each region was composed of small, randomly positioned lines of uniform orientation. Texture contrast was defined as the difference in the orientation of the line elements. The stimulus was presented in a randomized series of sampling positions relative to the V1 cells' classical receptive fields so that the temporal response of the neurons to different parts of the stimulus (0.5° steps over a 12° range) was measured one at a time. Fig. 13.3B shows the spatiotemporal response of a set of vertically oriented neurons to the stimulus in Fig. 13.3A. Several interesting observations can

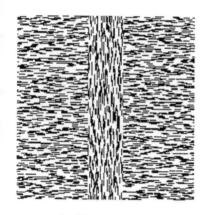

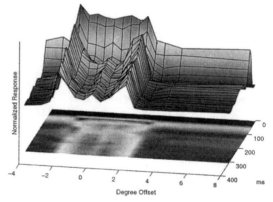

A. Texture strip   B. Spatiotemporal response

FIG. 13.3. (A) A texture strip with width of 4° visual angle. The strip is composed of short vertical line segments, and the background is composed of short horizontal line segments. (B) Spatiotemporal average response of a population of 14 V1 vertical neurons to a texture strip stimulus at different positions along a horizontal sampling line across the strip. The abscissa is the distance in visual angles from the RF center to the center of the strip. The texture boundary is located at −2.0° and 2.0° visual angles away from the center. The responses to the texture stimuli were initially uniformly high within the strip and low outside the strip corresponding to the the vertical orientation tuning of the cells. At 60 ms after stimulus onset, boundary signals started to develop at the texture boundaries. In the later stage, the responses in general were lower than the initial responses, but the responses at the boundaries were sharper and stronger relative to the rest of the image (see Lee, Mumford, Romero, & Lamme, 1998, for details).

be made. First, the initial neuronal response (35–70 ms poststimulus onset) was characterized by the response to local features (i.e., sensitivity to orientation of the line elements). Second, after the initial burst of response, there was a transient pause, followed by a more sustained response at a lower level. This phenomenon usually is considered an effect of intracortical inhibition, adaptation, or habituation. From a Bayesian framework, this decay, in response to the later period of V1 neurons' activity, could be considered a part of the explaining away by the higher order description. Third, the response at the texture boundary was significantly higher than the responses within the texture regions. This relative enhancement could be considered a consequence of the cells' resonance with the global percept of surface discontinuity. Fourth, orientation sensitivity of the cells was maintained at the later response, but the response was sustained at a very low level, suggesting a reduction in saliency but not in coding specificity. Thus, the lower level representations did not completely disappear but instead were maintained at a lower level. This is important because these activities might help to keep all irrelevant data for alternative hypotheses alive so that they might, at another moment, resurrect and support an alternative hypothesis (e.g., switching between the two percepts in the Necker cube). These observations are what one would expect from hierarchical Bayesian inference engine, though they potentially can also be explained by passive intracortical inhibition mechanisms (Li, 2001; Stemmler, Usher, & Niebur, 1995).

In the second experiment (Lee & Nguyen, 2001), my colleagues and I used a similar paradigm to examine how V1 neurons responded to the subjective contour of a subjective Kanizsa square (Fig. 13.4A and Fig. 13.4B). Over successive trials the illusory contour was placed at different locations relative to the center of the receptive field, 0.25° apart, spanning a range of 2.25°, as shown in Fig. 13.4B. Figures 13.4C–13.4J display examples of other control stimuli also tested in the experiment. In each trial, while the monkey fixated, a sequence of four stimuli was presented. The presentation of each stimulus in the sequence lasted for 400 ms. In the presentation of the Kanizsa figure, four circular discs were first presented and then abruptly turned into four partial discs, creating the illusion of a subjective square appearing in front of the four circular discs. Fig. 13.5A shows that the illusory contour response of a multiple unit occurred at precisely the same location of a real contour response, indicating the spatial precision of the response. Fig. 13.5B and Fig. 13.5C compare the temporal evolution of this unit's response to the illusory contour and the responses to a variety of real contours and controls. This unit responded significantly more to the illusory contour than to the amodal contour or to any of the rotated disc configurations (see Lee & Nguyen, 2001). For this neuron, as well as for the V1 populations in the superficial layer, the temporal onset of the response to illusory contour occurred about 100 ms after the abrupt onset of the illusory square, whereas the onset of the responses to the real contours occurred at about 40–50 ms (Fig. 13.5C and Fig. 13.5D). The response of V2 neurons to the same illusory contour occurred at about 65 ms after stimulus onset (Fig. 13.5E).

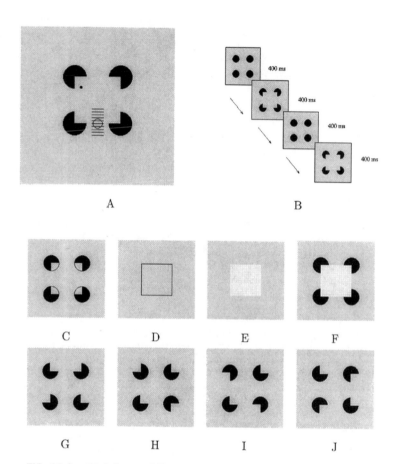

FIG. 13.4. (A) A figure of illusory contour and the 10 different parts (marked by lines) that were placed over the receptive field of a horizontally oriented neuron over successive trials during an experiment. (B) In a typical trial, the stimulus was presented in a sequence, 400 ms for each step. The first step displayed four circular discs, which then turned into four partial discs in the second step. The abrupt onset of the illusory square captures the attention of the monkey and makes the illusory square more salient. The third and fourth steps repeated the first and second steps. In each trial, the response of the cell to one location of the figure was examined. (C–J) Some examples of other stimuli that were also examined as controls. From "Dynamics of Subjective Contour Formation in the Early Visual Cortex," by T. S. Lee and M. Nguyen, 2001, *Proceedings of the National Academy of Sciences, 98*(4), 1908. Copyright 2001 by National Academy of Sciences. Reprinted with permission.

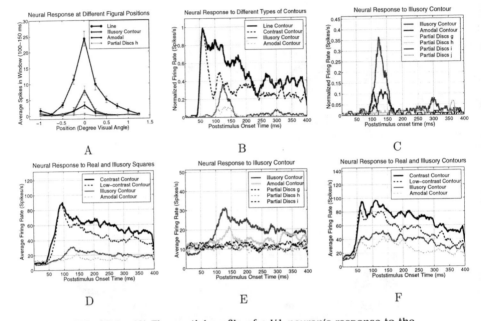

FIG. 13.5. (A) The spatial profile of a V1 neuron's response to the contours of both real and illusory squares in a temporal window 100– 150 ms after stimulus onset at the 10 different locations relative to the illusory contour. This cell responded to the illusory contour when it was at precisely the same location ($x = 0$), where a real contour evoked the maximal response from the neuron. This cell also responded significantly better to the illusory contour than to the amodal contour (T test, $p < 0.003$) and did not respond much when the partial discs were rotated. (B) The cell's response to the illusory contour compared with its response to the real contours of a line square, or a white square. The onset of the response to the real contours was at 45 ms, about 55 ms before the illusory contour response. (C) Temporal evolution of this cell's response to the illusory contour, the amodal contour, and the various rotated corner disc controls at the location where the real contour elicited the maximum response. The response to the illusory contour emerged at about 100 ms after the illusory square appeared. The cell responded slightly to the amodal contour and did not respond to any of the rotated corner discs. (D–E) Population averaged temporal response of 50 V1 neurons in the superficial layer to the real and illusory contours. (F) Population averaged temporal response of 39 V2 neurons in the superficial layer to the real and illusory contours. From "Dynamics of Subjective Contour Formation in the Early Visual Cortex," by T. S. Lee, and M. Nguyen, 2001, *Proceedings of the National Academy of Sciences*, *98*(4), 1908–1909. Copyright 2001 by National Academy of Sciences. Reprinted with permission.

These observations suggest that V2 could be detecting the existence of an illusory contour first by integrating information from a more global spatial context, forming a hypothesis of the boundary of the Kanizsa square. V2 neurons, because of their larger receptive fields, cannot provide a spatially precise representation of the sharp illusory contour; they can only inform the existence of a boundary at a rough location. V1 is recruited to compute and represent the precise location and orientation of the contour because it has the machinery for computing and representing precise curvilinear geometry efficiently or sparsely. The hypothesis of a Kanizsa square and its supporting illusory boundary are represented simultaneously by many visual areas, such as V1, V2, and even IT, where the concept of a square is represented. From this perspective, V1 does not simply perform filtering and edge detection and then forward the results to the extrastriate cortex for further processing (Hubel & Wiesel, 1962). Rather, it is an integral part of the visual system that continues to participate in all levels of visual reasoning insofar as the computations require the spatial precision and high resolution details provided by V1. This is the basic rationale underlying the high-resolution buffer hypothesis that Mumford and I (Lee et al., 1998; Mumford, 1996b) proposed a few years ago—a view now shared by many others (e.g., Bullier, 2001).

ATTENTION AS TOP-DOWN PRIORS

The hierarchical Bayesian framework discussed previously is appropriate for conceptualizing perceptual organization or interpretation of the input image. The feedback carries the contextual priors generated by the higher level description, directly related to what biologists call contextual processing (see Albright & Stoner, 2002, for review). Attention is another type of feedback that places priority or value in the information to be analyzed and makes perception purposeful. In fact, the dominant view in the biological community on the functional role of feedback is the mediation of selective attention (for reviews, see Desimone & Duncan, 1995; Itti & Koch, 2001). Because both attention and contextual priors use the same recurrent feedback pathways, it might be reasonable to consider attention in terms of priors and unify the two functions in a single framework.

People usually think of attention in terms of spatial attention, a spotlight that illuminates a certain location of visual space for focal visual analysis (Helmholtz, 1867; Treisman & Gelade, 1980). Attentive processing is usually considered a serial process that requires moving the spotlight around in the visual scene to select the location to be analyzed. There are in fact many types of attention. Feature or object attention is involved when we are searching for a particular feature or object in a visual scene (James, 1890). In spatial attention, selection is focused on the spatial dimension and dispersed (parallel) in the feature dimension, whereas in feature attention the selection is focused on the feature dimension and dispersed (parallel) in the spatial dimension. A generalization of feature attention is object attention, in which a configuration of features belonging to an object is searched. It was believed that conjunctive search operates in a serial mode (Treisman & Sato, 1990; Wolfe, 1998).

In recent years, a number of neurophysiological studies have shown that attention can modulate visual processing in many cortical areas (Desimone & Duncan, 1995) and even in the receptive fields of neurons (Connor et al., 1997; Tolias et al., 2001). The popular model for explaining the mechanism of attention is called biased competition (Deco & Lee, 2002; Desimone & Duncan, 1995; Duncan & Humphreys, 1989; Reynolds et al. 1999; Usher & Niebur, 1996). The basic idea is that when multiple stimuli are presented in a visual field, the different neuronal populations within a single cortical area activated by these stimuli will engage in competitive interaction. Attending to a stimulus at a particular spatial location or attending to a particular object feature, however, introduces a bias to influence the competition in favor of the neurons at the attended location and at the expense of the other neurons. The biased competition mechanism, formulated in terms of differential equations with roots in the connectionist models, has also been used in several models for explaining attentional effects in neural responses observed in the inferotemporal cortex (Usher & Niebur, 1996) and in V2 and V4 (Reynolds et al., 1999).

Conceptually, biased competition can also be formulated into a probabilistic framework. Recall that the hierarchical Bayesian inference in the visual system can be described as the process for finding the scene variables S_i, $\forall_i$ that maximize the joint probability

$$P(I, S_{lgn}, S_{v1}, \ldots, S_{it}) = P(I|S_{lgn})P(S_{lgn}|S_{v1})P(S_{v1}|S_{v2})$$
$$\cdot P(S_{v2}|S_{v4})P(S_{v4}|S_{it})P(S_{it}),$$

where $P(S_{it})$ is the prior on the expected frequency of the occurrence of various object categories.

Top-down object attention can be incorporated into this framework by including the prefrontal areas (area 46) in the hierarchy, as follows:

$$P(I, S_{lgn}, \ldots, S_{a46v}) = P(I|S_{lgn})P(S_{lgn}|S_{v1})P(S_{v1}|S_{v2})$$
$$\cdot P(S_{v2}|S_{v4})P(S_{v4}|S_{it})P(S_{it}|S_{a46v})P(S_{a46v}),$$

where ventral area 46 (a46v) is the area for executive control that will determine which object to look for and which object to remember. It integrates a large variety of contextual information and memory from the hippocampus, basal ganglians, cingulate gyrus, and many other prefrontal areas to make decisions and resolve conflicts (Miller & Cohen, 2001). It sets priority and endows value to make visual object processing purposeful and adaptive.

Because the hierarchy is reciprocally connected, this implies that attention, higher order contextual knowledge, and behavioral experience should be able to penetrate back to the earliest level of visual processing, at least as early as V1 and LGN. This was precisely what my colleagues and I observed in the following experiments.

BEHAVIORAL EXPERIENCE AND TASK DEMANDS

In this experiment (Lee, Yang, Romero, & Mumford, 2002), my colleagues and I studied the effect of higher order perceptual construct such as three-dimensional shape and behavioral experience on the neural processes in the early visual cortex (V1 and V2). We used a set of stimuli that allowed the dissociation of bottom-up low-level stimulus contrast from top-down higher order perceptual inference (Fig. 13.6). The stimuli included a set of shape from shading stimuli, which have been found to pop out readily (Braun, 1993; Ramachandran, 1988; Sun & Perona, 1996) and a set of two-dimensional contrast patterns, which do not pop out spontaneously, even though the latter have stronger luminance contrast and evoke stronger bottom-up raw responses in V1 neurons (see Fig. 13.6). The stronger pop-out of shape from shading stimuli in this case has been attributed to their three-dimensional interpretation. Therefore, we hypothesized that if we see a neural correlate of this stronger pop-out modulation due to shape from shading in V1, it would be a clear case of top-down modulation due to higher order percepts.

To evaluate the impact of behavior on early visual processing, we also divided the experiment into two stages; a prebehavior stage and a postbehavior stage. In both stages, monkeys performed the same fixation task (i.e., fixating on a red dot on the screen during stimulus presentation). In the prebehavior stage, the monkeys did not use the stimuli in their behavior. In the postbehavior stage, the monkeys used the stimuli in their behaviors for a period of time. Specifically, they were trained to detect the oddball of the various types and make a saccadic eye movement to it. Interestingly, V1 neurons were significantly sensitive to perceptual pop-out modulation in the postbehavior stage but not in the prebehavior stage. Pop-out modulation was defined by the enhancement of the neuronal responses to the oddball condition relative to the uniform condition, while the stimulus on the receptive field of the neurons was kept constant (see Fig. 13.6; Fig. 13.7). Furthermore, the pop-out modulation in V1, and similarly in V2, was a function of the stimuli, directly correlated with the subjective perceptual pop-out saliency we perceive in the stimulus. Fig. 13.7 shows that the lighting from above (LA) and lighting from below (LB) oddballs pop out strongly, the lighting from left (LL) and right (LR) oddballs pop out moderately, and the two-dimensional contrast oddballs do not pop out at all (Ramachandran, 1988). The figure also shows a strong correlation between the behavioral performance (reaction time and percentage correct) of the monkeys and the neural pop-out modulation in V1. Thus, the neural

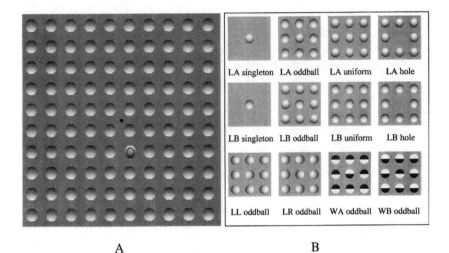

A   B

FIG. 13.6.   (A) A typical stimulus display was composed of 10 × 10
stimulus elements. Each element was 1° visual angle in diameter.
The diameter of the classical receptive field (RF) of a typical cell at
the eccentricities tested ranged from 0.4° to 0.8° visual angle. Displayed is the LA (lighting from above) oddball condition, with the LA
oddball placed on top of the cell's receptive field, indicated by the
open circle. The solid dot indicates the fixation spot. (B) There are
six stimulus sets. Each stimulus set had four conditions: singleton,
oddball, uniform, and hole. Displayed are the iconic diagrams of all
the conditions for the LA set, the LB set, as well as the oddball conditions for the other four sets. The center element in the iconic diagram
covered the receptive field of the neuron in the experiment. The surround stimulus elements were placed outside the RF of the neuron.
The comparison was between the oddball condition and the uniform
condition, and the singleton and the hole conditions were controls.
The singletons measured the neuronal response to direct stimulation
of the RF alone; the holes measured the response to direct stimulation of the extra-RF surround only. From "Neural Activity in Early Visual
Cortex Reflects Experience and Higher Order Perceptual Saliency," by
T. S. Lee, C. Yang, R. Romero, and D. Mumford, 2002, *Nature Neu-
roscience, 5*(6), 590. Copyright 2002 by *Nature Publishing Group.*
Adapted with permission.

modulation we observed in V1 could be considered a neural correlate of perceptual
saliency.

Apparently, the pop-out detection task forced the monkeys to see the stimulus
more clearly and to precisely localize the pop-out target in space. This is a task that
would engage V1's machinery according to the high-resolution buffer hypothesis.
Even though the monkeys were required only to fixate during the experiment,
having practiced the pop-out detection task for 2 weeks apparently made the early

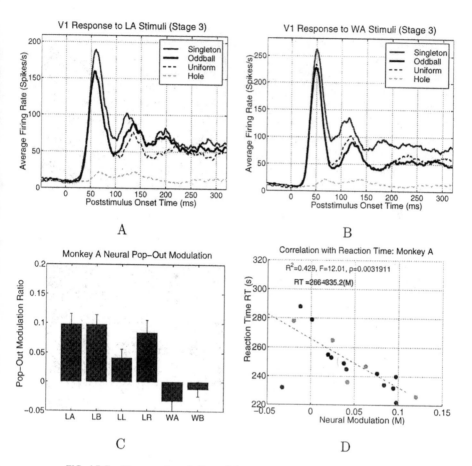

FIG. 13.7. Temporal evolution of the normalized population average response of 45 V1 units from a monkey to the LA set (A) and the WA set (B) at the postbehavior stage. Significant pop-out response was observed in LA (as well as LB, LL, and LR) starting at 100 ms after stimulus onset. No pop-out response was observed for WA (or WB). (C) Mean pop-out modulation ratios of 45 units for all six stimulus sets. Pop-out enhancements were statistically significant for stimuli LA, LB, LL, and LR but not for WA and WB. The pop-out modulation is computed as $(A - B)/(A + B)$, where A was the response to the oddball condition, and B was the response to the uniform condition. (D) Correlation between reaction time and V1 pop-out modulation for the six sets of stimuli. Data from three different stages (hence 18 points) are plotted. A significant negative correlation was observed between reaction time and pop-out modulation ratio. From "Neural Activity in Early Visual Cortex Reflects Experience and Higher Order Perceptual Saliency," by T. S. Lee, C. Yang, R. Romero, and D. Mumford, 2002, *Nature Neuroscience*, 5(6), 591, 593. Copyright 2002 by *Nature Publishing Group*. Adapted with permission.

pop-out processing more or less automatic. On the other hand, the pop-out effect could be greatly attenuated when the monkeys were asked to perform a very attention-demanding conflicting task. The pop-out signals emerged in V1 and V2 at roughly the same time (95 ms for V2 and 100 ms for V1). Interestingly, Bichot and Schall (1999) also found that the target selection/decision signal emerged in the frontal eye field during a visual search task at about the same time frame, around 100–130 ms, supporting the idea that interactive computation may not take place in a stepwise linear fashion iteratively but may occur interactively and concurrently between adjacent areas in the brain. The cycle time is much shorter under continuous dynamics. From this point of view, the 150 ms time frame reported by Thorpe et al. (1996) is quite sufficient for the whole hierarchy to settle down to a perceptual interpretation of the visual scene.

Perceptual pop-out has been thought to be an operation that is parallel, automatic, and preattentive. The findings discussed suggest that attention may be involved in the normal operation for early perceptual organization such as pop-out and grouping. The idea that attention may play a role in this parallel computation might seem to be at odds with conventional notions. However, recent psychological studies (Joseph, Chun, & Nakayama, 1997) suggest that attention may be critical for the detection of preattentive features and may, in fact, be necessary for overt perception of these stimulus features. These data suggest a stronger link between perceptual organization and attention, as well as behavioral experience.

OBJECT-BASED SPATIAL ATTENTION

Granted the signal my colleagues and I observed in the last experiment was related to perceptual saliency, what is the advantage of having the attentional highlighting signals going all the way to V1? Two observations help to reveal the important role of V1 in this computation. First, in the shape from shading pop-out experiment, we found that the pop-out enhancement could be found only at exactly the location of the oddball but not at the locations next to it, indicating that the highlighting effect is both spatially specific and stimulus specific. Second, when we examined the responses of V1 neurons to different parts of a texture square in a contrasting background (Fig. 13.8), my colleagues and I (Lee, Mumford, Romero, & Lamme, 1998) found that V1 neurons' responses were enhanced when their receptive fields were placed inside a texture-defined figure relative to when they were placed in a textured background and that this enhancement was uniform within the spatial extent of the figure, just as Lamme (1995) discovered earlier. Further, we also found that this highlighting signal is spatially bounded by the boundary response of the neurons (Fig. 13.8). Cortical organization beyond V1 is segregated according to more abstract attributes and is less topologically precise. Only in V1 could one find a spatially precise gridlike spatial topology, in Ullman's (1984) terms, to color the surface of an object clearly and precisely. This highlighting or coloring

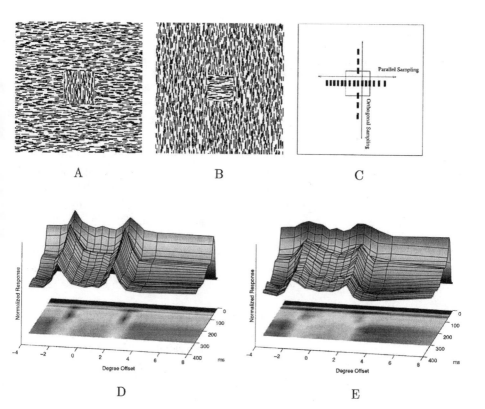

FIG. 13.8. Object-based spatial attention effect. V1 neurons' responses were found to be enhanced inside the figure relative to outside the figure. (A) and (B) show figures defined by texture contrast. (C) illustrates the placement of the receptive field when the neuron's preferred orientation is vertical. There are two sampling schemes: parallel sampling, when the preferred orientation of the cells is aligned with the orientation of the texture boundary, and orthogonal sampling, when the preferred orientation of the cells is orthogonal to the orientation of the texture boundary. (D) shows the population averaged response of 45 neurons in the parallel sampling scheme with the response to (A) and the response to (B) summed at each spatial location. (E) shows the population averaged response of 16 neurons in the orthogonal sampling scheme. In the parallel sampling scheme, my colleagues and I found a persistent and large texture edge response, which was absent in the orthogonal sampling scheme, suggesting that cells were sensitive to the orientation of the texture boundaries. The response inside the figure showed a definite enhancement at about the 15% level for both schemes. The response inside the figure in the orthogonal sampling scheme appeared as a plateau. The normalization exaggerated or dramatized the 15% enhancement effect. From "The Role of the Primary Visual Cortex in Higher Level Vision," by T. S. Lee, D. Mumford, R. Romero, and V. A. F. Lamme, 1998, *Vision Research, 38*, 2440. Copyright 1998 by Elsevier Science. Adapted with permission.

operation through attention might be the neural basis of object-based spatial attention (Behrmann, Zemel, & Mozer, 1998; Olson, 2001).

INTEGRATION OF OBJECT AND SPATIAL INFORMATION

The computation of perceptual pop-out saliency of the shape from shading stimuli is likely a product of three types of computation, bottom-up saliency, shape recognition (stimulus-evoked object attention), and spatial localization (stimulus-evoked spatial attention). It requires the interaction of the early visual areas with both the dorsal stream (e.g., lateral intraparietal area (LIP)) and the ventral stream (e.g., inferotemporal cortex (IT); see Logothetis, 1998). The top-down object attention and spatial attention feedback from both streams, coupled with intracortical contextual computation, produce the spatially precise higher order perceptual saliency effect.

So far I have only talked about the hierarchical inference of object forms, but the inference of space could also be formulated in the same way, only with a change of variable from S to S' to indicate the spatial aspects of the information and the assumption that spatial attention is initiated by an input from dorsal area 46.

$$P(I, S_{lgn}, \ldots, S'_{po}, \ldots, S'_{a46d}) = P(I|S_{lgn})P(S_{lgn}|S_{v1})P(S_{v1}|S'_{v2})$$
$$\cdot P(S'_{v2}|S'_{v3})P(S'_{v3}|S'_{po})$$
$$\cdot P(S'_{po}|S'_{a46d})P(S'_{a46d})$$

The scene variables S'_i in this case concern the spatial position encoding and spatial coordinate transforms. For simplicity, assume that the cross-talk between the higher areas in the different streams is relatively weak; then the activity of V1 is given by S_{v1} that maximizes

$$P(S_{v1}|S_{lgn}, S_{v2}, S'_{v2}, \ldots) = P(S_{lgn}|S_{v1})P(S_{v1}|S_{v2})P(S_{v1}|S'_{v2})/Z.$$

In the cortex, the what and where pathways are segregated into the ventral and the dorsal streams, respectively (Ungerleider & Mishkin, 1982). Their recurrent interaction in V1 therefore can integrate the spatial and object information. More generally, different aspects of information from each hypercolumn in V1 are channelled to visual modules or modular streams for further processing, and the feedback from these extrastriate modules to V1 carries the invariant information they inferred. V1, as the high-resolution buffer, is where all the higher order information can come back together to the same spatial locus to reintegrate all the broken features into a unified percept.

Deco and I (Deco & Lee, 2002) developed a neural dynamical model, which could be considered a deterministic approximation (Abbott, 1992; Amit & Tsodyks, 1991; Wilson & Cowen, 1972) of the statistical inference framework, to explore the possibility that V1 can serve as a buffer to coordinate the interaction between the dorsal stream and the ventral stream and to achieve feature integration in conjunctive visual search (Fig. 13.9). For simplicity, the model contains only three modules. The V1 module is directly and reciprocally connected to the IT module, which encodes object classes, and to the parietal-occipital area (PO) module, which encodes spatial location. The prefrontal areas can exert a top-down bias to a particular neuronal pool in IT to initiate object attention (what to look for) or to a particular neuronal pool in PO to initiate spatial attention (where to look at). V1 is modeled with a two-dimensional grid of hypercolumns, each with 24 pools of complex cells (eight orientations and three scales) modeled as power modulus of Gabor wavelets (Lee, 1996). PO is modeled by a two-dimensional grid of nodes. Each node (neuronal pool) indicates a particular spatial location and is connected to a small spatially contiguous subset of V1 hypercolumns in a reciprocal manner. Each IT neuron represents a particular object and is connected reciprocally to every V1 neuron. The pattern of connection is symmetrical and is learned by Hebbian learning, but the feedback weights are weaker than the feedforward weights (set to 60%; see Deco & Lee, 2002, for details). Within each module, there are inhibitory neurons to mediate competition.

When a single object is presented to the retina, a local region of V1 neurons are activated, which activate a number of IT neurons and a number of PO neurons. Competition within IT and within PO rapidly narrows down a winner cell in IT (corresponding to recognition of the identity of the presented object) and a winner cell in PO (corresponding to localization of the object in space). The coactivation of the specific pools of neurons in the three modules corresponds to the unified percept of identity, location, and features of the presented object (Fig. 13.10).

Visual search (object attention) is initiated by introducing a top-down positive bias to an IT neuron, presumably from the prefrontal cortex (Rao, Rainer & Miller, 1997). The IT neuron will project a top-down template of subthreshold activation to V1. Any subset of V1 hypercolumns whose response patterns match that of the top-down template will be selectively enhanced, as in resonance. These enhanced neurons exert a suppressive effect on other V1 neurons and provide a stronger bottom-up bias to the PO neuron corresponding to that location. Initially a number of PO neurons scattered in space will be activated by bottom-up V1 input. Over time, the lateral inhibition in PO will narrow the activation to a very localized set of neurons in PO, indicating the localization of the searched object. Interestingly, this model can produce the effect of both the parallel search and the serial search using one single mechanism. When the system is instructed to search for an L in a field of Xs, the time for the PO to converge in a single location is independent of the number of Xs, corresponding to parallel search. When the system is instructed to search for an L in a field of Ts, the search time increases linearly with the number

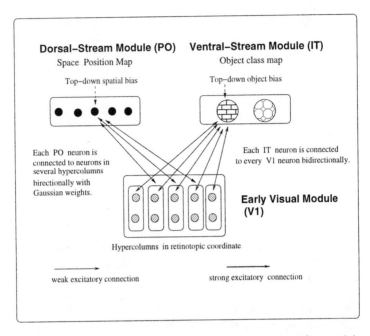

Dorsal–Stream Module (PO)
Space Position Map

Ventral–Stream Module (IT)
Object class map

Top–down spatial bias

Top–down object bias

Each PO neuron is
connected to neurons in
several hypercolumns
birectionally with
Gaussian weights.

Each IT neuron is connected
to every V1 neuron bidirectionally.

**Early Visual Module
(V1)**

Hypercolumns in retinotopic coordinate

weak excitatory connection

strong excitatory connection

FIG. 13.9.   A schematic diagram of the model. The simplified model contains three modules: the early visual module (V1), the ventral stream module (IT), and the dorsal stream module (PO). The V1 module contains orientation-selective complex cells and hypercolumns as in the primary visual cortex (V1). The IT module contains neuronal pools coding for specific object classes as in the inferotemporal cortex. The PO module contains a map encoding positions in spatial coordinates as in the parietal occipital cortex or posterior parietal cortex. The V1 module and the IT module are linked with symmetrical connections developed from Hebbian learning. The V1 module and the PO module are connected with symmetrically localized connections modeled with Gaussian weights. Competitive interaction within each module is mediated by inhibitory pools. Connections between modules are excitatory, providing biases for shaping the competitive dynamics within each module. Convergence of neural activation to an individual pool in the IT module corresponds to object recognition. Convergence of neural activation to a neuronal pool in PO corresponds to target localization. The V1 module provides the high-resolution buffer for the IT and the PO modules to interact. From "A Unified Model of Spatial and Object Attention Based on Inter-cortical Biased Competition," by G. Deco and T. S. Lee, 2002, *Neurocomputing, 44–46,* 771. Copyright 2002 by Springer-Verlag. Adapted with permission.

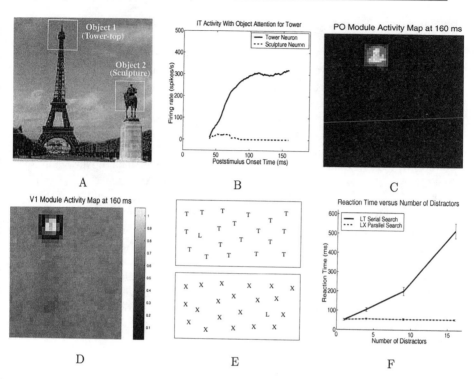

FIG. 13.10. (A) A Paris scene. (B) In a visual search task, the system functions in the object attention mode. For example, when the scene was presented to the retina, a top-down bias is imposed by the prefrontal area to a tower neuronal pool in the IT. This bias, when combined with the bottom-up excitation from V1, enables the tower neuron to dominate over the neurons encoding the other objects, such as the sculpture. (C) and (D) show that the activation of the PO map and the V1 map have converged to a single spatial locus at 160 ms after stimulus onset, indicating that the target (tower) has been localized. (E) The latter L can be instantly detected in a field of Xs but not in a field of Ts by humans. (F) The model system can detect L in a field of Xs in constant time, but the time required to detect L in a field of Ts increases linearly with the number of Ts. This shows that serial search and parallel search are in fact implemented by a single object-attention mechanism.

of distractors T. This is because when the target and the distractor are similar, the responses in the V1 hypercolumns (at least in feature level) to each are very similar, causing a confusion that requires constant interaction between V1 and IT to gradually resolve. Surprisingly, for reasons we do not completely understand, the time required to search for an ambiguous conjunctive target is linearly proportional to the number of distractors, as in serial search. Apparently, the phenomena of serial and parallel search emerge from the same parallel mechanism (see Deco & Lee, 2002, for details).

Spatial attention can be introduced by providing a bias (spatial prior) to a particular neuronal pool in PO. The interaction between PO and V1 acts in very much the same way except that the top-down bias from PO is spatial rather than featural. PO extracts only the spatial information from V1 to focus the competition on the spatial domain. This facilitates the convergence, or localization, of the winner in a visual search task. In the model my colleagues and I used, spatial attention serves a very useful purpose: The gating of information from V1 to IT is accomplished simply by PO's modulation of V1 activities rather than by modulating the feedforward connection weights as in other models (Olshausen, Andersen, & Van Essen, 1993; Reynolds et al., 1998). The system can serially channel visual information from different V1 hypercolumns to IT for object recognition simply by allocating the top-down spatial prior to different neuronal pools in PO. Another interesting observation is that a relatively small top-down modulation in V1 from PO is sufficient to relay a bias to IT to produce a winner in IT. This suggests that even though the top-down effect in the early visual areas is small, it could still be effective in coordinating the communication and information integration among multiple visual streams. Simple as it is, the model is sufficient to illustrate how the early visual cortex can coordinate and organize parallel and distributed computations in the visual system from a dynamical system perspective.

CONCLUSION

In this article, I propose that hierarchical probabilistic Bayesian inference, when coupled with the concept of efficient coding, provides a reasonable framework for conceptualizing the principles of neural computations underlying perceptual organization. I described a number of recent experimental findings from my laboratory providing evidence in support of this framework. Evidence from other laboratories (Albright & Stoner, 2002; Crist, Li, & Gilbert, 2001; Grosof, Shapely, & Hawken, 1993; Haenny & Schiller, 1988; Hupe et al., 1998; Ito & Gilbert, 1999; Lamme, 1995; Motter, 1993; Murray, Kersten, Olshausen, Schrater, & Woods, 2002; Ress, Backus, & Heeger, 2000; Roelfsema, Lamme, & Spekreijse, 1998; von der Heydt, Peterhans, & Baumgarthner, 1984; Zhou, Friedman, & von der Heydt, 2000; Zipser, Lamme, & Schiller, 1996) on the top-down contextual influences in the early visual areas also support the basic premise of this theory.

The hierarchical Bayes framework proposed here can reconcile some apparent contradictions between the predictive coding theory (Mumford, 1996a; Rao & Ballard, 1999) and adaptive resonance theory (Grossberg, 1987) in that it contains both the explaining away as well as the resonance components. Here, the top-down feedback of a higher level hypothesis does attenuate the saliency of the earlier representations that support it on the one hand but also suppresses even more severely the alternative evidence and hypotheses. This framework also unifies top-down attention and bottom-up perceptual inference into a single hierarchical system. Attention can be considered a variety of top-down priors (spatial, object, feature) for influencing the perceptual inference at the earlier levels.

Perceptual organization, such as grouping, segmentation, and figure-ground segregation, however, involves far more sophisticated computations than competitive interactions (e.g., August & Zucker, 2000; Blake & Zisserman, 1987; Grossberg, Mingolla, & Ross, 1994; Konishi, Yuille, Coughlan, & Zhu, in press; Lee, 1995; Shi & Malik, 2000; Tu & Zhu, 2002; Weiss, Simoncelli, & Adelson, 2002; Williams & Jacobs, 1997; Yu, 2003; Yu, Lee, & Kanade, 2002; Yuille & Bulthoff, 1996; Zhu, Lee, & Yuille, 1995). The hierarchy idea proposed here is deeply connected with the idea of compositional hierarchy from Bienenstock, Geman, and Potter (1997). With the addition of recurrent feedback of contextual and attentional priors, the proposed hierarchical framework provides a broader view on the nature of cortical computations of perceptual organization. Elucidating the varieties of Bayesian priors as a function of task demands and environmental statistics is important for understanding the computational and neural basis of attentive perceptual organization.

ACKNOWLEDGMENTS

This work is supported by NSF CAREER 9984706 and NIH Vision Research core grant EY08098 and Siemens, AG. The author extends his thanks to many of his colleagues, in particular David Mumford, Peter Schiller, Carl Olson, Gustavo Deco, My Nguyen, Cindy Yang, Rick Romero, Stella Yu, Brian Potetz, Victor Lamme, and Kae Nakamura for advice and assistance and to Marlene Behrmann and Steve Palmer for helpful comments on an earlier version of the manuscript. This paper is dedicated to the late Herb Simon.

REFERENCES

Abbott, L. (1992). Firing rate models for neural populations. In O. Benhar, C. Bosio, P. Giudice, & E. Tabet (Ed.), *Neural networks: From biology to high energy physics*. Pisa: ETS Editrice.

Albright, T. D., & Stoner, G. R. (2002). Contextual influences on visual processing. *Annual Review of Neuroscience, 25*, 339–379.

Amit, D., & Tsodyks, M. (1991). Quantitative study of attractor neural network retrieving at low spike rates: I. Substrate spikes, rates and neuronal gain. *Network, 2*, 259–273.

August, J., & Zucker, S. W. (2000). The curve indicator random field: Curve organization via edge correlation. In K. Boyer & S. Sarka (Ed.), *Perceptual organization for artificial vision systems* (pp. 265–288). Boston: Kluwer Academic.

Barlow, H. B. (1961). Coding of sensory messages. In W. H. Thorpe & O. L. Zangwill (Ed.), *Current problems in animal behavior* (pp. 331–360). Cambridge, UK: Cambridge University Press.

Behrmann, M., Zemel, R. S., & Mozer, M. C. (1998). Object-based attention and occlusion: Evidence from normal participants and a computational model. *Journal of Experimental Psychology: Human Perception and Performance, 24*(4), 1011–1036.

Bichot, N. P., & Schall, J. D. (1999). Effects of similarity and history on neural mechanisms of visual selection. *Nature Neuroscience, 2*(6), 549–554.

Bienenstock, E., Geman, S., & Potter, D. (1997). Compositionality, MDL priors, and object recognition. In M. C. Mozer, M. I. Jordan, & T. Petsche (Ed.), *Advances in neural information processing systems, 9* (pp. 838–844). Cambridge, MA: MIT Press.

Blake, A., & Zisserman, A. (1987). *Visual reconstruction.* Cambridge, MA: MIT Press.

Braun, J. (1993). Shape from shading is independent of visual attention and may be a "texton." *Spatial Vision, 7*(4), 311–322.

Bullier, J. (2001). Integrated model of visual processing. *Brain Research Review, 36*(2–3), 96–107.

Connor, C. E., Preddie, D. C., Gallant, J. L., & Van Essen D. C. (1997). Spatial attention effects in macaque area V4. *J. Neuroscience, 17*(9), 3201–3214.

Crist, R. E., Li, W., & Gilbert, C. D. (2001). Learning to see: Experience and attention in primary visual cortex. *Nature Neuroscience, 4*(5), 519–525.

Dayan, P., Hinton, G. E., Neal, R. M., & Zemel, R. S. (1995). The Helmholtz machine. *Neural Computation, 7*(5), 889–904.

Deco, G., & Lee, T. S. (2002). A unified model of spatial and object attention based on inter-cortical biased competition. *Neurocomputing, 44–46,* 769–774.

Desimone, R., & Duncan, J. (1995). Neural mechanisms of selective visual attention. *Annual Review Neuroscience, 18,* 193–222.

Duncan, J., & Humphreys, G. (1989). Visual search and stimulus similarity. *Psychological Review, 96,* 433–458.

Felleman, D. J., & Van Essen, D. C. (1991). Distributed hierarchical processing in the primate cerebral cortex. *Cerebral Cortex, 1,* 1–47.

Field, D. J. (1994). What is the goal of sensory coding? *Neural Computing, 6,* 559–601.

Grenander, U. (1976). *Lectures in pattern theory I: Pattern analysis.* New York: Springer-Verlag.

Grenander, U. (1978). *Lectures in pattern theory II: Pattern synthesis.* New York: Springer-Verlag.

Grenander, U. (1981). *Lectures in pattern theory III: Regular structures.* New York: Springer-Verlag.

Grosof, D. H., Shapley, R. M., & Hawken, M. J. (1993). Macaque V1 neurons can signal "illusory" contours. *Nature, 365*(6446), 550–552.

Grossberg, S. (1987). Competitive learning: from interactive activation to adaptive resonance. *Cognitive Science, 11,* 23–63.

Grossberg, S., Mingolla, E., & Ross, W. (1994). A neural theory of attentive visual search: Interactions at boundary, surface, spatial and object attention. *Psychological Review, 101*(3), 470–489.

Haenny, P. E., & Schiller, P. H. (1988). State dependent activity in monkey visual cortex. I. Single cell activity in V1 and V4 on visual tasks. *Experimental Brain Research, 69*(2):225–244.

Helmholtz, H. V. (1867). *Handbook of physiological optics.* Leipzig: Voss.

Hubel, D. H., & Wiesel, T. N. (1962). Receptive fields, binocular integration and functional architecture in the cat's visual cortex. *Journal of Physiology, 160,* 106–154.

Hupe, J. M., James, A. C., Payne, B. R., Lomber, S. G., Girard P., & Bullier, J. (1998). Cortical feedback improves discrimination between figure and background by V1, V2 and V3 neurons. *Nautre, 394* (6695), 784–787.

Ito, M., & Gillbert, C. D. (1999). Attention modulates contextual influences in the primary visual cortex of alert monkeys. *Neuron, 22,* 593–604.

Itti, L., & Koch, C. (2001). Computational modeling of visual attention. *Nature Review Neuroscience, 2*(3), 194–203.

James, W. (1890). *The principles of psychology.* New York: Henry Holt.

Joseph, J. S., Chun, M. M., & Nakayama, K. (1997). Attentional requirements in a "preattentive" feature search task. *Nature, 387,* 805–807.

Knill, D. C., & Richards, W. (1996). *Perception as Bayesian inference*. Cambridge, UK: Cambridge University Press.

Konishi, S. M., Yuille, A. L., Coughlan J. M., & Zhu, S. C. (in press). Statistical edge detection: Learning and evaluating edge cues. *IEEE Transactions on Pattern Analysis and Machine Intelligence*.

Lades, M., Vorbruggen, J. C., Buhmann, J., Lange, J., von der Malsburg, C., Wurtz, R. P., et al. (1993). Distortion invariant object recognition in the dynamic link architecture. *IEEE Transactions in Computers, 42*(3), 300–311.

Lamme, V. A. F. (1995). The neurophysiology of figure-ground segregation in primary visual cortex. *Journal of Neuroscience, 15*(2), 1605–1615.

Lee, T. S. (1995). A Bayesian framework for understanding texture segmentation in the primary visual cortex. *Vision Research, 35,* 2643–2657.

Lee, T. S. (1996). Image representation using 2D Gabor wavelets. *IEEE Transactions on Pattern Analysis and Machine Intelligence, 18*(10), 959–971.

Lee, T. S., & Mumford, D. (in press). Hierarchical Bayesian inference in the visual cortex. *Journal of Optical Society of America*.

Lee, T. S., Mumford, D., Romero, R., & Lamme, V. A. F. (1998). The role of the primary visual cortex in higher level vision. *Vision Research, 38*(15–16), 2429–2454.

Lee, T. S., & Nguyen, M. (2001). Dynamics of subjective contour formation in the early visual cortex. *Proceedings of the National Academy of Sciences, 98*(4), 1907–1911.

Lee, T. S., Yang, C., Romero, R., & Mumford, D. (2002). Neural activity in early visual cortex reflects experience and higher order perceptual saliency. *Nature Neuroscience, 5*(6), 589–597.

Lewicki, M. S., & Olshausen, B. A. (1999). Probabilistic framework for the adaptation and comparison of image codes. *Journal of Optical Society of America, A, 16*(7), 1587–1601.

Li, Z. (2001). Computational design and nonlinear dynamics of a recurrent network model of the primary visual cortex. *Neural Computation 13*(8), 1749–1780.

Logothetis, N. K. (1998). Object vision and visual awareness. *Current Opinions in Neurobiology, 8*(4), 536–544.

Marr, D. (1982). *Vision*. New York: W. H. Freeman.

McClelland, J. L., & Rumelhart, D. E., (1981). An interactive activation model of context effects in letter perception. Part I: An account of basic findings. *Psychological Review, 88,* 375–407.

Miller, E. K., & Cohen, J. D. (2001). An integrative theory of prefrontal cortex function. *Annual Review Neuroscience, 24,* 167–202.

Motter, B. (1993). Focal attention produces spatially selective processing in visual cortical areas V1, V2, and V4 in the presence of competing stimuli. *Journal of Neurophysiology, 70,* 909–919.

Mumford, D. (1992). On the computational architecture of the neocortex II. *Biological Cybernetics, 66,* 241–251.

Mumford, D. (1996a). Pattery theory: A unifying perspective. In D. C. Knill & W. Richards (Ed.), *Perception as Bayesian inference* (pp. 25–62). Cambridge, UK: Cambridge University Press.

Mumford, D. (1996b). Commentary on the article by H. Barlow. In D. C. Knill & W. Richards (Ed.), *Perception as Bayesian inference* (pp. 451–506). Cambridge, UK: Cambridge University Press.

Murray, S. O., Kersten, D., Olshausen, B. A. Schrater, P., & Woods, D. L. (2002). Shape perception reduces activity in human primary visual cortex. *Proceedings of the National Academy of Science, USA 99,* 15164–15169.

Olshausen, B. A., Andersen, C., & Van Essen, D. (1993). A neural model for visual attention and invariant pattern recognition. *Journal of Neuroscience, 13*(11), 4700–4719.

Olshausen, B. A., & Field, D. J. (1996). Emergence of simple-cell receptive field properties by learning a sparse code for natural images. *Nature, 381,* 607–609.

Olson, C. R. (2001). Object-based vision and attention in primates. *Current Opinion in Neurobiology, 11*(2), 171–179.

Palmer, S. (1999). *Vision science: Photons to phenomenology*. Cambridge, MA: MIT Press.

Palmer, S. E., Neff, J., & Beck, D. (1996). Late influences on perceptual grouping: Amodal completion. *Psychonomic Bulletin & Review, 3*(1), 75–80.

Peterson, M. A., & Gibson, B. S. (1991). The initial identification of figure-ground relationships: Contributions from shape recognition processes. *Bulletin of the Psychonomic Society, 29*(3), 199–202.

Prezybyszewski, A. W., Gaska, J. P., Foote, W., & Pollen, D. A. (2000). Striate cortex increases contrast gain of macaque LGN neurons. *Visual Neuroscience, 17*, 485–494.

Ramachandran, V. S. (1988). Perception of shape from shading. *Nature, 331,* 163–166.

Rao R., & Ballard, D. H. (1999). Predictive coding in the visual cortex: A functional interpretation of some extra-classical receptive-field effects. *Nature Neuroscience, 2*(1), 79–87.

Rao, S. C., Rainer, G., & Miller, E. (1997). Integration of what and where in the primate prefrontal cortex. *Science, 276,* 821–824.

Ress, D., Backus, B. T., & Heeger, D. J. (2000). Activity in primary visual cortex predicts performance in a visual detection task. *Nature Neuroscience, 3*(9), 940–945.

Reynolds, J., Chelazzi, L., & Desimone, R. (1999). Competitive mechanisms subserve attention in macaque areas V2 and V4. *Journal of Neuroscience, 19,* 1736–1753.

Roelfsema, P. R., Lamme, V. A. F., & Spekreijse, H. (1998). Object-based attention in the primary visual cortex of the macaque monkey. *Nature, 395*(6700), 376–381.

Rowley, H., Baluja, S., & Kanade, T. (1998). Neural network-based face detection. *IEEE Transactions on Pattern Analysis and Machine Intelligence, 20*(1), 23–38.

Schneiderman, H., & Kanade, T. (1998). Probabilistic modeling of local appearance and spatial relationships for object recognition. *IEEE Conference on Computer Vision and Pattern Recognition,* 45–51.

Shi, J., & Malik, J. (2000). Normalized cuts and image segmentation. *IEEE Transactions on Pattern Analysis and Machine Intelligence, 22*(8), 888–905.

Stemmler, M., Usher, M., & Niebur, E. (1995). Lateral interactions in primary visual cortex: A model bridging physiology and psychophysics. *Science, 269,* 1877–1880.

Sun, J., & Perona, P. (1996). Early computation of shape and reflectance in the visual system. *Nature, 379,* 165–168.

Thorpe, S., Fize, D., & Marlot, C. (1996). Speed of processing in the human visual system. *Nature, 381,* 520–522.

Tolias, A. S., Moore, T., Smirnakis, S. M., Tehovnik, E. J., Siapas, A. G., & Schiller, P. H. (2001). Eye movement modulate visual receptive fields of V4 neurons. *Neuron, 29*(3), 757–767.

Treisman, A., & Gelade, G. (1980). A feature-integration theory of attention. *Cognitive Psychology, 12,* 97–136.

Treisman, A., & Sato, S. (1990). Conjunction search revisited. *Journal of Experimental Psychology: Human Perception and Performance, 16,* 459–478.

Tu, Z. W., & Zhu, S. C. (2002). Image segmentation by data-driven Markov chain Monte Carlo. *IEEE Transactions on Pattern Analysis and Machine Intelligence, 24*(5), 657–673.

Ullman, S. (1984). Visual routines. *Cognition, 18,* 97–159.

Ullman, S. (1994). Sequence seeking and counterstreams: A model for bidirectional information flow in the cortex. In C. Koch & J. Davis (Ed.), *Large-scale theories of the cortex* (pp. 257–270). Cambridge, MA: MIT Press.

Ungerleider, L.G., & Mishkin, M. (1982). Two cortical visual systems. In D. J. Ingle (Ed.), *Analysis of visual behavior* (pp. 549–586). Cambridge, MA: MIT Press.

Usher, M., & Niebur, E. (1996). Modeling the temporal dynamics of IT neurons in visual search: A mechanism for top-down selective attention. *Journal of Cognitive Neuroscience, 8,* 311–327.

von der Heydt, R., Peterhans, E., & Baumgartner, G. (1984). Illusory contours and cortical neuron responses. *Science, 224*(4654), 1260–1262.

Weiss, Y., Simoncelli, E. P., & Adelson, E. H. (2002). Motion illusions as optimal percepts. *Nature Neuroscience, 5*(6), 598–604.

Williams, L., & Jacobs, D. (1997). Stochastic completion fields: A neural model of illusory contour shape and saliency. *Neural Computation, 9*(4), 837–858.

Wilson, H., & Cowan, J. (1972). Excitatory and inhibitory interactions in localised populations of model neurons. *Biological Cybernetics, 12,* 1–24.

Wolfe, J. M. (1998). Visual search: A review. In H. Pashler (Ed.), *Attention* (pp. 13–77). London: University College London Press.

Yu, S., Lee, T. S., & Kanade, T. (2002). A hierarchial Markov random field model for figure-ground segregation. *Lecture Notes in Computer Science 2134,* 118–133.

Yu, S. (2003). *Computational models of perceptual organization.* Unpublished doctoral dissertation, Robotics Institute, Carnegie Mellon University.

Yuille, A. L., & Bulthoff, H. H. (1996). Bayesian decision theory and psychophysics. In D. C. Knill & W. Richards (Ed.), *Perception as Bayesian inference* (pp. 123–162). Cambridge, UK: Cambridge University Press.

Zhou, H., Friedman, H. S., & von der Heydt, R. (2000). Coding of border ownership in monkey visual cortex. *Journal of Neuroscience, 20*(17), 6594–6611.

Zhu, S. C., Lee, T. S., & Yuille, A. (1995). Region competition: Unifying snakes, region growing and MDL for image segmentation. *Proceedings of the Fifth International Conference in Computer Vision, 416*–425.

Zipser, K., Lamme, V. A. F., & Schiller, P. H. (1996). Contextual modulation in primary visual cortex. *Journal of Neuroscience, 16,* 7376–7389.

Author Index

Note: *f* indicates figure; *n* indicates footnote.

A

Aaside, C. T., 367, *372*
Abbott, L., 449, *453*
Adams, J. L., 274, *274*
Adams, P. A., 64, *85*
Adelson, E. H., 4, *40,* 66*f, 83, 197,* 315, *334,*
  453, *456*
Adolph, K. E., 225, *230*
Agostini, T., 4, *41*
Albright, T. D., 306, 308, 311, 312, 313*f,* 314*f,*
  315, 317, 318, 319*f,* 320*f,* 323, 324*f,* 325,
  326*f,* 327*f,* 328*f,* 329*f,* 330*f,* 331, *332f, 334,*
  335, 441, 452, *453*
Allard, T., 239, *274*
Allman, J. M., 315, *334*
Alter, T., 419, *427*
Amirikian, B., 368, *372*
Amit, D., 449, *453*
Andersen, C., 452, *455*
Anderson, B. L., 4, *40,* 169, *197*
Anderson, D. I., 227, *230*
Anderson, J., 423, *427*
Anson, R., 416, *428*
Armel, C., 68, 69*f, 84*
Arterberry, M. A., 177*f,* 199
Arterberry, M. E., 274, *276*

Ashbridge, E., 92, *115*
Attneave, F., 6, 12, *40*
August, J., 453, *453*
Ault, S. J., 294, 296, *303*

B

Bachman, D. L., 339, *373*
Backus, B. T., 452, *456*
Badcock, C. J., 138, *149,* 349, *371*
Badcock, D. R., 138, *149,* 349, *371*
Bailllargeon, R., 208, 209, 210, 211*f,* 214, 215,
  216, 217*f,* 219, 225, *230, 231*
Bakin, J. S., 295, 298, *302*
Balint, R., 385*n, 396*
Ballard, D. H., 424, *428,* 432, 435, 436, 452, *456*
Baluja, S., 432, *456*
Banton, T., 181, *197*
Barbu-Roth, M. A., 227, *230*
Barlow, H. B., 6, *40,* 284*n, 302,* 436, *453*
Barrow, H. G., 160, 163, *197*
Barsalou, L., 238, *276*
Basri, R., 410, 419, *427, 428*
Bauchoud-Lévi, A.-C., 96, 97, *116*
Baumann, R., 295, *302*
Baumgartner, G., 452, *456*

Bavelier, D., 255, *278*
Baylis, G. C., 89, 94, *115,* 385, 386, 390, 392, 395, *396*
Baylis, L. L., 386, 392, *396*
Beck, D., 17, 19, 20, 30, 31*f,* 33, 35*f, 40, 42,* 118, *151, 374,* 431, *455*
Bednar, J. A., 240, *277*
Behrmann, M., 255, 262, 266, *275, 277, 278,* 341, *342f, 343f,* 344*f,* 345, *346f, 351f, 353f, 354f, 357f, 360f, 361f, 364f, 371, 372, 375,* 386, *396,* 448, *454*
Beller, H. K., 120, *149,* 351, *371*
Belliveau, J. W., 377, *399*
Ben-Av, M. B., 67*f, 83,* 118, 148, *149,* 338, *371*
Bender, D. B., 378, *397*
Benedek, G., 367, *373*
Bennett, P. J., 183, *198*
Benson, P. J., 379, *398*
Bertamini, M., 188, *197*
Bettucci, D., 379, *398*
Bialek, W., 424, *429*
Bichot, N. P., 446, *454*
Biederman, I., 160, *197,* 206, *230,* 235, 236, *275*
Bienenstock, E., 453, *454*
Bilsky, A. R., 147, *153*
Bisiach, E., 385, *396*
Bixby, J. L., 315, *335*
Black, S. E. E. E., 386, *396*
Blake, A., 69, *83,* 409, *427,* 453, *454*
Blake, R., 25, *40*
Blakemore, C., 284*n, 302*
Blasdel, G. G., 240, *277*
Bloch, B., 126, *151*
Blott, W., 384, *399*
Boer, L. C., 121, *149*
Bonato, F., 4, *41*
Born, R. T., 377, *399*
Bornstein, M. H., 207, 227, *230, 232*
Boucart, M., 362, 366, 369, *370, 371, 372, 373,* 380, 382*f,* 392, 393, *396, 397*
Boutsen, L., 387, 389, *396*
Braddick, O., 71, *83*
Brady, T. J., 377, *399*
Braun, J., 443, *454*
Bravais, A., 51*n, 83*
Brefczynski, J. A., 378, *396*
Breinlinger, K., 208, 214, *231*
Britten, K. H., 317, 322, 323, 325, 331, *334, 335*
Broadbent, D. E., 121, *149*
Brooks, J. L., 36, *42*
Brosgole, L., 27, 28*f, 42,* 118, *152,* 338, *375*

Brown, E., 222, *231,* 244, *277*
Brown, J. R., 136, *150*
Bruce, V., 234, *275*
Bruner, J. S., 234, *275*
Bruno, N., 188, *197*
Bucher, N. M., 80, 81*f, 84*
Buffart, H. F. J. M., 5, 10, *40,* 193, *197*
Buhmann, J., 432, *455*
Bullier, J., 149, *150,* 368, *371,* 441, 452, *454*
Bulthoff, H. H., 453, *457*
Burns, B., 243, 249, *275*
Burr, 159, *199*
Burt, P., 49*f,* 69, 71, 72, *83*
Butter, C. M., 341, *371,* 380, *396*

C

Campbell, F. W., 3, *40,* 159, *197*
Campos, J. J., 227, *230*
Capitani, E., 385, *396*
Carpenter, G., 424, *427*
Cattell, J. M., 243, *275*
Cavanagh, P., 64*f,* 65, 66, 68, 70, 71, *83, 84*
Chainay, H., 339, *372,* 384, *396*
Chambers, D., 158, *198*
Chandna, A., 361, 362*f, 373, 374*
Chatterjee, A., 341, 349, 368, *374*
Chelazzi, L., 101, *116,* 333, *334,* 433, 442, 452, *456*
Chellappa, R., 406, *428*
Chen, L., 118, 121, 147, 148, *150,* 338, 345, *372*
Choe, Y., 240, *277*
Chun, M. M., 446, *454*
Cicerone, C. M., 71, *83*
Cinel, C., 158, *198,* 387, 388, 389, 390, 391*f,* 393, 395, *398*
Clark, J. J., 25, *42*
Clark, S. A., 239, *274*
Cobb, S., 416, 419, *428*
Cohen, A., 385, *396*
Cohen, D. J., 395, *398*
Cohen, J. D., 442, *455*
Cohen, M. H., 71, *83,* 188, *199*
Connor, C. E., 101, *115,* 442, *454*
Cooper, A. C. G., 385, 386, 387, 392, *396, 397*
Cooper, G. F., 159, *197*
Corballis, P. M., 370, *372*
Corwin, J. V., 136, *152*
Coslett, H. B., 385, *399*

Coughlan, J. M., 453, *455*
Cowan, J., 449, *457*
Cowey, A., 377, *396, 398*
Crabbe, G., 169, 174, *199*
Craton, L. G., 214, 215, *230*
Creutzfelt, O. D., 393, *399*
Crick, F., 394, *397*
Crist, R. E., 452, *454*
Croner, L. J., 306, 322*f,* 323, 324*f,* 325, 326*f,*
    327*f,* 328*f,* 329*f,* 330*f,* 331, 332*f, 334*
Crook, J. M., 393, *399*
Csibra, G., 227, *230*
Czerwinski, M., 243, *275*

D

Dale, A. M., 393, *398*
Daugman, J. G., 13, *41*
Davidoff, J., 368, *371*
Davidson, D. L. W., 379, *398*
Davies, I. R. L., 235, *278*
Davis, G., 140, *150,* 338, *372,* 386, *398*
Dayan, P., 236, *276, 424, 428,* 432, 433, *454*
Deco, G., 433, 442, 449, 450*f,* 452, *454*
de Gelder, B., 96, 97, *116*
Dell' Acqua, R., 369, *372*
Dempster, A., 236, *275*
DeRenzi, E., 380, 385, *397*
Desimone, R., 101, *115, 116,* 300, *302, 303,*
    315, 333, *334,* 377, 378, *397, 398,* 433,
    441, 442, 452, *454, 456*
De Valois, K. K., 13, *41*
De Valois, R. L., 13, *41,* 294, *302*
De Weerd, P., 101, *115*
de Yoe, A. E., 378, *396*
Dobkins, K. R., 315, *334*
Doniger, G., 366, 367, *371*
Donk, M., 385, *397*
Donnelly, N., 132, *149,* 339, *371, 373,* 394, *396,*
    398
Dowling, W. J., 10, *41*
Driver, J., 89, 94, *115,* 140, *149,* 338, *372,* 385,
    386, 390, 392, 395, *396, 398, 399*
Dueker, G., 224, *231*
Duncan, J., 124, *150,* 386, 387, 393, 394, *397,*
    398, 433, 441, 442, *454*
Duncan, R. O., 311, 312, 313*f,* 317, 319*f,* 320*f,*
    334

E

Eagle, R. A., 69, *83*
Eckhorn, R., 378, *397*
Edelman, G. M., 297, *302, 304*
Edelman, S., 238, *275*
Efron, R., 341, *372*
Egeth, H. E., 119, 140, 148, *151,* 338, *374,* 395,
    399
Egly, R., 248, *275*
Eldracher, M., 240, *277*
Elliott, M. A., 378, *397*
Ellis, A. W. W. W., 392, *397*
Enns, J. T., 39, *42,* 124, 138, 140, 147, *150, 152,*
    345, 356, 363, *372, 374, 375,* 394, *397, 399*
Enroth-Cugell, C., 159, *197*
Eriksen, C. W., 248, *275*
Everett, B. L., 136, *150*

F

Fahle, M., 238, 239, *275,* 378, *397*
Fan, S., 121, *150*
Fant, G., 236, *276*
Farah, M. J., 93, *116,* 119, 147, *153,* 234, *275,*
    339, *372,* 379, 390, *399*
Feher, A., 367, *373*
Feldman, J., 369, *372*
Felleman, D. J., 432, *454*
Fendrich, R., 138, *150,* 349, 370, *372, 373*
Fenstemaker, S. B., 296, *303*
Field, D. J., 13, *42,* 179, 180, *197,* 436, *454,*
    455
Finkel, L. H., 181, *201,* 297, *302*
Finlay, B. L., *304*
Fischer, B., 159, *197*
Fischl, B., 393, *398*
Fize, D., 432, 446, *456*
Fleming, R. W., 169, *197*
Flude, B., 392, *397*
Flynn, C., 193, *200*
Fodor, J., 206, *230*
Foltin, B., 240, *277*
Foote, W., 433, *456*
Foster, C., 68, 69*f, 84*
Foxe, J. J., 366, 367, *371*
Frackowiak, R. S. J., 378, *399*
Frank, D. A., 233, *275*
Freeman, E., 140, *150, 372*
Freeman, T., 338, 339, *373*

Frey, B. J., 236, *276,* 424, *428*
Freyd, J. F., 68, *84*
Friedman, H. S., 149, *153,* 282, 283*f,* 284*n,* 285*f,*
    286*f,* 287*f,* 289, 290, 292*f,* 293*f,* 295*f,* 296,
    297, 300, *303, 304,* 368, *375,* 452, *457*
Friedman-Hill, S., 147, *153,* 385, 386, 387, *397,*
    399

G

Gade, A., 341, *372, 374*
Gallant, J. L., 442, *454*
Gallogly, D. P., 180, *198*
Gannon, T., 384, *399*
Garner, W. R., 5, 8, *41, 83,* 242, 249, *275*
Garraghty, P. E., 239, *275*
Garrigan, P., 183, 185, *199*
Gaska, J. P., 433, *456*
Gasser, M., 250, *278*
Gattass, R., 315, *334*
Gauthier, I., 243, 244, *275,* 341, 368, *372*
Gazzaniga, M. S., 370, *372*
Gegenfurtner, K. R., 296, *303*
Geiger, D., 419, *428*
Geisler, W. S., 180, *198*
Gelade, G., 242, *278,* 379, *399,* 431, 441, *456*
Gelatt, C. D., 263, *276*
Geman, D., 404, 409, *428*
Geman, S., 404, 409, *428,* 453, *454*
Genovese, C., 341, *374*
Georgopoulos, A. P., 368, *372*
Georgopoulos, M. S., 368, *372*
Gepshtein, S., 70, 72, 74, *76f, 77f, 83*
Gerhardstein, P. C., 96, 97, *116*
Gerlach, C., 341, 367, *372, 374*
Getty, D. J., 325, *335*
Ghahramani, Z., 236, 237*f,* 240, 267, *275*
Gibson, B. S., 89*f,* 91, 92, 93, 94*f,* 95, 96, 97,
    103*n,* 104*n,* 105*f,* 107*f,* 109, 110, *113n,*
    115, 116, 119, 147, *152,* 161, 166, *200,*
    431, *456*
Gibson, E. J., 238, 241, *275*
Gibson, J. J., 7, 13, *41,* 159, 169, *198,* 206, *230*
Giersch, A., 362, 366, *372,* 380, 382*f,* 392, 393,
    397
Gilbert, C., 384, 393, *397*
Gilbert, C. D., 296, 298, *302,* 452, *454*
Gilchrist, A., 4, *41*
Gilchrist, I., 386, 387, 389, 392, *397*
Gillam, B., 158, *198*

Ginsburg, A. P., 349, *372*
Ginsburg, P. A., 138, *150*
Girard, P., 452, *454*
Gish, K., 138, *152,* 349, 369, *375*
Gizzi, M., 315, *334*
Gold, J. M., 183, *198*
Goldmeier, E., 121, *150,* 355, *372*
Goldstone, R. L., 238, 239, 241, 244, 246*f,* 247*f,*
    248*f,* 250, 251*f,* 252, 253*f,* 255, 256*f,* 257*f,*
    258, 261*f,* 265, 266, 267, 272, 273, *275,*
    276, 277
Goodale, M. A., 228, *231,* 377, 379, *398*
Goodrich, S. J., 386, 392, *397, 399*
Gormican, S., 118, 124, *152*
Göttschaldt, K., 95, *115*
Gowdy, P. D., 71, *83*
Grabbé, G., 71, *84*
Grabowecky, M., 386, *399*
Grainger, J., 369, *372*
Grant, P., 119, 139, *152*
Gray, C. M., 25, *41,* 378, *399*
Green, D. M., 325, *335*
Greenberg, M. E., 233, *275*
Gregory, R. L., 181, *198,* 297, *303*
Grenander, U., 433, 435, *454*
Grimes, D., 424, *428*
Grosof, D. H., 393, *397,* 452, *454*
Gross, C. G., 315, *334,* 378, *397*
Grossberg, S., 13, *41,* 158, 181, *197, 198,* 259,
    276, 297, 298, *303,* 395, *397,* 419, 424,
    428, 432, 435, 452, 453, *454*
Grünbaum, B., 53*n, 83*
Gurvits, L., 419, *428*
Guttman, S. E., 158, 181, 194, *198, 199*
Guy, G., 419, *428*

H

Hadad, B., 119, 134, 135*f, 151,* 206, *231*
Haenny, P. E., 452, *454*
Hajnal, V. J., 378, *399*
Hall, D. G., 227, *231,* 385, 386, 387, 392,
    397
Hall, G., 238, *276*
Halle, M., 236, *276*
Han, S., 118, 121, 147, 148, *150,* 338, 345,
    372
Hanson, A., 413, *429*
Hardy, D., 49, *83*
Harris, C. S., 243, *278*

Harris, J. P., 181, *198*
Harvey, E. H., 91, 92, 97, *116*
Harvey, E. M., 300, *304*
Hawken, M. J., 393, *397,* 452, *454*
Haxby, J. V., 378, *399*
Hayes, A., 179, 180, *197*
He, Z. J., 147, *150,* 297, *303*
Heeger, D. J., 452, *456*
Heeley, D. W., 379, *398*
Heitger, F., 160, 181, *198,* 295, 298, *303, 304*
Heitger, R., 419, *428*
Helmholtz, H. V., 433, 441, *454*
Hemenway, K., 10, *42*
Hepler, N., 294, *302*
Hertenstein, M. J., 227, *230*
Hespos, S. J., 224, *230*
Hess, R. F., 179, 180, *197*
Hesse, R. I., 65, *83*
Heywood, C. A., 377, *398*
Higgins, B. A., 367, *371*
Hildreth, E. C., 27, *41,* 64, 65, *83,* 159, *199*
Hillyard, S. A., 378, *398*
Hinton, G. E., 13, *41,* 96, *115,* 236, *276,* 424, *428,* 432, 433, *454*
Hochberg, J., 49, *83,* 104, 111, *115, 116*
Hochhaus, L., 136, *150*
Hoffman, D. D., 71, *83,* 134, *150,* 176, 179, *198,* 200, 218, *230*
Hofstadter, D. R., 264, *276*
Hogervorst, M. A., 69, *83*
Holcombe A. O., 57, 59, 72, *83*
Hollier, J., 395, *398*
Homa, D., 248, *275*
Hopfield, J. J., 13, *41*
Horn, B., 408, *428*
Horn, B. K. P., 6, *41*
Howard, I. P., 110, *115*
Hubbard, E. M., 227, *230*
Hubel, D. H., 3, 13, *41,* 118, *150,* 159, *198,* 228, *231,* 309f, 315, *334,* 441, *454*
Hughes, H. C., 138, *150,* 349, 369, *373*
Hummel, J. E., 235, *276*
Humphreys, G. W., 23, *41,* 118, 124, 132, 147, 148, *149, 150,* 158, *198,* 338, 339, 341, 342, 345, 348, 355, 362, 367, 369, 370, *371, 372, 374, 375,* 379, 380, 382f, 384, 385, 386, 387, 388, 389, 390, 391f, 392, 393, 394, 395, *396, 397, 398, 399,* 442, *454*
Hupe, J. M., 452, *454*

I

Ito, M., 384, *397,* 452, *454*
Itti, L., 441, *454*
Ivry, R., 138, *150,* 369, *373, 375*

J

Jacobs, D., 403, 404, 410, 411, 412, 413, 416, 423, 424, *428, 429,* 453, *457*
Jacobson, K., 208, 214, *231*
Jagadeesh, B., 101, *115*
Jain, A., 406, *428*
Jakobson, R., 236, *276*
James, A. C., 452, *454*
James, W., 441, *454*
Jankowiak, J., 339, *373*
Javitt, D. C., 366, 367, *372*
Jeannesod, M., 377, *398*
Jenkins, W. M., 239, *274*
Job, R., 369, *372*
Johansson, G., *198*
Johnson, M. H., 228, *230*
Johnson, S. P., 206, *230,* 244, *276*
Johnston, R. S., 379, *398*
Jolicœur, P., 92, *115*
Jones, V., 384, *399*
Jordan, T. R., 379, *398*
Joseph, J. S., 446, *454*
Judd, S. A., 67, 68f, *84*
Julesz, B., 65, *83,* 147, *151,* 159, *199*

K

Kaas, J. H., 239, *275, 276,* 315, *334*
Kahn, S., 119, 139, 142, 148, *151,* 338, *374*
Kaiser, M. K., 68, *84*
Kanade, T., 432, 453, *456, 457*
Kanizsa, G., 14, *41,* 71, *83,* 169, 193, *198,* 295, *303*
Kapadia, M. K., 384, 393, *397*
Kaplan, G. A., 71, *83,* 159, *198*
Karizsa, G., 412, *428*
Karlin, S., 406, *429*
Karnath, H.-O., 386, *398*
Karni, A., 238, *276*
Kartsounis, L., 341, 367, *373*
Kastner, S., 101, *115*
Kaufman, J., 213, 219, *230, 231*

Kaufman, L., 214, 216, 218, *231*
Kawaguchi, J., 195, *198*
Kay, P., 234, *276*
Kellman, P. J., 6, 10, *41,* 71, *83, 84,* 127, *150,*
   152, 157*f,* 158, 159, 160, 163, 165, 166,
   167*f,* 168, 170, 171, 173, 176, 177*f,* 178,
   179, 181, 183, 185, 187, 188, 189, 192*f,*
   194, 196, *198, 199, 200, 201,* 206, *230,*
   274, *276,* 356, 367, *373, 375,* 393, *398, 399*
Kemler, D. G., 250, *276, 278*
Kennedy, J. M., 89, *115*
Kersten, A., 244, 255, *276*
Kersten, D., 452, *455*
Kestenbuam, R., 206, 221, *231*
Keuss, P. J. G., 121, *149*
Kienker, P. K., 13, *41,* 96, *115*
Kim, J., *199*
Kim, J. H., 97, 98*f,* 99*f,* 101, 108, *116*
Kim, J. S., 71, *83*
Kim, S. G., 367, *371*
Kimchi, R., 11, *42,* 118, 119, 120, 121, 122*f,*
   123*f,* 124, 125*f,* 126, 128*f,* 129*f,* 130, 131*f,*
   132, 133*f,* 134, 135*f,* 140, 141*f,* 143*f,* 144*f,*
   145*f, 150, 151, 152,* 206, *231,* 338, 341,
   342*f,* 343*f,* 345, *346f,* 349, 351*f,* 354*f,* 353*f,*
   355, 357*f,* 358, 360*f,* 361*f,* 364*f, 371, 373*
Kingstone, A., 124, 138, *150,* 345, *372*
Kinsbourne, M., 339, *373*
Kiper, D. C., 296, *303*
Kirkpatrick, S., 263, *276*
Kleffner, D. A., 147, *151*
Klempen, A., 158, *198*
Klempen, N., 387, 388, 389, 390, 391*f,* 393,
   395, *398*
Knight, R. T., 370, *374*
Knill, D. C., 433, *455*
Knoll, J. K., 99*f, 115*
Koch, C., 441, *454*
Koffka, K., 117, 140, *151,* 161, 169, 193, *199,*
   243, *276,* 281, *303,* 338, *373*
Köhler, W., 12, *41,* 95, *115,* 117, *151*
Kohonen, T., 238, *276*
Kojo, I., 188, *199*
Kolers, P. A., 69, *83,* 240, *276*
Konishi, S. M., 453, *455*
Korte, A., 71, *83*
Kosko, B., 404, 424, *428*
Kossyfidis, C., 4, *41*
Kovács, I. 147, *151,* 361*f,* 362*f,* 367, *372, 373,*
   380, 382*f,* 392, 393, *397, 398*
Kozma, P., 366, *373*

Kramer, P., 70, *83*
Krantz, D. H., 49, *83*
Kroll, J. K., 99
Kübler, O., 160, 181, *198,* 295, 298, *303*
Kubovy, M., 51*n,* 52*f,* 53, 54*f,* 55*f,* 56, 57*f,* 58*f,*
   59, 70, 72, 74, *76f, 77f,* 78, 79, *83, 84,* 395,
   398
Kuhn, T. S., 233, *276*
Kumada, T., 386, *398*
Kumaran, K., 419, *428*
Kurylo, D. D., 118, 148, *151,* 338, *373*
Kwong, K., 377, *399*

L

LaBerge, D., 243, *276*
Lades, M., 432, *455*
Laird, N., 236, *275*
Lamb, M. R., 138, *151,* 347, 349, 370,
   374
Lamme, V. A. F., 148, *151,* 298, *303, 304,* 367,
   374, 432, 437, 441, 446, 447*f,* 452, *455,*
   456, 457
Lampignano, D. L., 101, 108, *116*
Lange, J., 432, *455*
Lasaga, M. I., 126, *151*
Law, I., *372*
Lawson, R., 341, *374,* 380, *398*
Lee, T. S., 149, *151,* 298, *303,* 367, 368, *374,*
   432, 433, 437, 438, 439*f,* 440*f,* 441, 442,
   443, 444*f,* 445*f,* 446, 447*f,* 449, 450*f,* 452,
   453, *454, 455, 457*
Leeuwenberg, E., 193, *197*
Leeuwenberg, E. L. J., 5, 10, *40, 41, 43,* 193,
   201
Lehky, S. R., 13, *41*
Leslie, A. M., 227, *232*
Leventhal, A. G., 294, 296, *303*
Levi, D. M., 181, *197*
Levitin, D., 19, *42*
Levitt, J. B., 296, *303*
Levy, J., 347, 349, *375*
Lewicki, M. S., 436, *455*
Li, C. C., 183, *199*
Li, W., 452, *454*
Li, Z., *455*
Lightfoot, N., 243, *275, 277*
Liinasuo, M., 188, *199*
Lin, E. L., 256, *276*
Linnell, K., 395, *398*

Linnet, C. M., 119, 139, *152*
Lippa, Y., 241, *276*
Liu, A. K., 393, *398*
Liu, D., 294, 296, *303*
Liu, Z., 403, 404, 410, *428*
Livingstone, M., 228, *231*
Lockhead, G., 224, *231*
Logothetis, N. K., 70, *84, 448, 455*
Lomber, S. G., 452, *454*
Lorenceau, J., 369, *371*
Loukides, M. G., 168, *199*
Lourens, T., *201*
Lovegrove, W. J., 138, *149,* 349, *371*
Lu, Z. -L., 26, *41*
Lucchelli, F., 380, *397*
Luce, R. D., 49, *84*
Luck, S. J., 378, *398*
Luzzatti, C., 385, *396*

M

Machado, L. J., 183, 185, *199*
Mack, A., 119, 139, 142, 148, *151, 152,* 338, *374*
Mackintosh, 241, *278*
Macomber, J., 208, *231*
Macuda, T. J., 289, 297, *304*
Malach, R., 377, *399*
Malik, J., 26*f,* 27, 42, 453, *456*
Mareschal, D., 228, *230*
Markman, A. B., 235, *276*
Marks, L. E., 249, *277*
Marlot, C., 432, 446, *456*
Marotta, J. J., 341, 344, *374*
Marr, D., 9, 13, 27, *41,* 90, 118, 134, 147, *151,* 159, 162, 180, *199,* 282, *303,* 338, *373,* 432, *455*
Marstrand, L., 341, *373*
Martin, G. E., 53*n, 84*
Mather, G., 64*f,* 65, 66, *83*
Mattingly, J. B., 386, *398*
Mattock, A., 222, *231,* 244, *277*
Maunsell, J. H. R., 315, *334, 335*
Mazziota, J. C., 378, *399*
McBeath, M. K., 68, *83*
McClelland, J. L., 12, *41,* 61, *84,* 147, *151,* 274, *276,* 404, 423, *428,* 432, 435, *455*
McDaniel, C., 234, *276*
McKeeff, T. J., 344, *374*
McLeod, P., 390, 395, *396*

Medin, D. L., 241, 267, *276, 278*
Medioni, G., 419, *428*
Melara, R. D., 249, *277*
Mendola, J. D., 393, *398*
Mennemeier, M., 97, *116*
Merikle, P. M., 121, *152,* 347, *374*
Merzenich, M. M., 239, *274*
Metzger, F., 14, *41*
Metzger, W., 281, *303*
Michotte, A., 26, *41,* 71, *84,* 169, 179, *199*
Miikkulainen, R., 240, *277*
Miller, E., 449, *456*
Miller, E. K., 442, *455*
Miller, J., 121, *151*
Milner, A. D., 228, *231,* 377, 379, *398*
Milner, P. M., 25, *41*
Mingolla, E., 13, *41,* 158, 181, *198,* 395, *397,* 419, *428,* 453, *454*
Mishkin, M., 101, 108, *115, 116,* 228, *232, 235,* 315, *335,* 385, *399,* 448, *456*
Mitchell, M., 264, *276*
Moore, C. M., 119, 140, 148, *151,* 338, *373*
Moore, T., 442, *456*
Moran, J., 300, *303,* 378, *398*
Mordkoff, J. T., 395, *399*
Morgan, M., 238, 239, *275*
Morikawa, K., 68, *84*
Morison, V., 222, *231,* 244, *277*
Morrone, 159, *199*
Mortara, F., 379, *398*
Moscovitch, M., 386, *396*
Motter, B., 452, *455*
Motter, B. C., 300, *303,* 333, *334*
Movshon, J. A., 66*f, 83,* 296, *303,* 316, 317, 322, 323, 325, 331, *334*
Mozer, M. C., 255, 262, 266, *275, 277, 278,* 386, *396,* 424, *428,* 448, *454*
Muller, H. M., 339, *373,* 378, *397*
Mumford, D., 298, *303,* 404, 408, 411, 413, 415, 416, *428,* 432, 433, 435, 437, 441, 443, 444*f,* 445*f,* 446, 447*f,* 452, *455*
Munakata, Y., 258, *277*
Murphy, G. L., 256, *276*
Murphy, T. D., 248, *275*
Murray, M. M., 366, 367, *371*
Murray, R. F., 183, *198*
Murray, S. O., 452, *455*
Mutani, R., 379, *398*
Myers, G. R., 378, *399*

N

Nakayama, K., 4, *41,* 70, 71, *84,* 147, *150,* 161, 181, *200,* 295, 297, 298, *302, 303,* 308 *335,* 446, *454*

Navon, D., 120, 121, *151,* 345, 354, *373*

Neal, R., 424, *428*

Neal, R. M., 236, *276,* 432, 433, *454*

Needham, A., 206, 208, 210, 211*f,* 213*f,* 214, 215*f,* 216, 217*f,* 218, 219, 220, 221, 222, 223*f,* 224, 225, *230, 231,* 244, *277*

Neff, J., 30, 31*f, 42,* 118, *151, 373,* 431, *455*

Neisser, U., 27, *42,* 63, *84,* 124, 134, *151,* 338, *373*

Nelson, J., 345, *371*

Nelson, R., 17, 32*f, 33, 42*

Newcombe, F. A., 339, *374*

Newsome, W. T., 317, 322, 323, 325, 331, *334, 335*

Nguyen, M., 149, *151,* 438, 439*f,* 440*f, 455*

Niebur, E., 433, 438, 442, *456*

Nijhawan, R., 16, 28, 29*f, 42,* 118, *152,* 338, *375*

Nitzburg, M., 413, *428*

Norcia, A. M., 361, 362*f, 373, 374*

Nosofsky, R. M., 241, *277*

Nowak, L. G., 149, *150,* 368, *371*

Nyberg, L., 425, *428*

O

Obermayer, K., 240, *277*

O'Connell, D. N., 64, *85*

Olofsson, U., 425, *428*

Olson, A., 158, *198,* 386, 387, 388, 389, 390, 391*f,* 393, 395, *398*

Olson, C. R., 448, *455*

Olshausen, B. A., 13, *42,* 436, 452, *455*

Ooi, T. L., 297, *303*

Oram, M. W., 92, *115*

O'Regan, J. K., 25, *42*

O'Reilly, R. C., 93, 96, *116,* 147, 148, *153,* 258, *277,* 298, *304*

Orlansky, J., 69, *84*

Ormsbee, S. M., 220, *231*

Oyama, T., 69, *84*

P

Pacquet, L., 347, *374*

Palm, G., 424, *429*

Palmer, E. M., 170, 188, 189, 196, *199, 200*

Palmer, S. E., 4, 5, 10, 11*f,* 12, 14, 15*f,* 16, 17, 19, 20, 21, 22, 26, 28*f,* 29*f,* 30, 31*f,* 32*f,* 33, 34, 35*f,* 36, 39, *40, 42,* 80, 81*n, 84,* 111, *115,* 118, 120, 121, 134, 147, *151, 152,* 162, 191, 193, *200,* 206, *231,* 255, *277,* 338, 352, 355, *373, 374,* 431, 432, 433, *455, 456*

Palmeri, T. J., 240, *277*

Pantle, A. J., 70, *84*

Pare, E. B., 317, 322, 323, 325, *334*

Paquet, L., 121, *152,* 347, *374*

Pashler, H., 239, *277*

Pasupathy, A., 101, *115*

Paulson, O. B., *372*

Pavel, M., 67, *84*

Payne, B. R., 452, *454*

Pearl, J., 404, 420, 421, *428*

Peled, A., *151*

Pennefather, P. M., 361, 362*f, 373, 374*

Penrod, S. D., 235, *277*

Perani, D., 385, *396*

Pereira, F., 424, *429*

Perona, P., 443, *456*

Perrett, D. I., 92, *115,* 379, *398*

Perry, J. S., 180, *198*

Pessoa, L., 395, *397*

Peterhans, E., 160, 175, 181, *198, 200,* 295, 298, *302, 303, 304,* 367, *375,* 393, *399, 456*

Peterson, M. A., 88, 89*f,* 91, 92, 93, 94*f,* 95, 96, 97, 98*f,* 99*f,* 101, 103, 104*f,* 105*n,* 107*f,* 108, 109, 110, 113*n, 115, 116,* 118, 119, 147, 148, *152,* 161, 166, *200,* 206, *231,* 300, *304,* 431, 452, *456*

Petter, G., 172, 173, 175, *200*

Pettigrew, J. D., 284*n, 302*

Pevtzow, R., 255, 256*f,* 257*f,* 258, 261*f,* 265, 266, *277*

Phillips, A., 214, *231*

Picciano, L., 70, *84*

Pick, H. L., 241, *277*

Pinker, S., 92, *116*

Plamer, S. E., 118, *152,* 338, *374*

Poggio, G. F., 159, *197*

Polat, U., 361, 362*f, 373, 374*

Pollen, D. A., 433, *456*

Pomerantz, J. R., 78, 79, *84,* 126, *152,* 347, 356, *374*

Postman, L., 234, *275*

Potter, D., 453, *454*

Potter, M. C., 99*f, 115*

Potts, B. C., 249, *277*

Preddie, D. C., 442, *454*
Prezybyszewski, A. W., 433, *456*
Price, C. J., 339, *373*
Prinzmetal, W., 389, 390, 395, *399*
Pristach, E. A., 356, *374*
Pylyshyn, Z., 95, *116*

Q

Qui, F. T., 289, 297, *304*
Quinlan, P. T., 339, *373,* 394, *398*

R

Rafal, R., 94, *115*, 385, 386, 392, *396*
Rainer, G., 449, *456*
Rajaram, S., 424, *429*
Ramachandran, V. S., 68, 69*f, 84,* 147, *151,*
    419*f, 428,* 443, *456*
Rao, R., 424, *428,* 432, 435, 436, 452, *456*
Rao, S. C., 393, *399,* 449, *456*
Rapcsak, S. Z., 96, 97, *116*
Ratcliff, G., 339, *374*
Razpurker-Apfeld, I., 140, 141*f,* 143*f,* 144*f,*
    145*f, 151, 152,* 338, 364, *373*
Redies, C., 393, *399*
Rensink, R. A., 25, 39, *42,* 124, 147, *150, 152,*
    356, *374,* 394, *397, 399*
Reppas, J. B., 377, *399*
Ress, D., 452, *456*
Restle, F., 193, *197*
Reuter-Lorenz, P., 138, *150,* 369, *373*
Reynolds, H. N., 159, *198*
Reynolds, J., 433, 442, 452, *456*
Reynolds, J. H., 101, *116,* 333, *334*
Rho, S. H., 389, 390, 395, *399*
Ricci, R., 341, 349, 368, *374*
Richards, W., 433, *455*
Richards, W. A., 134, *150,* 218, *230*
Richter, W., 368, *321*
Riddoch, J., 23, *41*
Riddoch, M. J., 132, *149,* 339, 341, 342, 348,
    356, *372, 373, 375,* 379, 380, 384, 386,
    387, 389, 390, 392, 393, 394, *397, 398, 399*
Ringach, D. L., 170, 183, *200*
Rissanen, J. J., 6, *42*
Robertson, L. C., 138, *150,* 347, 369, *370, 373,*
    374, 375, 385, 386, 387, *397, 399*
Robson, J. G., 3, *40*

Rocha-Miranda, C. E., 378, *397*
Rochat, P., 220, *231*
Rock, I., 11*f,* 12, 14, 16, 19, 22, 26, 27, 28*f,* 29*f,*
    36, *42,* 67, 71, *84,* 118, 119, 134, 139, 140,
    142, 147, 148, *151, 152, 200,* 206, *231,*
    297, *304,* 338, 363, *373, 375,* 416, *428*
Rodet, L., 240, 267, *277*
Rodman, H. R., 317, *335*
Rodriguez, J., 234, *275*
Roediger, H. L., 240, *276,* 425, *429*
Roelfsema, P. R., 367, *374,* 452, *456*
Rogers, B. J., 110, *115*
Rogers-Ramachandran, D., 416, 419*f, 428*
Rokers, B., 403, 404, *428*
Roling, P., 235, *278*
Romani, C., 386, 387, 393, *398*
Romero, R., 298, *303,* 432, 437, 441, 443, 444*f,*
    445*f,* 446, 447*f, 455*
Rosen, B. R., 377, *399*
Rosenthaler, L., 160, 181, *198,* 295, 298, *303*
Ross, W., 453, *454*
Rovamo, J., 188, *199*
Rowley, H., 432, *456*
Rubin, E., 87, 90, *116,* 161, *200,* 236, *275*
Rudra, A., 403, 404, 423, 424, *428*
Rumelhart, D., 404, 423, *428*
Rumelhart, D. E., 147, *151,* 258, 259, 267, 274,
    276, 277, 432, 435, *455*
Ruskin, D., 416, 419*f, 428*
Russell, C., 140, *150,* 338, *372*
Russo, T., 158, *198*

S

Saffran, E., 385, *399*
Sager, L. C., 126, *152*
Sagi, D., 118, 148, *149,* 238, *276,* 338, *371*
Sajda, P., 297, *302*
Sakoda, W. J., 138, *152,* 349, 369, *375*
Salzman, C. D., 322, *335*
Sambin, M., 409, *429*
Sandhofer, C., 250, *278*
Sanocki, T., 369, *375*
Sato, S., 442, *456*
Schacter, D. L., 240, *277*
Schafer, R. P., 234, *277*
Schall, J. D., 446, *454*
Schank, R., 236, *277*
Schiller, P. H., 148, *153,* 298, *304,* 442, 452,
    454, 456, 457

Schmidhuber, J., 240, *277*
Schmidt, H., 124, *152,* 385, *399*
Schneiderman, H., 432, *456*
Schrater, P., 452, *455*
Schroeder, C. E., 367, *372*
Schumacher, L. E., 13, *41,* 96, *115*
Schyns, P. G., 240, 241, 267, *277*
Sejnowski, T. J., 13, *41,* 96, *115,* 240, *277*
Sekuler, A. B., 120, *152,* 183, 193, *198, 200,* 352, *374*
Sekuler, E., 345, *371*
Sellers, E., 369, *375*
Sha'ashua, A., 417, *429*
Shadlen, M. N., 331, *334*
Shaeffer, M. M., 241, *276*
Shalev, R. S., 339, *373*
Shallice, T., 385, *399*
Shannon, C., 406, 424, *429*
Shapiro, P. N., 235, *277*
Shapley, R. M., 170, 183, *200,* 370, *372,* 393, *397,* 452, *454*
Sharma, J., 393, *399*
Shepard, G. C., 53*n, 83*
Shepard, R. N., 67, 68*f, 84,* 206, *231*
Shepp, B. E., 243, 249, 250, *275*
Sheth, B. R., 393, *399*
Shi, J., 26*f,* 27, 42, 453, *456*
Shiffrar, M., 67*f,* 68, *83, 84*
Shiffrin, R. M., 241, 243, *275, 276, 277*
Shimojo, S., 4, *42,* 161, 181, *200,* 297, *303,* 308, *335*
Ship, S., 378, *399*
Shipley, T. F., 6, 10, *41,* 71, *84,* 127, *150, 152, 157f,* 159, 160, 163, 165, *167f,* 168, 170, 171, 173, 176, 177, 178, 179, 181, 183, 185, 186, 187, 188, 189, 191, 196, *199, 200, 201,* 356, 367, *373, 375,* 393, *398, 399*
Shiu, L., 239, *277*
Shulman, G. L., 138, *152,* 349, 369, *375*
Siapas, A. G., 442, *456*
Sigman, E., 71, *84*
Silverman, G. H., 161, 181, *200,* 308, *335*
Silverstein, A., 49, *83*
Simizu, M., 69, *84*
Simon, H. A., 8, 11, *42*
Simoncelli, E. P., 453, *456*
Singer, W., 25, *41,* 378, *399*
Singh, M., 169, 179, *197, 200*
Sirosh, J., 240, *277*
Skow Grant, E., 101, 108, *116*
Slater, A., 222, *231,* 244, *277*

Smirnakis, S. M., 442, *456*
Smith, L. B., 250, *276, 278*
Snodgrass, J. G., 136, *152,* 367, *372*
Snodgrass, S. G., 345, *375*
Somers, M., 222, *231,* 244, *277*
Sommer, F., 424, *429*
Sowden, P. T., 235, *278*
Spekreijse, H., 148, *151,* 298, *303,* 452, *456*
Spelke, E. S., 8, *42,* 206, 207, 208, 214, 221, 230, *231*
Spencer-Smith, J., 244, 255, *276*
Sperling, G., 26, *41,* 49*f,* 69, 71, 72, *83*
Spillman, L., 148, *152*
Sporns, O., 297, *304*
Srinivas, K., 425, *429*
Stark, M., 385, *399*
Stemmler, M., 438, *456*
Stevyers, M., 244, 250, 251*f,* 252, 253*f,* 255, 272, *276, 278*
Stoever, R. J., 126, *152*
Stoner, G. R., 306, 311, 312, 313*f,* 317, 318, 319*f, 334, 335,* 441, 452, *453*
Sugita, Y., 148, *152,* 366, *374*
Sullivan, M. A., 138, *152,* 349, 369, *375*
Sun, J., 443, *456*
Super, B. J., 180, *198*
Super, H., 148, *151*
Suppes, P., 49, *83*
Sur, M., 393, *399*
Sutherland, N. S., 241, *278*
Swets, J. A., 325, *335*

T

Tagaris, G. A., 368, *372*
Tanaka, J., 243, *275*
Tang, B., 119, 139, 142, 148, *151,* 338, *374*
Tarr, M. J., 92, *116,* 243, *275,* 341, 344, 368, *372*
Taylor, D., 222, *231,* 244, *277*
Taylor, H., 406, *429*
Tehovnik, E. J., 442, *456*
Teller, D. Y., 227, *232*
Temesvary, A., 170, 196, *199*
Tenenbaum, J. B., 236, *278*
Tenenbaum, J. M., 160, 163, *197*
Terazzi, E., 379, *398*
Termine, N., 206, 221, *231*
Ternes, J., 70, *84*
Thibaut, J., 241, 267, *277*
Thinès, G., 71, *84,* 169, 179, *199*

Thompson, K. G., 294, 296, *303*
Thornber, K., 409, *429*
Thorpe, S., 432, 446, *456*
Tishby, N., 424, *429*
Tolias, A. S., 442, *456*
Tononi, G., 297, *304*
Tootell, R. B. H., 377, 393, *398, 399*
Tozawa, J., 69, *84*
Treiman, R., 389, 390, 395, *399*
Treisman, A., 27, *42*, 118, 124, 134, *152*, 242, 278, 338, *375*, 379, 385, 386, 387, *397, 399*, 431, 441, *456*
Tremoulet, P. D., 227, *231*
Trick, L. M., 140, *152*, 362, *375*
Trobe, J. D., 341, *371*, 380, *396*
Tse, P. U., 68, 70, 71, *84*
Tsodyks, M., 449, *453*
Tu, Z. W., 433, 453, *456*
Tudor, L., 16, 28, 29f, *42*, 118, *152*, 338, *375*
Tuma, R., 119, 139, 142, 148, *151*, 338, *374*
Turatto, M., 140, *150*, 338, *372*
Tversky, A., 49, *83*
Tyler, C., 416, 419, *428*

U

Udesen, H., 341, *374*
Ugurbil, K., *372*
Ullman, S., 63, 64f, 65, 71, *85*, 404, 408, 417, 424, *429*, 432, 446, *456*
Ungerleider, L. G., 101, 108, *115, 116*, 228, *232, 235*, 315, *335*, 377, 378, 385, *397, 399*, 448, *456*
Usher, M., 433, 438, 442, *456*

V

Vaishnavi, S., 341, 348, 368, *374*
Van der Helm, P. A., 5, *43*, 193, *201*
Vanderwart, M. A., 345, *375*
van der Zwan, R., 295, *302*
Van Essen, D. C., 315, *334, 335*, 432, 442, 452, *454, 455*
van Lier, R. J., 166, 193, *200, 201*
Vecchi, M. P., 263, *276*
Vecera, S. P., 93, 96, *116*, 119, 147, 148, *153*, 298, *304*, 379, 390, *399*
Vogel, E. K., 378, *398*
Volman, S. F., *304*

von der Heydt, R., 149, *153*, 160, 175, 181, *198, 200*, 282, 283f, 284n, 285f, 286f, 287f, 289, 290, 292f, 293f, 295f, 296, 297, 298, 300, *303, 304*, 367, 368, *375*, 393, *399*, 419, *428*, 452, *456, 457*
von der Malsburg, C., 26, *43*, 432, *455*
von Helmholtz, H., 7, *43*, 71, *85*
Vorbruggen, J. C., 432, *455*

W

Wagemans, J., 53, 54f, 55f, 56, 57f, 58f, 59, 74, *83*
Wallach, H., 64, *84*, 311, *335*
Waltz, D., 10, *43*
Wang, K., 368, *372*
Ward, L. M., 121, *153*
Ward, R., 386, 392, *397, 399*
Warren, W. H., 69, *85*
Warrington, E. K., 341, 367, 369, *372, 373*, 385, *399*
Watson, J. D. D., 378, *399*
Weber, J., 10, *43*
Weidenbacher, H. J., 300, *304*
Weidenbacher, H. L., 91, 92, 97, *116*
Wienberger, N. M., 238, *278*
Weiss, Y., 453, *456*
Weisstein, N., 243, *278*
Weisz, A., 64, *85*
Wertheimer, M., 5, 15f, 26, *43*, 61, 63, 65, *85*, 117, *153*, 179, *201*
Westheimer, G., 148, *153*, 367, *375*, 384, 393, *397*
Wheeler, D. D., 273, *278*
Wheeler, K., 159, *198*
Whitworth, F. A., 138, *149*, 349, *370*
Whorf, B. L., 234, *278*
Wickens, T., 158, 181, 193, *199*
Wierzbicka, A., 236, *278*
Wiesel, T. N., 3, 13, *41*, 118, *150*, 159, *198*, 309f, 315, *334*, 393, *397*, 441, *454*
Wilcox, T., 227, *232*
Williams, C. K. I., 262, 266, *277*
Williams, L., 403, 404, 409, 413, 416, *429, 457*
Williams, P., 243, *275*, 341, *375*
Wilson, H., 449, *457*
Wilson, J., 138, *152*, 349, 369, *374*
Wisniewski, E. J., 267, *278*
Witherington, D., 227, *230*

Wolfe, J., 158, *198,* 387, 388, 389, 390, 391*f,*
    393, 395, *398*
Wolfe, J. M., 147, *153,* 441, *457*
Woods, D. L., 452, *455*
Woods, R. P., 378, *399*
Wouterlood, D., *197*
Wurtz, R. P., *201,* 432, *455*

Y

Yang, C., 443, 444*f,* 445*f, 455*
Yang, Y, 25, *40*
Yantis, S., 70, *83,* 395, *399*
Yarbus, A. L., 158, 165, *201*
Yen, S. C., 181, *201*
Yin, C., 163, 165, 170, 171, 173, 185, 187, *199,*
    201
Young, A. W., 392, *397*
Young, M. P., 108, *116, 375*
Yovel, G., 347, 349, *375*
Yovel, I., 347, 349, *375*
Yu, S., 453, *457*

Yuille, A. L., 453, *455, 457*
Yund, E. W., 138, *151,* 294, *302,* 349, *374*

Z

Zeki, S., 377, 378, *399*
Zeki, S. M., 315, *335*
Zemel, R. S., 255, 262, 266, *275, 277, 278,* 432,
    433, 448, *454*
Zhou, H., 282, 283*f,* 284*n,* 285*f,* 286*f,* 287*f,* 289,
    290, 292*f,* 293*f,* 295*f,* 296, 297, 300, *304,*
    368, *375,* 452, *457*
Zhou, Y., 121, 149, *150, 153,* 294, 296, *303*
Zhu, S., 404, *429*
Zhu, S. C., 433, 453, *455, 456, 457*
Zihl, J., 377, *398*
Zipser, D., 258, 259, 267, *277*
Zipser, K., 148, *153,* 298, *303, 304,* 452,
    457
Zisserman, A., 409, *427,* 453, *454*
Zucker, S. W., 453, *453*
Zweck, J., 416, *429*

Subject Index

A

Agnosia
  integrative, 339–345, 348–349, 365, 379–380
Amodal completion, 30, 114, 168–169, 411
  see also Identity hypothesis
  see also Interpolation
Aperture problem, 64–67
Apparent motion, *see* Motion
Apparent shapelessness, 90, 96–98, 102
Area
  see Configural cues
  see Figure-ground
Attention, 33, 118–119, 124–126, 139–146, 148, 207, 226, 241–244, 248–254, 300–302, 338, 378–379, 385, 391–395, 431–453
  selective, 241, 249–250, 252, 254, 395, 433, 441
Attraction function, 60
Awake behaving monkey, 296

B

Balint's syndrome, 23, 385, 387–392
Bayesian inference, 433–435, 438, 442
Belief propagation, 404, 412, 420–421, 423
Bigram, 405–406, 412, 420–425
Binocular depth cues, *see* Depth
Border ownership, 281–302
  time course of, 292–294, 298
Boundary assignment, 156, 161–162, 165–168, 181

C

Categorization
  network modeling and, 237, 258–272
  perceptual learning and, 238, 241, 243–257, 273–274
Choice probability, 56
Closure
  see Configural cues
  see Figure-ground
  see Grouping
Connectedness, 166, 227, 392
  see also Grouping
Collinearity, *see* Grouping
Color and pattern, 217–220, 228–229
Color vision, 285–286, 288, 290, 294, 296–300, 377
Common fate, *see* Grouping
Competitive model, 101
Conceptual learning, 273
Configural cues, 89, 91–93, 96–97, 101, 108, 111–114
  see also Figure-ground
Contour assignment, 89–90, 101, 114
Contour completion, 112, 187, 412–419, 384
  see also Interpolation
Contour interpolation, *see* Interpolation
Convexity, 11, 89, 92, 97, 101, 111, 290–291, 410–411
  see also Configural cues
Corners, 67, 160, 162, 176, 178, 191, 289–290, 405, 409–410, 413
Correspondence tokens, 46
Correspondence problem, 63–64
Cue competition, 93–96
Curve of least energy, 408

D

Denotivity, 89–110
   high-denotative regions, 91–94, 97, 105–106,
     108–110
   low-denotative regions, 92–95, 106, 108–110
Depth, 6, 11–12, 26–28, 35–36, 38–39, 67, 69,
     89–90, 92–93, 101, 106–111, 113–115,
     158–165, 168, 172–175, 183, 185–187,
     295, 297–298, 300, 310–313, 317–319,
     333, 337, 339, 349, 384
   binocular cues, 103–111, 159, 182, 187,
     310–311
   monocular cues, 89, 92
   see also Figure-ground
Differentiation, 238, 249–258, 270, 272–273
Distributed cortical network model, 297
Dorsal pathway, 109, 227–228
   see also 'what' and 'where' pathways
Dynamic superposition, 71

E

Early visual cortex, *see* Visual cortex
Enclosure, 91–92, 111
   see also Configural cues
Entropy, 56–59
Exploration skills, 221–223, 227, 229
Extrastriate visual areas, *see* Visual
     cortex

F

Familiarity, 68, 97, 134–136, 147–148, 161,
     166, 195, 243, 300, 392
   see also Past experience
   see also Object memory
Feedback, 12, 34–35, 40, 147, 166, 168, 235,
     237, 250, 252, 273, 297–298, 350,
     378–379, 432–433, 435, 441, 448–449,
     452–453
Feedforward, 34, 118, 147, 166, 274, 368, 424,
     431–432, 435, 449, 452
Figure-ground, 10–11, 14, 36–38, 87–115, 119,
     142, 146, 161, 166, 281–302, 384, 431,
     453
   depth and, 11, 36, 38, 90–93, 106–115
   global and local mechanisms in,
     289–292

surface completion and, 87–115
   see also Configural cues
Fragments, 65, 68, 149, 157, 162, 165, 167, 176,
     180, 188–191, 197, 384, 393, 410–413,
     417, 420, 422

G

Gap, 67, 126–137, 147, 172–174, 177, 342,
     356–360, 411, 416, 420, 436
Gestalt
   Approach, 5–6, 12–13, 170
   see also Grouping
   see also Figure-ground
Gestalt lattice, 50–61
Global and local processing, 119–127, 130,
     138–139, 146–147, 191–196, 345–349,
     350, 352–355, 362–363, 365–370
   attention and, 125–126
Good continuation, *see* Grouping
Grouping, 3–40, 45–82, 117–119, 126–149,
     273–274, 321–333, 338, 345, 351–370,
     379–395, 411–412, 431, 446, 453
   by closure, 117, 126–127, 130, 132, 139,
     147–148, 356, 358–359, 362, 365–370,
     408, 411
   by connectedness, 19–23, 126–139, 147–149,
     355–358, 389
   by collinearity, 126–127, 130, 132, 134, 139,
     147–149, 178, 348, 356, 358–362, 366,
     368, 370, 381, 384, 392, 395
   by common fate, 8, 19, 23, 36–37, 39, 63,
     65–66, 117
   by common region, 19–22, 30, 34
   by good continuation, 118, 127, 177, 179,
     262, 408, 415–416
   by similarity, 5, 7, 14–15, 17–18, 20, 28,
     30–31, 37, 39, 48–49, 66, 140–146,
     363–366, 379
   by spatial proximity, 14–15, 17, 22, 27–28,
     34, 46, 48–50, 60–61, 63, 65–66, 69–74,
     77–78, 117–118, 126–127, 130, 132,
     139, 338, 359, 363–366, 379, 411
   by spatiotemporal proximity, 46, 48, 61, 63,
     65–72, 74–75, 78
   by synchrony, 23–25
   recursive, 64–65
   strength, 49, 56–57
   time course of, 118–149, 338, 350–365

H

Hangman, 423–427
Hierarchical model, 298
Hierarchical statistical inference, 449
Hierarchical stimuli, 119–139, 345–365
Hierarchy of information, 224, 227–228
High-denotative regions, *see* Denotivity

I

Indifference curve, 49–50
Identity hypothesis, 168–181, 191, 195
    see also Interpolation
Illusory contours, 12, 32–33, 165, 168–170,
        173–174, 176, 181–183, 193–194, 295,
        370, 393, 403–405, 409–410, 412–413,
        420, 427, 440
    see also Interpolation
    see also Modal completion
Imprinting, 239–241, 272–273
Image segmentation, 27, 119, 147, 162
Infant perception, 205–229
Inhibition, 97–101, 114, 123, 127, 130, 438, 449
Inflection point, 410
Integrative agnosia, *see* Agnosia
Interpolation
    contour, 56, 156, 163–194, 359–363
    global and local processing in, 191–196
    spatiotemporal, 168, 188–191
    surface, 163–194
    three-dimensional, 181–191
    see also Amodal completion
    see also Identity hypothesis
    see also Modal completion
    see also Occlusion
Interposition, 92–93, 111
Intrinsic and extrinsic edges, 161–163
Iterative algorithm, 297–299, 423
Inferotemporal cortex, *see* Visual cortex
Inverted, 92–95, 134–137, 147, 243, 299

J

Junctions, 71, 158, 160–164, 176, 181, 191, 291,
        383, 412, 436
    contour, 160–164
    L-junctions, 176, 290–291, 295
    T-junctions, 71, 160–161, 176, 291, 383

L

Learning and perception, 205–229
    see also Perceptual learning
Lesions, 23, 337–370, 384, 386–387, 391–392,
        395
Low-denotative regions, *see* Denotivity

M

Markov Models, 404–422, 424
Matching units, 46, 48, 61–74
Memory, 403–427, 442
    perceptual completion and, 403–427
    see also Object memory
Microgenesis, 117–149, 350, 352–360, 365
Modal completion, 168–169
    see also Identity hypothesis
    see also Illusory contours
    see also Interpolation
Models of motion perception, 61–63
    interactive, 61–78
    sequential, 61, 77
Monocular depth cues, *see* Depth
Motion, 5, 11, 22–23, 25–26, 36–38, 46, 61, 64,
        66, 70–77, 156, 158–161, 188, 206,
        226–227, 294, 306–333, 377
    apparent, 61
    common motion, 25, 206, 226, 322
    element-motion (e-motion), 46, 70–72,
        74–77
    group-motion (g-motion), 46, 70–72, 74–77
    second-order, 64, 66
    see also Models of motion perception
Motion lattices, 72–77

N

Neural coding, 281–302
Neural mechanisms, 160, 181, 187, 339
Neural networks, 240, 257–273, 423
Non-rigid transformations, 65

O

Object-based spatial attention, *see* Attention
Object boundaries, 159, 206, 208, 210, 219–223,
        227–229, 409, 416

Object segregation
  infancy and, 205–229
Object features, 26, 206, 214, 216, 221–224,
    224, 227–229
Object knowledge, 225, 289
Object memory, 89–113, 134, 136, 147–149,
    158, 168, 183, 195, 297, 300, 302, 345,
    369
Object perception, 155–197, 244, 377
  infancy and, 205–229
Object recognition, 92, 134, 148, 160, 166,
    193–195, 236, 243, 301, 338–339, 341,
    344–345, 365–370, 378, 380, 392–393,
    403, 419, 427
Occlusion, 163, 165–166, 171, 175–176, 180,
    191–195, 282, 295, 299, 308, 310, 312,
    337, 382, 386, 411–413, 417, 419
  infancy and, 224
  kinetic, 71
  see also Interpolation
Orientation effects, 92, 95, 97

P

Parallel Interactive Model of Configural
    Analysis (PIMOCA), 96–102, 109,
    113–114
Past experience, 119, 134–137, 147
Perceptual completion,
  see Interpolation
  see Memory
Perceptual learning, 233–274
  attention and, 241, 243, 249–254
Perceptual saliency, 444, 446, 448
Perceptual work, 81–82
Persistence, 188–189, 191
Petter's Effect, 172–173, 175
Phenomenology, 16–17, 19, 21, 78–82, 170,
    175
Phenomenological report, 17, 82
Primary visual cortex, see Visual cortex
Primate electrophysiology, 281–302, 305–333,
    431–453
Primate visual cortex, 281–302, 305–333,
    431–453
Primed matching, 119–120, 122, 126, 128–129,
    131, 133–134, 142, 144–145, 351
Prior experience, 224
Prosopagnosia, 344

Psychophysics, 3, 297
  traditional, 80–81
  phenomenological, 45–82
Pure distance law (the), 57–61

R

Randon-dot cinematogram, 63
Random-dot stereogram, 103–104, 110–111,
    289, 302
Receptive field, 13, 101, 148, 284–287, 289–291,
    293–294, 296, 308–309, 315–317, 320,
    325–326, 378, 438–439, 443–444, 447
Recognition, see Object recognition
Redundancy, 425–427
Relatability, 127, 156, 176–181, 183, 185–194,
    197, 356, 365
  see also Identity hypothesis
  see also Interpolation
Representation, 237–273
  componential, 237, 249, 271
  configural, 243, 271, 273

S

Segmentation, 27, 119, 147, 156–158, 160, 162,
    166, 179, 197, 255–256, 258, 298, 330,
    341, 380, 383, 453
  attention and, 394–395
  networks, 262–272
Selective attention, see Attention
Self-splitting objects, 172–173, 176
  see also Interpolation
Shape, 87, 89–91, 93–94, 97, 99, 101–103, 108,
    111, 113, 114
Shape-from-motion, 65
Shaped apertures, 111–114
Similarity, see Grouping
Single-cell recording, see Primate
    electrophysiology
Simultanagnosia, 385, 387
Solidity, 208, 228
Spatial frequency, 181, 349–351, 361, 365,
    369–370
  channels, 138–139, 349
  spatial filtering, 138–139
Spatial layout, 188, 213
Spatiotemporal information, 156

Spatiotemporal interpolation, *see* Interpolation
Stereoscopic vision, 289, 297
Stochastic completion field, 413–414, 416–417, 419, 421, 427
Structure, 5–8, 10, 38, 40
Structural simplicity, 5–6, 9–10
Subjective, 45–46, 78–82
  as phenomenal, 45–46, 79
  as idiosyncratic, 79
Superghost, 420, 423–427
Support, 208, 210–211, 228
Suppression, 101, 108, 315
Surface completion, 87–114
  see also interpolation
Surface perception, 282, 289, 296–298
Symmetry, 10–11
  in global completion, 191, 193–196
  see also Configural cues

T

Tangent discontinuity, 160, 163, 165, 176–179, 186, 191–192
  see also Junctions
Tasks
  direct vs. indirect, 78–82
  correct/incorrect, 78–82
  "objective" vs. "subjective", 14, 17–19, 78–82
  phenomenological, 78–82
T-junctions, *see* Junctions
Ternus display, 70–71
Temporal lobe, 341–342
Three-dimensional displays, 90–91, 103–114
Three-dimensional information, 181
Top-down and bottom–up processing, 34, 45, 118, 134–135, 147, 149, 156, 166–168, 194, 206, 258, 260, 300–301, 368, 404, 424, 431, 433, 435, 441–443, 448–449, 451–453
Transparency, 29–30, 39, 102, 114, 160–161, 168
Two-dimensional displays, 90–102, 113–114, 181, 183, 185, 188

U

Uniform connectedness, 11, 26–27, 118, 123, 132, 137, 147, 162
Unitization, 238, 243–249, 254–258, 270, 273
Upright, 92–95, 134–137, 147, 243, 339

V

Ventral pathway, 108, 228
  see also 'what' and 'where' pathways
Virtual objects, 72, 74–77
Visible regions representation, 158, 161–166
  see also Interpolation
Visual agnosia, *see* Agnosia
Visual binding, 377–396
  attention and, 378–379, 384–385, 390–392, 394–395
Visual cortex, 13, 282–300, 308–333, 361–363, 367, 393, 416, 435–452
  area V2, 27, 159, 175, 284–292, 294–298, 300, 367, 370, 393, 435, 438, 440–441
  area V4, 27, 101, 284, 287–288, 292, 294, 298, 300, 333, 377, 435, 442
  extrastriate areas, 284, 296–298, 314, 441, 448
  inferotemporal cortex (area IT), 442, 448, 450
  medial temporal cortex (area MT), 159, 298, 300, 314–321, 323, 325, 328, 333, 377
  primary visual cortex (area V1), 3–4, 13, 27, 40, 148, 159, 175, 180, 238–240, 284, 287–288, 292, 296, 298, 300, 308–309, 314–315, 367, 370, 384, 393, 435–438, 440–441, 443–452
Visual search, 138, 394, 446, 449, 451–452
  attention and, 124–126

W

'What' and 'where' pathways, 228, 448
Word memory, 403–404, 425